Nages Nagaratnam • Kujan Nagaratnam
Gary Cheuk

Diseases in the Elderly

Age-Related Changes and Pathophysiology

Springer

Nages Nagaratnam
Sydney Medical School (Westmead)
The University of Sydney
North Rocks
Australia

Kujan Nagaratnam
Norwest Specialist Medical Group
Bella Vista
New South Wales
Australia

Gary Cheuk
Blacktown-Mt Druitt Hospital
Blacktown
New South Wales
Australia

ISBN 978-3-319-25785-3 ISBN 978-3-319-25787-7 (eBook)
DOI 10.1007/978-3-319-25787-7

Library of Congress Control Number: 2016931332

Springer Cham Heidelberg New York Dordrecht London

Printed on acid-free paper

Springer International Publishing AG Switzerland is part of Springer Science+Business Media (www.springer.com)

Diseases in the Elderly

The Authors

Nages Nagaratnam, OAM, MD, FRACP, FRCPA, FRCP, FACC, FCCP, is clinical associate professor at the Sydney Medical School, the University of Sydney, and was a conjoint associate professor in the School of Medicine, College of Health and Science at the University of Western Sydney, Australia. He graduated and obtained the doctorate in medicine from the University of Ceylon and was for many years consultant physician in internal medicine in Sri Lanka and senior physician at the General Hospital, Colombo, the premier teaching hospital. He is a founding fellow of the National Academy of Sciences of Sri Lanka and was president of the Sri Lanka Association for the Advancement of Science, Section A. In Australia he was consultant physician in geriatric and internal medicine at the Blacktown-Mt Druitt and Westmead Hospitals. He has a lifelong commitment to training and guiding the careers of generations of young doctors. He has authored more than 200 scientific publications in both national and international journals. His interests spanned many fields of medicine with continuous clinical research throughout his career. In the last two decades his interests are in geriatrics, rehabilitation, stroke and stroke rehabilitation.

Kujan Nagaratnam, MBBS (UNSW), FRACP, graduated in medicine from the University of New South Wales in 1988. He did his internal medical training and advanced training in geriatric medicine and stroke medicine at Westmead and Royal Prince Alfred Hospitals, Sydney. He obtained his fellowship of the Royal Australasian College of Physicians (FRACP) in 1997. He held senior staff specialist appointments in geriatric and stroke medicine at Westmead Hospital and Blacktown-Mt Druitt Hospitals until 2012. He is also a visiting consultant physician at the Norwest Private and Westmead Private Hospitals in Sydney. He is currently the chairman and head of the Department of Geriatric and Stroke Medicine, Norwest Private Hospital, Sydney. His academic interests includes teaching both undergraduate and postgraduate medical students. He is a clinical senior lecturer in medicine at the University of Sydney. His special interests are stroke medicine, cognitive impairment and dementia, neurological diseases in the elderly and peri-operative medical management of elderly patients.

Gary Cheuk, MBBS(UNSW), FRACP, graduated from the University of New South Wales in 1985 with honours. He commenced basic physician training in Dunedin (New Zealand) and St George Hospital (Sydney). He underwent advance training in geriatric medicine at Concord and Westmead Hospitals and was granted fellowship of the Royal Australasian College of Physicians in 1993. In the following year he became the director of Rehabilitation and Aged Care Service at Blacktown-Mt Druitt Hospital, a position he occupies until 2015. Dr Cheuk has been involved in undergraduate and postgraduate teaching for many years. Service planning and development are areas of interest for Dr Cheuk, and he was instrumental in the establishment of the Stroke Unit at Blacktown Hospital and the building of the Rehabilitation Hub at Mt Druitt Hospital. His clinical interests include dementia care, Parkinson's disease and related disorders, stroke medicine and musculoskeletal diseases in the older persons.

Disclaimer

Continuous development and research in the fields of medicine, science technology and health care result in ongoing changes in the domains of clinical practice as evidence continues to evolve rapidly. We have taken reasonable care and effort to provide material which are current, accurate and balanced at the time of publication.

We and the publishers do not accept responsibility or liability for any errors in the text or any consequences arising from the information. The information provided is neutral and for general education and does not replace interaction with the practising clinicians. Clinicians should depend on their own experience when providing advice or treatment.

We have acknowledged the sources and works of the cited sites at the appropriate locations in the text and references. We have utilised the source materials in the sense of fair use and extend our apology for any oversight. Readers are advised to cross-reference and confirm points relevant to them.

Preface

The elderly have been categorised as young old between the ages of 65 and 74 years, old old between 75 and 84 years and oldest old those above 85 years and over. Current demographic data predicts an increase in the elderly population worldwide. The oldest old group is said to be a rapidly growing segment of the population and is expected to grow nearly 4 % per annum in Australia. In the United States the oldest old is projected to double from 4.3 to 9.6 million by 2030. This trend has resulted in the alarming increase in prevalence of disease, patients with multiple pathologies and the alarming rise of care-demanding conditions such as dementia. As age advances there are innumerable problems confronting the elderly. The perception that all old people require care over extended periods of their lives is at variance with known facts. The majority of old people remain independent for the remaining years of their life. Several studies have highlighted the divergent attitudes between the health professionals towards elderly people, and many tend to discriminate against people because they are old. This has often compromised the quality of care older people receive.

Epidemiological data emphasise the value of studies which compel the need to broaden and disseminate knowledge about age-related problems especially in the very old. Understanding the ageing process and its consequences is of prime importance in identifying the health-care challenges posed by the growing elderly population. A proper understanding of the changes relating to ageing and their significance is necessary to develop appropriate corrective/remedial strategies. *Diseases in the elderly: Age-related Changes and Pathophysiology* provides a comprehensive overview of the two important issues relating to disease in elderly. The book has a strong focus on age-related changes and the pathophysiology of the disease in the elderly. Adequate knowledge of the structural and physiological changes that occur with ageing and the underlying pathophysiology of diseases in the elderly is a prerequisite for the proper understanding and forms a rational basis for the diagnosis and treatment of disease in the elderly. Apart from providing intense information on a given subject, it also provides means for self assessment which is composed of multiple-choice questions, short answer questions and extended matching questions. The questions have been largely based on the text. Since readers' time is often restricted, this book provides a bulleted box with key points at the end of each section.

The book contains 19 chapters which are arranged by organ system and structured to cover the specific areas. Many sections follow a common pattern with headings and subheadings. The text offers the primary care physician, junior hospital doctors, medical undergraduates and specialist nurses and others working in aged-care settings a systematic approach to geriatric medicine. The intent is to provide information where interest demands, extending the 'aims and scope' of the book to anatomy and physiology and beyond. We strive to be concise and thorough in our approach to the stipulated areas.

Sydney, North Rocks, Australia — Nages Nagaratnam
Bella Vista, NSW, Australia — Kujan Nagaratnam
Blacktown, NSW, Australia — Gary Cheuk

Acknowledgements

We thank Mrs Sheila Nagaratnam (line drawings), Mr Yogan Nagaratnam (for his help in numerous ways), Mr Panjan Nagaratnam (for photographs), Sai Nagaratnam (for checking the references) and Manisha Nagaratnam (for her help with the figures and tables). Thanks to Drs John Sarks and Derek Davies for the illustrations and for reviewing the relevant sections, to Norvatis Company Archives for the illustrations and to Prof David Harris, Dr Logan Kanagaratnam, Mr Brian Lucas, Prof Nicholas Manolios and Dr Mohan Nagarajah for their help.

Contents

Cardiovascular Disease and Related Disorders in the Elderly

1

1.1 Anatomical and Physiological Changes with Ageing

Tissue integrity and competency of systolic and diastolic function normally depends on the extracellular collagen concentration [1]. With ageing, there is an abnormal increase in the extracellular fibrillar collagen which contributes to myocardial stiffness [1] and decrease in compliance [2]. Normal early diastolic function is compromised and diastolic pressures increase leading to left ventricular diastolic dysfunction [3]. Animal studies and cultured cardiac fibroblasts have indicated that myocardial fibrosis is associated with chronic mineralocorticoid excesses relative to sodium intake and excretion [4]. Aldosterone plays a crucial role in the development of cardiac fibrosis [5].

Although there is a loss of myocytes with advancing age, the left ventricular wall thickens with age in both men and women due to increase in size of remaining cardiac myocytes [6], but there is no increase in the left ventricular mass [7]. As age advances, about 35 % of myocytes are lost [8]. The left ventricular (LV) diastolic filling rate decreases to a 50 % of the peak rate by the age of 80 [9]. The LV end-diastolic volume does not reduce with age due to the forceful contractility of the left atrium and this enhanced atrial contribution to ventricular filling is associated with left atrial hypertrophy. Resting left ventricular systolic function (ejection fraction and/or stroke volume) is not altered by ageing nor is the resting cardiac output [10]. The maximum heart rate decreases during exercise with age [10–12]. Furthermore, significant changes occur in cardiovascular function in ageing healthy adults during exercise [12]. There is resetting of the baroreceptor reflex in the elderly.

The beta-adrenergic responsiveness decreases with age limiting the maximum achievable heart rate (HR) [2]. Due to the reduced maximal heart rate and the limit to increase contractility in response to beta-adrenergic blockade in the elderly, the exercise cardiac output may be reduced and the heart partially compensates for this by exercise-induced dilatation of the left ventricle [13]. Both at rest and on exercise, the incidence of cardiac arrhythmias increases with age [14]. Numerous alterations

N. Nagaratnam et al., *Diseases in the Elderly: Age-Related Changes and Pathophysiology*, DOI 10.1007/978-3-319-25787-7_1

occur in the heart and vessels as a result of deregulation of molecular longevity pathways resulting in compromised function [15]. About 80 % of old people have aortic valvular sclerosis and moderate to severe aortic incompetence is present in 16 % [16]. Mitral annular calcification increases with advancing age [17]. The blood supply of the tissues and cardiovascular function is influenced by structural changes to the peripheral vessels with ageing [13]. Some researchers had advocated cautious interpretation of these age-associated changes in cardiac performance since they may be age-related diseases rather than primarily the ageing process [17]. It is likely that cardiovascular ageing involves mechanisms which are the result of a variety of insults such as oxidative stress, inflammation, non-enzymatic glycation and changes in the cardiovascular genes [18].

Normal ageing is associated with both physiological and structural changes in the arterial vasculature which have functional implications. There is increase in the size of the lumen and increased wall thickness with stiffening mainly involving the arteries [19]. With age, arterial calcification together with changes in the elastin collagen balance leads to generalised thickening of the conduit arteries [20]. The stiffening of the vasculature results in an age-related shift of the velocity of the reflected pulse wave from diastole to late systole [20]. This leads to increased systolic workload for the heart, decreased coronary perfusion and transmission of higher pressures to the end organs [21]. The stiffening leads to left ventricular hypertrophy, renal impairment and cerebrovascular disease [21]. With age, the walls of the peripheral vessels become thicker and stiffer [22]. Likewise, the walls of the veins become thicker due to increase in the connective tissue and calcium deposits [22]. Table 1.1 summarises the anatomical and physiological changes with ageing.

Box 1.1. Key Points. Cardiovascular Changes with Ageing

- Increase in extracellular fibrillar collagen [1].
- Loss of myocytes and increase in size of remaining myocytes [6, 8].
- Fibrous tissue of the skeleton of the heart becomes sclerotic and calcifies ([4, 5] and Table 1.1).
- Left ventricular wall thickens, left atrium hypertrophies, valves calcify [17, 21].
- Fibrous tissue in the conducting system increases (see Table 1.1).
- Beta-adrenergic responsiveness decreases [2].
- Large artery walls thicken [22].

1.2 Heart Failure

Introduction

Heart failure is a progressive disorder, acute or insidious in onset, due to ventricular dysfunction resulting from a decline in pump failure [26]. In the population all over the world, heart failure is most prevalent in the 75 years and over age group [27]. Heart failure is the major cause of disability in the elderly and increasing age itself is a risk factor in its development. The incidence of congestive heart failure among

Table 1.1 Anatomical and physiological cardiac changes with ageing

Anatomical	Physiological	Results
Myocardium		
Cardiac myocytes increase in size	Afterload increased, early diastolic filling impaired	Reduced up to 50 % by 80 years
changes in collagen and left ventricular thickness	Increased atrial contractility	Hypertrophy of atrium
	End-diastolic volume increased at rest	
Fibrous skeleton – sclerotic, calcifies		Mitral annular calcification and aortic valve calcifies
Amyloid deposition	Systolic and diastolic dysfunction	Arrhythmias, conduction defects, restrictive myocardial changes
Pacemaker		
Increased elastic and collagen tissue in conducting system	Beta-adrenergic responses to the heart decreased	Maximal HR is limited
		Decreased contractility of myocardium, cardiac output decreased
	Duration of contractility lessened, spill over of catecholamines responses to beta-adrenergic receptor stimulation	Further reduction of contractility of myocardium
Valves		
Collagen tissues – sclerotic + calcification of cardiac skeleton aortic and mitral annulus – nodular thickenings at closure lines of valves and summit of intraventricular septum. Valves calcify and/or become myxomatous	Aortic sclerosis mitral insufficiency AV conduction abnormalities	Aortic sclerosis, mitral incompetence, AV node, AV bundle, bifurcation, proximal L and R BB may be affected
Arterial system		
Intimal hyperplasia and thickening	Decrease in compliance	Increased stiffness
Increased peripheral vascular resistance	Increase in blood pressure	Systolic and diastolic hypertension
Elastic content decreases	Increase in systolic pressure	Systolic hypertension
Endothelial dysfunction	Structural changes	Reduced endothelium-dependent vasodilatation

Information sources: Aalami et al. [2]; Burlew [3]; Olivetti et al. [4]; Lakata [15, 21, 22]; Esler et al. [23]; Taddei et al. [24]; Stamato et al. [25]

community-dwelling elderly is 7–8 % after the age of 75 [28]. Its prevalence is likely to increase over the next few decades with the increase in world population, and in the over 65 years. The elderly are inclined to developing chronic heart failure as a result of age-related changes in the cardiovascular system and high prevalence of coronary heart disease and hypertension [29].

Age-related cardiovascular changes
With ageing, there is abnormal increase in the extracellular fibrillar collagen giving rise to increased myocardial stiffness adversely affecting myocardial elasticity leading to systolic and diastolic dysfunction [30]. Age-related changes in the cardiovascular system and function may lower the threshold at which cardiac disease becomes evident [31]. Many changes occur in the cardiovascular system such as decreased heart rate, reduced cardiac output and systolic hypertension. Due to age-related changes in the sarcoplasmic reticulum, myocardial relaxation is slowed [32]. There is increased thickness of the muscle wall of both ventricles due to the increased myocyte size [33]. The heart rate is unchanged at rest and early diastolic filling is reduced; however, an enhanced atrial contraction helps to maintain ventricular filling at a normal volume. With exercise, there is an age-related reduction in heart rate [34, 35], but the cardiac output is maintained during exercise by an augmentation of stroke volume brought about by cardiac dilatation at end diastole and end systole. However, many studies concluded that the cardiac output decreases with advancing age [36]. There is a decreased responsiveness to beta-adrenergic modulation [31], and beta-adrenergic stimulation enhances the strength of contraction but decreases its duration thus permitting relaxation and proper filling. Decreased conservation of sodium and changes in the baroreceptor reflex function may bring about postprandial and orthostatic hypotension in some individuals [32]. The maximum exercise level (VO_2 max) decreases with age, and this is largely due to decrease in the skeletal muscle mass [37]. In addition to these, there are changes in hepatic and renal function with advancing age.

Pathophysiology of chronic heart failure
In heart failure, the ventricular dysfunction results in an inability of the ventricles either to eject or to fill [38]. Thus, there are two types of heart failure, one as a result of the systolic dysfunction resulting in systolic heart failure with ejection fraction less than 40 % and the other diastolic dysfunction resulting in diastolic heart failure with normal ejection fraction. The term diastolic heart failure is now largely replaced by the more favoured term, heart failure with preserved ejection fraction (HF-PEF). In many patients, both systolic and diastolic dysfunction coexist.

The ventricular end-diastolic pressure increases as a result of both systolic and diastolic dysfunction, thereby enhances the force of contraction and consequently the stroke volume [39]. With progression of systolic and diastolic dysfunction, the ability of this mechanism is enfeebled and the stroke volume can decline considerably resulting in reduction of the cardiac output [26]. Diastolic heart failure is the result of altered ventricular relaxation and abnormal ventricular filling.

Several compensatory neurohormonal mechanisms are activated with the reduction in the cardiac output [40]. Although these compensatory mechanisms provide benefit for the heart in normal physiological situations, they can intensify the progression of chronic heart failure [39, 40]. The neurohormonal mechanisms include increase in sympathetic activity, the renin-angiotensin-aldosterone system [28, 37], the antidiuretic hormone-vasopressin system and atrial natriuretic peptide [39, 40]. The eventual result of these responses is arterial and venous constriction [39].

Angiotensin II is a strong vasoconstrictor of renal and systemic circulation leading to release of aldosterone which causes retention of sodium and water and increased loss of potassium [40]. The natriuretic peptides (atrial, brain and C-type) exert a wide range of effects on the heart, kidneys and the central nervous system [40].

Box 1.2. Key Points. Heart Failure in the Elderly

- With ageing, heart rate decreases, cardiac output reduces, systolic BP elevates.
- Decreased responsiveness to beta-adrenergic modulation [2, 31].
- Maximum exercise level (VO_2 max) decreases [37].
- Ventricular end-diastolic pressure increases following systolic and diastolic dysfunction [39].
- Several compensatory neurohormonal mechanisms are activated which can intensify the progression of chronic heart failure [40].
- Combined right and left ventricular failure most common.

1.3 Cardiac Arrhythmias in the Elderly

Introduction

Cardiac arrhythmias comprise any abnormality that hinders the initiation and/or progression of normal activation of the myocardium [41]. Cardiac arrhythmias are a large concern among the elderly, and they occur so frequently that they are often regarded as "normal" and inevitable part of the ageing process [42]. Not only are cardiac arrhythmias more frequent than in the younger age group, they are influenced by certain aspects of aetiology, pathophysiology, diagnoses and treatment [43].

Ageing and the conduction system

A number of characteristic morphological, histological and biochemical changes are associated with ageing of the heart [44]. Both the sinus and AV nodes decrease in size [45]. There is a reduction in the number of cells with increase in collagen fibres which is more evident in the SA node and less so in the AV node and the bundle of His [46]. There is a reduction in the number of myocytes of the conduction tissue with development of cardiac fibrosis [44]. The electrical characteristics of the conducting system also change with age together with cardiac calcium regulation [47]. There is a slow inward current caused by calcium and alterations in potassium conductance resulting in transmembrane electrical ageing changes [45]. The heart rate (HR) is generally not affected by ageing, but the responsiveness to stress and exercise especially is decreased limiting the maximum achievable heart rate. The atrial depolarisation results in the P wave. Normally, the cardiac impulse is physiologically delayed in the AV node thereby the ventricles are protected from being depolarised, during supraventricular tachycardia. With healthy ageing, the time of conduction through the AV node is increased and hence the P-R interval increases with age.

Pathophysiology
The conducting system consists of three parts, the sinoatrial (SA) node, the atrioventricular (AV) node and bundle of His, bundle branches and the Purkinje network. The conducting system is composed of specialised myocytes [48] which are capable of generating and conducting the cardiac impulse from the atria to the ventricular chambers [49]. The myocytes are connected to each other by intercalated discs and play an important role in the electrical conducting system [50]. The SA node initiates the conduction of the cardiac impulse [51]. There are no specialised conducting tracts between sinus node and AV node [52]. The bundle of His originates from the distal portion of the AV node [53] which consists of specialised cells surrounded by a fibrous collar [54] that penetrates the right fibrous trigone [48] and courses through the membranous septum and bifurcates into the right and left bundle branches. The left bundle branch in turn bifurcates into the left anterior and posterior fascicles [51], and the bundle branches end in the Purkinje system of both the ventricles. The Purkinje fibres are long strands of barrel-shaped cells called Purkinje myocytes.

The cardiac impulse originates in the SA node and activates both atria which depolarises spontaneously resulting in the P wave on the electrocardiogram (ECG). The impulse travels through the right atrium after some delay [55] to the AV node resulting in the P-R interval on the ECG. It is then conducted through the AV node to the bundle of His and bundle branches to the Purkinje system and activates both ventricles. The conducting system of the heart is innervated by both the sympathetic and parasympathetic nervous system. Sympathetic stimulation increases the automaticity and enhances conduction. The parasympathetic (vagal) stimulation decreases sinus node automaticity and slows atrioventricular conduction [50]. There is considerable variation in the resting heart rate among healthy asymptomatic population.

There is an increase risk and severity of arrhythmias with increasing age [47]. The common conditions affecting the conducting system by altering impulse formation or impulse propagation or both are age-related degeneration, myocardial infarction, procedural complications of drug toxicity [56]. The dysregulation of intracellular calcium probably plays an important role in producing electrical instability [47]. The reason for the increased incidence of atrial and ventricular ectopic beats is unclear. This increase may be related in part to increase in atrial size in the occurrence for the atrial arrhythmias and the increase in ventricular beats to the age-associated increase in the left ventricular mass and catecholamine levels [57]. Two different fundamental disturbances, namely, alterations in impulse formation (automaticity) or alterations of impulse propagation, can result in bradyarrhythmias and tachyarrhythmias [57]. Focal or nonfocal mechanisms may be involved [19], and an abnormal impulse initiation can result from either automaticity caused by normal or abnormal automatic mechanisms (focal mechanism) or by triggered activity [41, 58]. Nonfocal mechanisms are diverse forms of re-entry due to circus movement [58]. The bradyarrhythmias are the result of abnormalities of the intrinsic automatic behaviour or conduction which impair sinoatrial or the atrioventricular conduction causing partial or total conduction block [57]. The tachyarrhythmias may arise from altered automaticity (occurring in ordinary atrial or ventricular myocardium) or triggered activity (due to early or delayed afterdepolarisations) [41, 57, 58] and re-entry [58]. Most clinically significant tachyarrhythmias are probably due to re-entry.

Box 1.3. Key Points. Cardiac Arrhythmias in the Elderly

- Reduction of myocytes of the conduction tissues with development of cardiac fibrosis [44, 46].
- Electrical characteristics of the conducting system change [47].
- Alterations in impulse formation (automaticity) and impulse propagation [50].
- Common conditions affecting the conducting system are age-related degeneration, myocardial infarction and procedural complications and drug toxicity [56].
- Supraventricular ectopics may be related to age-related atrial size and increase in ventricular beats to age-related increase in left ventricular mass and catecholamines [57].
- Tachyarrhythmias may rise from altered automaticity or triggered activity and re-entry [41, 8].
- Bradyarrhythmias result from abnormalities of intrinsic automatic behaviour or conduction [57].

1.4 Infective Endocarditis in the Elderly

Introduction

Infective endocarditis can be defined as an infection of the endocardium which may affect the valves and involve the myocardium. The incidence of infective endocarditis (IE) is increasing in older patients. This is due to an increase in the life expectancy and general ageing of the population, longer survival of patients with congenital and valvular disease of the heart, the use of intravenous catheters and prosthetic devices [59], proliferation of invasive procedures [60] and higher prevalence of hospital-acquired bacteraemia [61, 62]. More than 50 % of the cases with IE occur in persons over the age of 60 with high-risk profile.

Pathophysiology and pathogenesis

It is customary to categorise IE into acute and subacute forms based largely on the severity of the disease and its course [63]. There is often no clear distinction between the typical acute IE which is usually abrupt in onset and rapidly progressive affecting even normal hearts and the subacute IE which usually begins insidiously and progresses over weeks to months [64] and where the heart has some underlying pathology. This subdivision however still has clinical value.

The development of infective endocarditis giving rise to vegetations occurs in areas of increased turbulence and eddy currents (on the atrial side of the atrioventricular valves and on the ventricular surface of the semilunar valves) or in lower pressure side of the defect in non-valvular congenital defects [63]. For example, atrial septal defect or in the case of mechanical prosthesis, the vegetations occur usually along the margin of the sewing ring causing a ring abscess and sometimes paravalvular perforation [63]. *Streptococci* adhere to the cardiac valves with pre-existing endothelial lesions [65], whereas Staphylococcus aureus not only settle on the damaged endothelium but also invade intact endothelium [65, 66]. These interactions are mediated by several surface adhesins [65]. The inflamed endothelia produce cytokines, integrins and tissue factor which in turn draw monocytes, platelets and integrins, and the bacteria attaching to these structures become embedded and protected from host defences [66]. The vegetations in acute IE tend to be larger and more often involve the normal valves and may cause perforation of the valve leaflet and sometimes erode into the underlying myocardium to produce paravalvular abscesses [63]. In a study of 44 elderly patients with IE, the mitral valve was affected in 45 %, aortic in 32 % and both in 5 % [67].

Streptococcus sp. is the most common cause and accounts for 25–75 % of endocarditis cases, *S. viridans* is less prevalent in older patients and *S. bovis*, a non-enterococcal group D streptococcus, is the causative organism in up to 25 %. In approximately 80 % of cases, the predominant organisms in the elderly population are *streptococci* and *staphylococci* [68]. *Staphylococcus aureus* has become the primary pathogen of endocarditis with the present-day use of intravascular devices [69, 70], and elderly diabetic patients are at increased risk of bacteraemia and IE [71]. Recently, many studies have shown a trend towards increasing incidence of *Staphylococcus aureus* IE [72, 73]. *Enterococci* can account for 25 % in the elderly and some studies have noted a high prevalence in the elderly [74]. Other commonly encountered organisms are the HACEK organisms (*Haemophilus parainfluenzae, Haemophilus aphrophilus, Actinobacillus actinomycetemcomitans, Cardiobacterium hominis, Eikenella species* and *Kingella species*) [75].

The portal of entry and subsequent consequences of microbiology show specific features of IE in the elderly as compared with younger patients [76, 77]. Manipulations or procedures of oral cavity, genitourinary tract (prostatic and vesical disease) and gastrointestinal tract (colonic lesions) commonly produce transient bacteraemia involving streptococci and staphylococci.

Box 1.4. Key Points. Infective Endocarditis in the Elderly

- *Streptococcus* spp. is the most common cause in older patients [68].
- *Staphylococcus aureus* is increasing with present-day use of intravascular devices [72, 73].
- *Enterococci* accounts for 25 % in the elderly [74].
- Portal of entry – manipulations or procedures of oral cavity, genitourinary tract, gastrointestinal tract is commonly associated with *streptococci* or *staphylococci* bacteraemia [76, 77].

1.5 Coronary Artery Disease in the Elderly

Introduction

Coronary artery disease is characterised by the presence of atherosclerosis of the epicardial coronary arteries. Coronary artery disease (CAD) is the most common form of heart disease in the world today. Its prevalence increases with age affecting about two-third of men and women in the sixth decade and accounts for significant morbidity and mortality in the elderly. CAD accounted for 51 % of all cardiovascular deaths and half of them were from acute myocardial infarction [78].

Pathophysiology

Atherosclerosis is by far the commonest cause of coronary artery disease. Age is an important risk factor. Atherosclerosis is primarily typified by the formation of intimal plaques called *atheroma.* A chain of events leads to the formation of plaque. The endothelium has critical roles, preventing intravascular clotting and regulating vascular tone and endothelial permeability. Several theories have been proposed to explain the initial and subsequent growth of the atheromatous plaque. Many of the events are linked to at least initially to chronic injury of the endothelium [79]. The endothelial dysfunction may be triggered by factors such as sheer stress and turbulent flow [80], oxidative stress, hyperlipidaemia, hypertension, smoking among others [79, 81]. Insudation of the lipoproteins, mainly the low-density lipoprotein (LDL) into the intima undergoes modification and initiates monocyte migration to localise in the intima and promotes differentiation of monocytes into macrophages. The lipoproteins are taken up by the monocytes to become lipid-filled foam cells, the hall mark of atherosclerosis [82, 83]. Further plaque progression involves more macrophages and formation of a core of extracellular lipid and cholesterol within the plaque and expanding the plaque size. The endothelial cells, macrophages and smooth muscle cells (SMCs) release chemotactic growth factors which stimulate proliferation of SMC of intimal or medial origin. A fibrotic cap is formed separating the plaque from the lumen.

The macrophages also produce abundant tissue factor. It is believed that the main prothrombotic stimulus in the plaque is the tissue factor which activates coagulation [84, 85]. As the plaque evolves, denudation of the endothelium occurs followed by platelet deposition giving rise to the release of platelet-derived growth factor (PDGF) which further enhances the proliferation of SMC [86]. Thrombi are formed over the plaque as a result of (1) loss of endothelium, The thrombus could be superficial when it is formed on the plaque surface or deep when is formed within the plaque following plaque rupture. The fibrous cap of the plaque tears to expose the lipid core containing large amounts of cholesterol crystals, fragments of collagen and tissue factor, and thrombus forms rapidly within the plaque itself [87].

Injury (erosion/denudation) to the endothelium exposes the collagen allowing platelets to adhere to it. With continuing platelet-to-platelet adhesion, the platelet mass grows using the IIb/IIIa receptor and fibrinogen as binder. The early platelet mass is unstable, but with the conversion of fibrinogen to fibrin, it becomes secure [88]. Damage to the tissue results in the release of tissue factor and activates factor X which in turn activates the generation of thrombin from prothrombin. Thrombin converts fibrinogen to fibrin. Enhanced exposure and activity is the final common pathway of clot formation [87]. Activated platelets release two substances which contribute to increased expression of IIb/IIIa receptor. One is thromboxane A2 (TXA2) which can be blocked by aspirin and the other is adenosine diphosphate (ADP) which also stimulates platelet recruitment and is inhibited by clopidogrel [89]. Under high shear-stress conditions, von Willebrand factor (vWF) appears to play an important role in both platelet adhesion and aggregation [90].

The plaque (1) may undergo patchy or massive calcification and some lesions in acute coronary syndromes tend to have less calcification and hence more softness of the plaque resulting in an increase in vulnerability to shear force [91]. (2) The fissured or ulcerated lesions may develop superimposed thrombus, (3) macrophages may release metalloproteinases and other proteolytic enzymes that can weaken the fibrous cap and make them more vulnerable to rupture [81, 92]. The loss of endothelial integrity may invoke haemorrhage either an influx of blood from the vessel lumen or result from intraplaque neovascularisation which can trigger acute clinical events [93]. The haemorrhage could cause sudden expansion of the plaque [94, 95] and cause its rupture. Damage to the underlying media may result in atherosclerotic aneurysm (Fig. 1.1) [80].

The plaque instability leads to development of clinical events. Attention has been drawn recently that the fibrous cap is a strong determinant of the likelihood of plaque rupture which in turn leads to thrombosis followed by either plaque

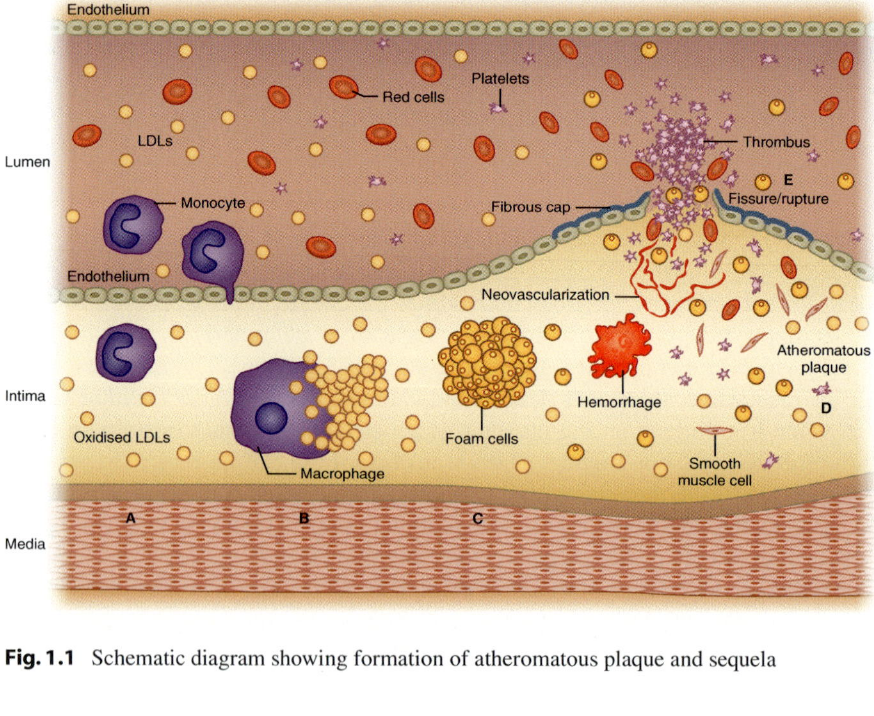

Fig. 1.1 Schematic diagram showing formation of atheromatous plaque and sequela

expansion or occlusion [96, 97]. The process of rupture is believed to underlie most acute coronary syndromes including unstable angina, ST-elevated myocardial infarction (STEMI) and non-ST elevation myocardial infarction (non-STEMI) [98, 99]. There are three forms of unstable angina [100].

1. Unstable angina can result from non-occlusive thrombus on pre-existing plaques [100]. Disruption of the fibrous cap allows aggregating platelets into the coronary circulation [101]
2. Coronary vasoconstriction resulting in dynamic obstruction and four subgroups has been recognised [100]. The first and second are called prinzmetal angina and characterised by ST-segment elevation accompanying rest pain [100]
3. Progressive mechanical obstruction resulting from severe organic narrowing of the lumen can occur with [100] or without previous intracoronary procedures [102].

There is increasing evidence in recent years that inflammation may play an important role in atherogenesis [100, 103, 104], and the inflammatory response is an immune-mediated process [103]. Seroepidemiological studies have shown raised antibody titres against several organisms [104], namely, *Chlamydia pneumoniae* [104, 105], *Helicobacter pylori* [106] and *cytomegalovirus* [107] in patients with atherosclerosis. An association between coronary artery disease and high titres of antibodies to *Chlamydia pneumoniae* has been documented [103–105] and the organism has been identified in atherosclerotic plaques [100, 105] and implicated in plaque instability [104]. Raised serological antibody titres against toxoplasmosis were seen in 12 patients and members of their families [108]. There were evidence of myocardial [109], pericardial [110] and vascular involvement such as a sudden 'stroke' or arteritis [109]. The more usual picture was chronic heart disease [109]. The electrocardiogram showed disturbances of rate, rhythm, conduction defects or abnormalities such as ventricular hypertrophy, Q waves and low electrical complex [108].

Box 1.5. Key Points. Coronary Artery Disease in the Elderly

- The endothelium has critical roles [79].
- The atheromatous plaque may undergo calcification, fissure, ulcerate or haemorrhage [91].
- The fibrous cap is a strong determinant of the likelihood of plaque rupture [96, 97].
- The process of rupture is believed to underlie most acute coronary syndromes [98, 99].
- Increasing evidence that inflammation may play an important role in atherogenesis [100, 103, 104].

1.6 Valvular Heart Disease in the Elderly

Introduction

Valvular heart disease is characterised by involvement of one or more valves of the heart, congenital or acquired by any disease process. With the increase in the number of elderly population, valvular heart disease due to degenerative calcification, myxomatous degeneration, papillary muscle dysfunction, infective endocarditis among others is increasing and (Table 3.1) is becoming significant cause of mortality and morbidity in this age group worldwide [111]. Many elderly have either mitral or aortic valvular disease due to degenerative valvular disease. Two to three per cent of the 75 years and older are affected with calcific aortic stenosis, and of the 1–2 % of the population with bicuspid aortic valves, about half develop aortic stenosis and one-third develop aortic regurgitation [112]. In the elderly, calcific aortic stenosis and mitral incompetence due to mitral valve prolapse are the most frequently occurring lesions although rheumatic mitral stenosis and aortic incompetence are not uncommon [113, 114].

Pathophysiology

Aortic stenosis increases in frequency with age and the important causes are the degenerative calcifying valves, congenital abnormalities and rheumatic heart disease.

Calcific degenerative disease: Although calcific aortic valve disease is common in the older age group, it is not a consequence of ageing [115–117]. Aortic valve stenosis is not invariably present among the elderly for 25–45 % of the 80-year-old group have no evidence of aortic calcification [115]. It was considered as a passive degenerative process over the years, but now, it is considered as an active process akin to atherosclerosis with chronic inflammatory cell infiltration, lipoid deposition and active calcification of the leaflets [112, 117, 118]. It is often accelerated by the presence of congenital bicuspid valves, and patients with bicuspid valves tend to present with significant aortic stenosis or regurgitation in the fifth or sixth decade of life [118].

Aortic valve sclerosis: Aortic valve sclerosis (AVS) in the absence of flow obstruction is common in the elderly. It is believed that the initial lesion in calcific aortic valve disease appears to implicate an active process with some likeness to atherosclerosis including lipid deposition [117], macrophage infiltration and formation of osteopontin and other proteins [119]. It is assumed to be benign and perhaps antecedent to aortic valve stenosis.

Congenital: Abnormal aortic bicuspid and aortic tricuspid valve abnormalities give rise to stenosis by their incomplete formation and fusion of the leaflets resulting in a reduced lumen. The valves eventually lead to fibrosis, rigidity and calcification. The bicuspid valve comes to attention in the younger elderly (fifth or sixth decade) [118, 120] and the aortic tricuspid later. *Rheumatic*: In aortic stenosis of rheumatic origin, there are adhesions, and fusion of the commissures and cusps with progressive fibrosis of the cusps, calcification and scarring and retraction of the leaflet and the valve orifice is reduced.

Aortic regurgitation (AR) could present in an acute or chronic form and due to aortic root disease or leaflet pathology [121, 122]. About 8–14 % of unselected patients aged 50–60 years had evidence of aortic regurgitation on echocardiography, and this rose to 24–33 % in those above the age of 70 years [123, 124]. Infective endocarditis, trauma or aortic dissection may cause acute regurgitation. The most common cause of chronic aortic regurgitation is isolated severe AR from aortic root/annular dilatation presumably resulting from medial disease as in Marfan's disease [112], rheumatoid arthritis, ankylosing spondylitis or syphilis [125]. Other causes include rheumatic heart disease, congenital bicuspid valve, previous infective endocarditis, myxomatous degeneration and various forms of aortitis, autoimmune and connective tissue disorders [125].

Moderate-to-severe mitral regurgitation MR is present in approximately 10 % of the general population over the age of 75 years [126]. The prevalence of MR increases with age, and the types of MR in the elderly are degenerative and result from myxomatous degeneration, mitral valve prolapse, calcified mitral annulus and ischaemic [127]. Mitral regurgitation (MR) can be acute or chronic. Acute MR in elderly patients is due to chordal rupture associated with myocardial infarction, infective endocarditis or mucoid degeneration of the valve cusps [118, 128]. Chronic MR may result from disruption or injury of these elements, namely, the annulus, valve leaflets, chordae, papillary muscles and left ventricle [118, 128]. Mitral annular calcification occurs predominantly in women and MR is rarely haemodynamically significant, but extension of the calcification may give rise to conduction abnormalities. In the elderly, myxomatous degeneration of the valves is an important cause of mitral valve prolapse and is more common in men. Chordal rupture is common and may result in sudden severe MR [118].

Mitral stenosis is predominantly due to rheumatic heart disease and is usually identified before old age. A rare cause is mitral annular calcification and is more common in elderly women than men. Little more than half the patients with rheumatic heart disease do not give a history of rheumatic fever or chorea. The mitral and aortic valves are usually involved.

Box 1.6. Key Points. Valvular Disease in the Elderly

- Calcific aortic valve disease is not a consequence of ageing, now considered an active process akin to atherosclerosis with chronic inflammatory cell infiltration, active calcification of the leaflets and lipoid deposition [115–117].
- Aortic valve sclerosis is perhaps antecedent to aortic valve stenosis.
- Common cause of aortic regurgitation is isolated severe AR from aortic root/annular dilatation [112].
- Types of mitral regurgitation in the elderly are degenerative and result from myxomatous degeneration, primary floppy valves, calcified mitral annulus and ischaemic [127].

1.7 Hypertension and Hypertensive Heart Disease in the Elderly

Introduction

High blood pressure is by definition a repeatedly elevated blood pressure, a systolic blood pressure above 140 mmHg with a diastolic blood pressure above 90 mmHg. According to the Joint National Committee (JNC) VI criteria, more than 50 % of people over the age of 60 years especially women are hypertensive [129]. The Framingham Study indicated that the lifetime risk of developing high blood pressure in men and women who are free of hypertension at 55 years through 80 years is 95 % and 91 %, respectively [130].

Pathophysiology and ageing

With normal ageing, there is intimal thickening of the arteries together with microscopic changes in the media and its elastic content diminishes. This gives rise to decreased compliance (vascular elasticity) [131] and increased stiffness [131–134]. Apart from atherosclerotic changes, the vascular endothelium becomes dysfunctional [135, 136] contributing further to stiffness of the arterial walls. Age-related changes in the nitric oxide and angiotensin II pathways have important roles in vascular ageing [134]. The endothelium-derived relaxing factor (EDRF) which is nitric oxide may be decreased and endothelin which is a potent vasoconstrictor may be increased resulting in endothelial dysfunction [137, 138].

Arterial blood pressure depends on the peripheral vascular resistance as well as the central artery stiffness. Increase in the peripheral vascular resistance leads to increase in systolic and diastolic pressures, while central artery stiffness leads to elevation of systolic pressure and reduction of diastolic. With ageing, the systolic blood pressure increases well into the 80s, while the diastolic blood pressure peaks in the 50s and subsequently declines [139] which manifests as a widened pulse pressure [133, 140]. Isolated systolic hypertension is the most common form of hypertension in the elderly [141, 142] and is due to arterial stiffness [143].

Box 1.7. Key Points. Hypertension in the Elderly

- With normal ageing, there is intimal thickening.
- Decrease compliance (vascular elasticity) [131].
- Central artery stiffness leads to elevation of systolic pressure and reduction of diastolic [139].
- Isolated systolic hypertension is most common form in the elderly and is due to arterial stiffness [141, 142].

1.8 Peripheral Arterial Disease

Introduction

Peripheral arterial disease (PAD) is the term used to denote reduced blood flow from narrowing or obstruction of the blood vessels to the lower limbs and is largely due to atherosclerosis. A population-based Western Australian study found the prevalence of PAD increases with age, 10.6 % in men aged 65–69 to 23.3 % in men aged 75–79 years [144]. Most epidemiological studies report the prevalence of PAD to be about 10–25 % in both genders over 55 years [145].

Pathophysiology

Atherosclerosis is by far the commonest pathological feature of PAD. It is caused by the formation of intimal plaques called atheroma which consists of lipid foam cells, macrophages and monocytes. Overlying the lipid core is a fibrous cap. In the lower limbs, high-risk plaques are stenotic and fibrous [146]. The stenotic lesions lead to narrowing of the lumen resulting in arterial insufficiency or complete occlusion of the vessel. Reduction in arterial flow may eventuate in the development of collateral vessels. The plaque can fissure or rupture forming a nidus for thrombus formation which can occlude the vessel triggering an acute syndrome.

Box 1.8. Key Points. Peripheral Arterial Disease

- Atherosclerosis is the commonest pathological feature of PAD.
- In the lower limbs, high-risk plaques are stenotic and fibrous.
- Stenotic lesions lead to arterial insufficiency or may completely occlude the vessel.
- The plaque can fissure or rupture forming a nidus for thrombus formation – triggering an acute syndrome [146].

1.9 Carotid Artery Disease

Introduction

Imaging of the extracranial and intracranial vasculature had become significant part of the evaluation of patients with stroke or transient ischaemic attack (TIA). Extracranial carotid artery disease is the cause of stroke in 14–40 % of patients, and artery-to-artery embolism is the main mechanism of ischaemic stroke [147]. An understanding of the distribution of the blood vessels to the brain and the extracranial to intracranial collateral pathways, the pial-to-pial collateral pathways and the variability of the circle of Willis is necessary to appreciate what happens in a stroke or TIA.

Pathophysiology

The carotid artery can be involved by a number of pathologies, atherosclerotic carotid artery disease, carotid artery stenosis, spontaneous carotid artery dissection, carotid artery tortuosity and kinking and atherosclerotic aortic arch disease, traumatic occlusion and inflammatory arteriopathies [148]. The internal (ICA) and external (ECA) branches of the common carotid artery are the common sites for plaque formation in the cerebrovascular system. The carotid bifurcation and the proximal ICA are the most frequently involved. The distal carotid artery and the origin of the middle cerebral artery and the carotid siphon may also be affected.

Carotid disease results from atherosclerosis leading to plaque formation, plaque ulceration, narrowing of the vessels in the thromboembolism and carotid embolic disease. Fusler et al. [149] proposed a pathophysiological classification representing stages in the pathogenesis of vascular diseases. Type I consists of functional changes in the endothelial cell without substantial morphological changes, type II consists of denudation of the endothelium and intimal damage and type III consists of denudation of the endothelium with damage to the intima and media. Endothelial dysfunction begins and is triggered by factors such as shear stress [150], turbulent flow [151], oxidative stress [152, 153], hyperlipidaemia, smoking, and impaired glucose metabolism among others [154].

Thrombi may form in the plaque as a result of loss of endothelium and within the plaque as result of plaque rupture. The plaques may undergo calcification, form fissured or ulcerated lesions and the ruptured plaque exposes highly thrombogenic substances which encourage thrombus formation and release emboli in the blood stream [155]. High-grade stenosis may occur in the absence of calcification, or on the other hand, dense calcification may be seen in the absence of high-grade stenosis.

In patients older than 50 years, carotid artery disease is strongly and independently associated with coronary artery disease [156]. Increase in the thickness of the intima and media of the carotid artery is directly associated with increased risk of myocardial infarction in older adults without a history of cardiovascular disease [157]. Haemostatic factors Factor VIIc and Factor VIIIc activity was higher in patients with carotid artery disease and may be related to carotid artery disease in the elderly. Low concentrations of folic acid and vitamin B_{12} with high plasma homocysteine concentrations are associated with increased risk of extracranial carotid artery disease in the elderly [158]. The pathophysiology of watershed infarction in internal carotid artery disease is due to low flow and microembolism, and recent postulates state that emboli and hypoperfusion play a synergistic role [159].

Box 1.9. Key Points. Carotid Artery Disease

- The carotid bifurcation and the proximal ICA are the most frequently involved.
- Carotid disease results from atherosclerosis leading to plaque formation, plaque ulceration, narrowing of the vessels in the thromboembolism and carotid and carotid embolic disease.
- In older patients, carotid artery disease is strongly and independently associated with coronary artery disease [156].
- High plasma homocysteine concentrations are associated with increased risk of extracranial carotid artery disease in the elderly [158].
- The pathophysiology of watershed infarction in internal carotid artery disease is due to low flow and microembolism and recent postulates state that emboli and hypoperfusion play a synergistic role [159].

1.10 Related Disorders

1.10.1 Syncope

Introduction

Syncope is a transient loss of consciousness and accompanied by loss of postural tone due to inadequate cerebral perfusion and followed by rapid and spontaneous recovery [160, 161]. In pre-syncope, there is no loss of consciousness. Syncope is common, can be dangerous, disabling and difficult to diagnose. About 3 % of the population is affected [162]. A retrospective analysis of very old institutionalised patients (mean age 87 years) revealed that over a 10-year period the prevalence of syncope was 23 % and 1-year incidence was 7 % [163]. In a prospective study, the incidence of syncope in nursing home residents was 6 %, and 30 % of these patients had at least one recurrent episode [163]. Syncope had been reported in 1 % of medical admissions and 3 % of the emergency department visits to a general hospital [164]. The Framingham study data suggested that annually 3 % of men and 3.5 % of women have syncope [165]. Furthermore, it indicated an annual incidence of 6 % for at least one episode for those over the age of 75 in men in comparison with only 0.7 % in the age group 35–44 [165].

Cardiovascular causes of syncope are more prevalent in the elderly as compared to the young and occur in 33.8 % in the elderly compared to 16.8 % in the young [166]. In one population study of syncope, the history and physical examination in elderly persons revealed a 40 % yield in the diagnosis [167] and when additional specific tests such as electrocardiogram or cardiac catheterisation were included a further 15 %. Cardiogenic syncope is associated with higher rates of morbidity and mortality than other causes [168]; the 1-year mortality for patients with cardiac syncope was 30 % in comparison to 12 % in those with noncardiac causes [169].

Pathophysiology

Normally, blood pressure is maintained by cardiovascular and neuroendocrine mechanisms. The *cardiac output* (CO) is the amount of blood that is pumped by the heart per unit time, measured in litres per minute. The amount of blood that is put out by the left ventricle of the heart in one contraction is the *stroke volume* (SV). Stroke volume X *heart rate* = cardiac output. The resistance offered by the arterioles and capillaries to the flow of blood from the arteries to the veins is the peripheral resistance (PR). *Venous return* (VR) can be defined as the volume of blood returning to the right heart (VR = CO when averaged over time). Cardiac output X *peripheral resistance* = *blood pressure.* The ability to maintain normal blood pressure declines with age as does heart rate response to change of position. This could lead to reduction in the capacity to maintain adequate cerebral blood flow leading to syncope. Any cause or circumstance that reduces blood pressure either by peripheral vasodilatation or decrease cardiac output may produce syncope. Cardiac output could be transiently compromised by myocardial, anatomical or electrical abnormalities (Fig. 1.2). Age- and disease-related abnormalities that impair the ability to respond to physiological stress subject the elderly to increased risk of syncope which would

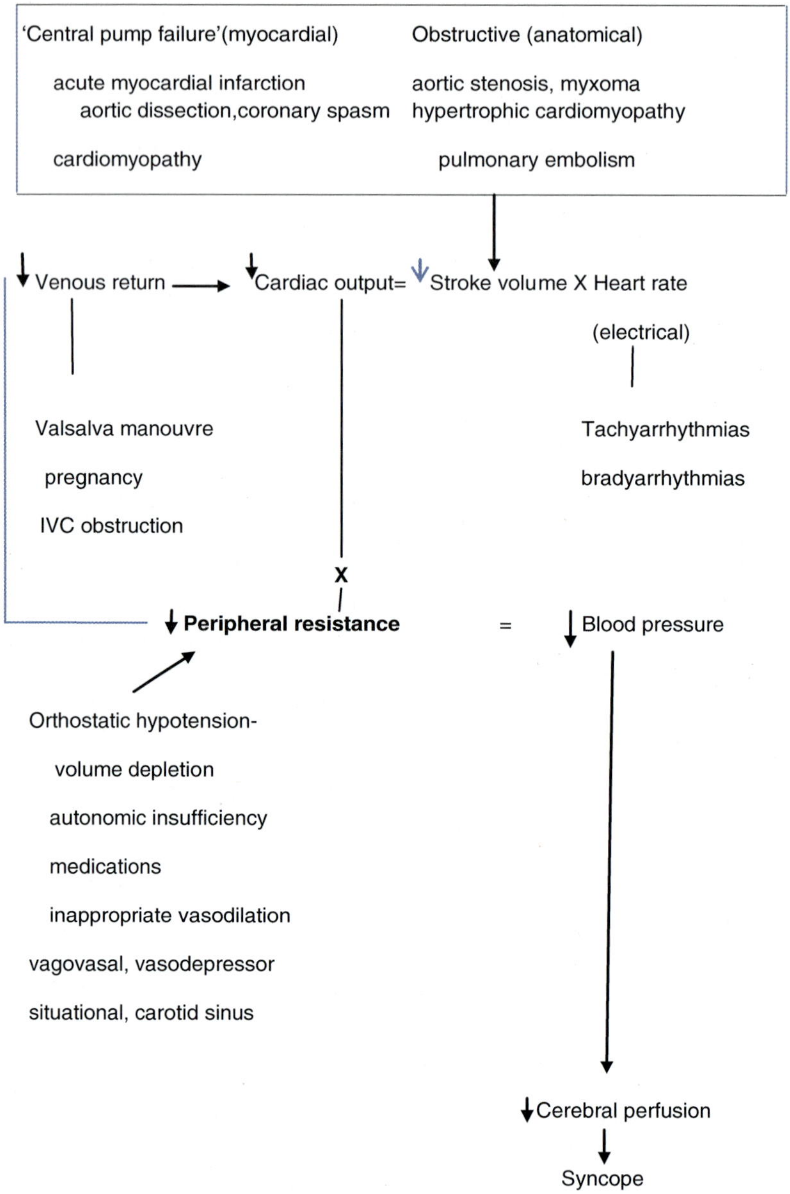

Fig. 1.2 Pathophysiology of syncope

normally not cause syncope [163]. The common causes of syncope are the neurally mediated syndromes, cardiac and orthostatic.

With the neurally mediated syndrome, there is acute vasodilatation of the vascular beds with pooling in the lower extremities and it provokes vasovagal response through the Bezold-Jarisch mechanism leading to hypotension and bradycardia

[170]. They are normal reflexes and may be exaggerated in some and blunted in other situations [171]. The term neurocardiogenic syncope has been used for vasovagal syncope for the triggers are said to arise from the heart [172]. The neutrally mediated syncope includes vasovagal syncope, situational syncope and carotid hypersensitivity syncope. Almost half of cognitively normal elderly patients seen in the emergency with non-accidental falls have carotid sinus hypersensitivity [173]. When pressure is applied over the internal carotid artery in the region of the carotid sinus, the normal response is slowing of the heart rate with an impaired atrioventricular node conduction. In carotid sinus syncope, accidental mechanical manipulation such as tight collars or head turning this reflex is exaggerated. The reflex response has two components, namely, cardioinhibitory giving rise to asystole lasting for more than 3 s and a vasodepressor component causing a fall in blood pressure of 50 mmHg or more or the response may be mixed [174].

In orthostatic syncope, changing from supine to erect position results in venous pooling of blood. With the change in position, the baroreceptors precipitate an increase in medullary sympathetic outflow resulting in vasoconstriction of the systemic resistance vessels and splanchnic vessels, a compensation for the orthostatic stress. Orthostatic hypotension occurs when the autonomic nervous system is impaired and may occur with change in position or with hypovolaemia. It occurs in primary and secondary autonomic failure and with medications. The increased susceptibility of older person to syncope is due to age-related physiological changes to cerebral blood flow and baroreceptor response and heart rate response to orthostatic stress [175] together with multiple diseases [175, 176]. Renal sodium conservation and intravascular volume maintenance are impaired by age-related decreases in basal and stimulated renin levels and aldosterone production with increases in atrial natriuretic peptide in the elderly and predispose to syncope. The elderly are more likely to become dehydrated. They may have a severe response to diuretics leading to rapid volume depletion, postural hypotension and to syncope.

The cardiac causes can be subdivided into mechanical and electrical [171]. In the former, blood flow is abruptly impeded leading to systemic hypoperfusion and syncope. The electrical causes manifest in the form of arrhythmias [171]. Arrhythmias as a result of loss of compensatory reflex peripheral vasoconstriction cause hypotension resulting in syncope.

The cause could be determined in less than 50 % of the patients [177]. In a study, 510 patients (4.5 %) had syncope of unknown origin [178], but the reported incidence of syncope of unknown origin varies. In another study, approximately half of the patients admitted with syncope were similarly classified [169]. Broadly, syncope can be categorised as cardiac or noncardiac. The latter includes neurally mediated reflex syncope (situational syncope – micturition, postprandial, cough, etc.) (carotid sinus, vasovagal) and orthostatic (postural) due to autonomic failure. The cardiac causes result from structural heart abnormalities (mechanical) and arrhythmias (electrical).

Many daily situations such as micturition, defecation, postural changes and eating were found to be associated with syncope in 20 % of institutionalised elderly patients [163, 179]. Similarly other situations included were strenuous coughing, laughing or swallowing. Postprandial hypotension is also common among the elderly and could occur during or after a meal and produce syncope [180].

Carotid sinus hypersensitivity was seen in more than half of the cognitively normal older persons presenting to the accident and emergency with non-accidental falls [173]. A lesion in the bifurcation of the carotid, a tight collar or tumour could produce syncope (carotid sinus syncope) by stimulation of the baroreceptors in the carotid sinus [181]. Carotid massage has its greatest usefulness in the elderly patients [167, 182, 183] and appears to be safe if it is done in patients who do not have carotid bruits, recent stroke, myocardial infarction or a history of ventricular tachycardia [184]. Baroreflex sensitivity decreases with age. When the vagus nerve is stimulated by, for instance, pain, fright or nausea, syncope (vasovagal syncope) could result.

Orthostatic hypotension is an important factor and is common in the elderly and is an important risk factor for syncope. The causes include age-associated physiological changes, medications and autonomic insufficiency syndromes (idiopathic orthostatic hypotension, Shy-Drager syndrome). Arrhythmias are more frequently diagnosed in the elderly than in younger patients. In a study comparing community-dwelling elderly patients with young persons, arrhythmias were found in 28 % of the elderly and only 13 % of the young persons [166] and several other entities such as aortic stenosis, transient ischaemic attack, myocardial infarction and carotid sinus syncope were primarily found in elderly persons [166].

Box 1.10. Key Points. Syncope in the Elderly

- Syncope is common, can be dangerous, disabling, difficult to diagnose and can cause sudden cardiac death.
- Cardiovascular causes are more prevalent in the elderly in 38.8 % [166].
- The prevalence of ventricular arrhythmias in over 60 years age group is about 70–80 %.
- The neurally mediated syncope includes vasovagal syncope, situational syncope and carotid hypersensitivity syncope [170].
- Many daily situations such as micturition, defaecation, postural changes and eating associated with syncope in 20 % of institutionalised elderly patients [163, 179].
- Carotid sinus hypersensitivity was seen in more than half of the cognitively normal older persons presenting with non-accidental falls [173].
- Orthostatic hypotension is an important risk factor for syncope [175].

1.10.2 Leg and Foot Ulcers in the Elderly

Introduction

An ulcer is characterised by a breach in the skin followed by erosion of the subcutaneous tissues which could extend deeper to involve the muscle and bone. Population studies have shown the prevalence of leg ulcers in the aged 65 years and older to be between 0.12 % [185] and 1.02 % [186]. The prevalence of venous ulcers varies from 0.1 to 1 % [187–189] and accounts for almost 80 % of all leg ulcers [190]. The prevalence of chronic venous insufficiency ranges from 5 to 8 % [189] and is responsible for 70 % of chronic ulcers of the lower limbs [191]. Arterial ulcers account for 10–25 % of lower limb ulcers [192]. The prevalence of pressure ulcers ranges from 9.2 % in acute hospitals [193] to 17.4 % in nursing homes at the time of admission [194], and the presence of high-grade ulcers occurs in 4 % in the elderly in nursing care facilities [185].

Pathophysiology
Any condition that affects the circulation, sensation or structure of the feet will place the individual at risk of developing ulcers. The name of the ulcers highlights their primary cause, for example, ischaemic, venous, neuropathic and pressure.

1. Ischaemic ulcers
Chronic ischaemia from peripheral obliterative arterial disease results in reduced perfusion decreasing tissue resilience and viability, and as ischaemia worsens, ulceration may appear especially after local trauma. Three mechanisms are said to be involved, extramural strangulation, mural thickening and intramural restriction of blood flow [196]. The reduced blood flow impedes healing by curtailing the oxygen and other soluble mediators necessary for the repair process [197]. Limb-threatening foot ulcers may develop in a patient with relatively mild symptoms of arterial insufficiency, and it is known that the blood supply needed for healing an ulcer is very much more than that needed for maintaining intact skin integrity [198]. Factors that worsen leg and foot ulcers include smoking, hypertension, diabetes, advanced age, coronary artery disease and arthritis (Fig. 1.3).

2. Venous stasis ulcers
Deep vein insufficiency and/or occlusion are complications of deep vein thrombosis and the long-term problems arising from them are venous ulcers [199] which are an important cause of leg ulcers in older people. Acute thrombus is associated with mediators of inflammation and the venous recanalisation [200]. Recanalisation

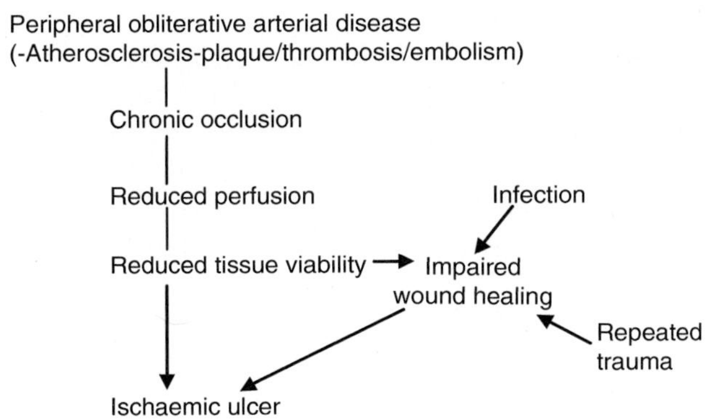

Fig. 1.3 Sequence of events in ischaemic ulcer (Information sources: Hopkins and Wolfe [199]; Kahn and Ginsberg [200])

following deep vein thrombosis results in destruction of the valves resulting in deep vein insufficiency [200]. If recanalisation fails, the chronic venous occlusion leads to the development of a collateral circulation which is also without valves. Either event has a deleterious effect on the function of the calf pump resulting in high venous pressure or venous hypertension [199, 201] in the leg and foot. The exact mechanism leading from venous hypertension to venous ulceration remains unclear [187, 202]. It is now believed that the pathogenesis is associated with abnormalities in the microcirculation and inflammatory reaction [187, 191]. There are several theories as to the direct cause of the ulceration. Venous hypertension leads to local venous dilatation and pooling [188]. Furthermore, there is decreased flow in the capillaries resulting in trapping of the white blood cells which may release proteolytic enzymes that destroy the tissues [188, 203]. Another hypothesis is that venous hypertension results in venous pooling which induces the deposition of fibrin and other macromolecules causing trapping of the growth factors which are necessary for wound repair [188, 204, 205]. Calf muscle pump failure may be another factor resulting in stasis of blood and increased venous pressure [206].

With chronic venous insufficiency, oedema and dilated superficial veins appear, and with time, skin pigmentation occurs on the medial and sometimes on the lateral aspects of the ankle and leg. This is followed by stasis dermatitis and ulceration. There is a strong case for routine and long-term use of thromboprophylaxis particularly in high-risk patients. Factors which aggravate venous ulcers include congestive heart failure, obesity, diabetes, fracture or injury and physical inactivity (Fig. 1.4).

3. Neuropathic ulcers

In neuropathy, the motor, sensory and autonomic fibres are involved. With sensory disturbance, there is a loss of protective sensation which is a key factor in the development of an ulcer [207]. Motor fibre involvement gives rise to wasting of the intrinsic muscles of the feet [192] with collapse of the arch and loss of stability. Overaction of the extrinsic muscles tends to depress the metatarsal heads with 'cocked-up' toes [208]. These changes results in abnormal pressure points, increased shearing and greater friction on the feet [198]. Diminished sweating, dryness and fissuring and cracking of the skin results from involvement of the autonomic fibres. Break in the skin barrier predisposes to infection (Fig. 1.5).

4. Pressure ulcers

Pressure ulcers have also been referred to as bed sores and decubitus ulcers. Pressure over the bony prominences that exceeds the blood pressure causes not only cessation of blood supply to the skin but also has an intense effect on the muscle and fat adjacent to the bone even before there is evidence of damage to the skin. Pressure is a key factor in the causation of ulcer [209], and there is a relationship between pressure intensity and duration [210]. Immobility and multiple co-morbidities contribute largely to pressure ulcers [195, 211].

Other important pathogenic factors are shearing, friction and moisture [209]. Shearing which is the applied force that causes an opposite parallel sliding motion in the planes of an object is the second key factor [210]. It cuts off large areas of

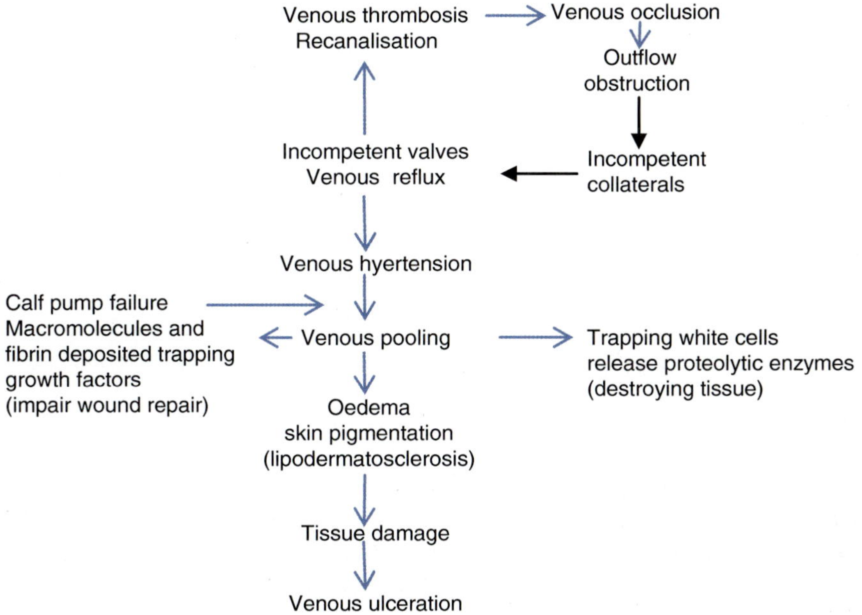

Fig. 1.4 Sequence of events giving rise to venous ulceration (Information sources: Trent et al. [188]; Hopkins and Wolfe [199]; Kahn and Ginsberg [200]; Coleridge-Smith et al. [203]; Rudolp and Shannon [204]; Falanga and Eaglstein [205])

Fig. 1.5 Sequence of events in neuropathic ulcers (Information sources: Boike and Maier [192]; Sumpio [198])

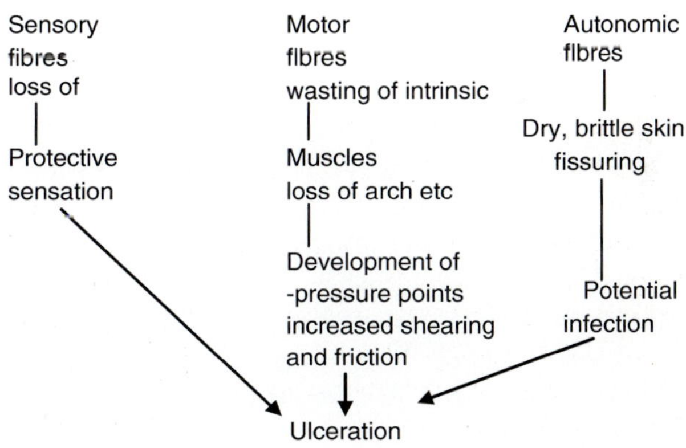

vascular supply. Friction occurs between the skin and bed surface as the patient slides down from a semi-recumbent position and increases the susceptibility to ulceration [210]. Other factors predisposing to ulceration are the reduction of spontaneous movements in hospitalised patients and moisture secondary to incontinence and perspiration resulting in skin maceration. Nicotine has a peripheral vasoconstrictive action which increases the risk of ulceration. Table 1.2 shows the location, appearances and other characteristics of leg ulcers (Fig. 1.6).

Table 1.2 Ulcers defined by their location, appearance and other characteristics

	Arterial	Venous	Neuropathic	Pressure
Location	Feet-on heels tips of toes, between toes	Below knee medial aspect just above ankle	Both feet at increased pressure points	Sacrum, ischium, trochanter, ankles, heels
Appearance	Base yellow/ brown or grey/ blackened colour	Base usually yellow, fibrous tissue yellow, if infected pink-brown	Base variable circulation	Depending on stage (NPUAP): Stage I. Erythema of intact skin. Stage II. Partial thickness skin loss Stage III. Full thickness of skin Stage IV. Full thickness
Margins	Punched out	Irregularly flat border	Punched out	Varies according to the stage
Surrounding skin	Skin – shiny redness if foot is dangling; pale if elevated	Calloused tight, brown pigmentation sclerotic	Rim of hyperkeratotic tissue	With extensive destruction of tissue, necrosis and damage to deeper tissue
Other characteristics	Painful especially at night	Pain relieved by rest and elevation	Burning, tingling or numbness	Infection – induration purulent discharge
Clinical features	History of cardiovascular cerebrovascular disease, limb claudication absent pulses, skin, nail changes	Deep vein thrombosis or deep vein insufficiency or occlusion post-phlebitic syndrome	Gait abnormalities, deformities of feet, motor strength reflexes and sensation reduction	Immobilisation or immobilised body part, hospitalised patients have poor nutritional status, incontinence, co-morbidities

Information sources: Spentzouris and Labropoulos [212]; Hart [213]

Box 1.11. Key Points. Leg and Foot Ulcers in the Elderly

- Any condition that affects the circulation, sensation or structure of the feet will place the individual at risk of developing ulcers.
- Vein insufficiency or occlusion or both are complications of deep vein thrombosis and the long-term problems arising from them are venous ulcers [199].
- Mechanisms leading to venous hypertension to venous ulceration remain unclear, but may be associated with abnormalities in the microcirculation and an inflammatory response [187, 202].
- In neuropathy, the motor, sensory and autonomic fibres are involved [192, 207].
- Pressure is a key factor in the causation of ulcer, and there is a relationship between pressure intensity and duration [209].

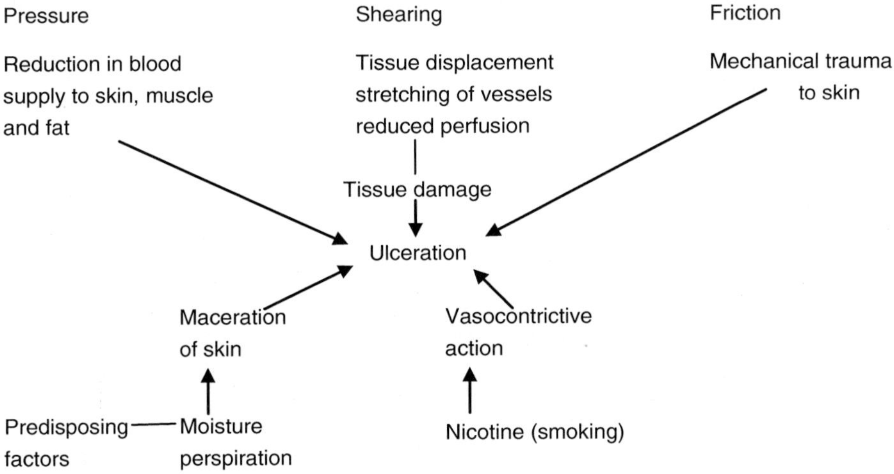

Fig. 1.6 Sequence of events in pressure ulcers (Information sources: Anders et al. [195]; Goode and Allman [209]; Yarkony [210])

Multiple Choice Questions

1. The following changes in the heart due to ageing are true, EXCEPT:
   A. There is loss of cardiac myocytes with advancing years and the left ventricular wall thickens.
   B. In ventricular systolic and diastolic dysfunction, the stroke volume is maintained by augmented contraction due to higher ventricular end-diastolic pressure.
   C. The beta-adrenergic responsiveness decreases with age limiting the maximum achievable heart rate (HR).
   D. The left ventricular diastolic filling rate decreases to a 20 % of the peak rate by the age of 80 years.
2. The following are true in heart failure, EXCEPT:
   A. In the elderly, there is a shift from coronary heart disease to hypertension as the most common aetiology in the development of heart failure.
   B. In heart failure with preserved ejection fraction (HFPEF), there is impaired relaxation and reduced compliance of the myocardium.
   C. In individuals with heart failure and left ejection fraction, more than 40 % have systolic heart failure.
   D. Certain non-steroidal anti-inflammatory drugs such as ibuprofen and indomethacin can precipitate heart failure.
3. The following in relation to coronary artery disease are true, EXCEPT:
   A. Atherosclerosis is the commonest cause of coronary artery disease.
   B. The fibrous cap is a strong determinant of the likelihood of plaque rupture.

C. Unstable angina can result from a non-occlusive thrombus in pre-existing plaques.
D. There is no evidence that inflammation plays a role in atherogenesis.

4. The following are true relating to infective endocarditis (IE), EXCEPT:
   A. Presently, *staphylococcus aureus* is the primary pathogen causing IE.
   B. Transient bacteraemia is commonly produced by manipulations or procedures of oral cavity, gastrointestinal tract and genitourinary tract.
   C. A new or changing murmur is heard in 30–52 % of patients with IE, and the murmurs are heard much more frequently in the elderly.
   D. In the elderly, non-specific symptoms may lead to incorrect diagnosis.
5. The following are true in chronic valvular disease, EXCEPT:
   A. Aortic valve sclerosis is perhaps antecedent to aortic valve stenosis.
   B. All patients with rheumatic heart disease give a history of rheumatic fever or chorea.
   C. Abnormal aortic bicuspid and tricuspid valves can give rise to aortic stenosis.
   D. Acute mitral incompetence in the elderly is due to chordal rupture due to myocardial infarction.
6. An 80-year-old male was seen in the ED following a syncopal episode in the shopping centre. He was said to have been unconscious and pulseless but recovered promptly. He has had similar episodes at least on five occasions in the past one year and had had chest pain on effort. Examination revealed an ejection systolic murmur in the aortic area and which radiated to both sides of neck and towards the apex. The electrocardiogram shows left ventricular hypertrophy. What is the diagnosis?
   A. Vasovagal syncope
   B. Aortic stenosis
   C. Ventricular arrhythmia
   D. Drop attack
7. A 75-year-old woman is seen following an episode of syncope. She has been in reasonably good health. She had been seated for several hours and on rising to the ground and momentarily lost consciousness. The blood pressure was 140/90 mmHg supine and 110/70 mmHg on standing. The CNS was grossly intact. What is the diagnosis that best describes the findings?
   A. Transient ischaemic attack
   B. Postural hypotension
   C. Partial (focal) epileptic seizure
   D. Syncopal attack
8. The following are true of neuropathic ulcers, EXCEPT:
   A. The foot is red when dangling but pale when elevated.
   B. The sensation is reduced.
   C. The ulcers are on pressure points.
   D. The reflexes are diminished.

Extended Matching Questions (EMQ)

THEME: Repeated syncopal attacks

A. Stokes-Adam attacks
B. Hypertrophic cardiomyopathy
C. Aortic stenosis
D. Vertebrobasilar insufficiency
E. Carotid sinus hypersensitivity
F. Postprandial hypotension
G. Multisystem atrophy (Shy-Drager)
H. Ventricular tachycardia
I. Left atrial myxoma

1. A 65-year-old man was seen with repeated syncopal attacks. He had dyspnea and angina and has had about five episodes of syncopal attacks in the past 1 year. On examination, he had an ejection systolic murmur in the aortic area radiating on both sides of neck and towards the apex and a slow rise pulse. The ECG showed left ventricular hypertrophy. Cardiac catheterisation revealed a peak-to-peak aortic valve gradient of 36 mmHg and aortic valve size of 0.8 cm^2.
2. A 68-year-old was accompanied by his wife who was the informant. She had noticed that over the past 3–4 months her husband had what she called 'turns', in that he abruptly becomes pale and lose consciousness and recovers in a few seconds and on recovery he appeared flushed. Sometimes, there was twitching if the unconsciousness lasted longer. During this, he is pulseless but his breathing is normal. These happen anytime of the day and on two occasions when he was sleeping.
3. An 80-year-old man presented with several episodes of transient loss of consciousness. These happen within an hour of beginning a meal. It had been recorded that his blood pressure dropped to 20 mmHg during the incident.
4. A 72-year-old man was seen with recurrent episodes of syncope. The patient himself had noticed that these happen whenever he wears a tight collar or suddenly turns his head. Initially, he feels lightheaded, becomes pale, often accompanied by sweating and nausea followed by fainting.
5. A 70-year-old man presented with breathlessness on exertion and orthopnoea. He complained of dizziness and has had three syncopal episodes. He complained of joint pains and had lost weight. He had no past history of rheumatic fever. Symptoms changed with change of position. Physical examination revealed an elevated JVP. The first sound was loud and a diastolic rumble was heard.
6. A 75-year-old man noted pain in his right thigh and calf on walking about 100 m over the past 8 weeks making him to stop walking. He becomes free of pain in 3–4 min after he had stopped walking. He also said of an ulcer on his right foot which was painful especially at night and not healing. He was obese,

hypertensive, diabetic and had been smoking about 30 cigarettes for 40 years. On examination, there were skin and nail changes and an ulcer on the tips of the second and third toes of his right foot. The pulses were normal in the inguinal region. Pulses could not be felt distally.

Answers to MCQs

1 = D; 2 = C, 3 = D; 4 = C; 5 = B; 6 = B; 7 = B; 8 = A
EMQ: 1 = C; 2 = A; 3 = F; 4 = E; 5 = I

References

Anatomical and Physiological Changes with Aging

1. Burlew BS, Weber KT. Connective tissue and the heart. Functional significance and regulatory mechanisms. Cardiol Clin. 2000;18(3):435–42 (abstract).
2. Aalami OO, Fang TD, Sang HM, Nacamuli RP. Physiological features of aging persons. Arch Surg. 2003;138:1068–76.
3. Burlew BS. Diastolic dysfunction in the elderly-the interstitial tissue. Am J Geriatr Gerontol. 2004;13(1):29–38 (abstract).
4. Olivetti G, Melissari M, Canasso I, Anversa P. Cardiomyopathy of the aging human heart. Myocyte loss and reactive cellular hypertrophy. Circ Res. 1991;68:1560–8.
5. Ganau A, Saha PS, Roman MJ, de Simone G, Realde G, Devereux RB. Ageing induces left ventricular remodelling in normotensi-ve subjects. J Hypertens. 1995;13:1818–22.
6. Anversa P, Palarkal T, Sonnenblick FH, Olivetti G, Meggs LG, Capasso JM, et al. Myocyte cell loss and myocyte cellular hyperplasia in the hypertrophied aging rat heart. Circ Res. 1990;67:871–85.
7. Lakatta EG, Levy D. Arterial and cardiac aging: major shareholders in cardiovascular disease enterprise; the aging heart in health: links to heart disease. Circulation. 2002;107: 346–54.
8. Morley IF, Reece SS. Clinical implications of the aging heart. Am J Med. 1989;86:77–86.
9. Lakatta EG. Cardiovascular aging in health. Clin Geriatr Med. 2000;16:419–44.
10. Malbut-Shennan K, Young A. The physiology of physical performance and training in old age. Coron Artery Dis. 1999;10:37–42.
11. Fleg JL, O'Connor F, Gerstenblith G, Becker LC, Clulon J, Schulman SP, et al. Impact of age on the cardiovascular response to dynamic up exercise in healthy men and women. J Appl Physiol. 1995;78:890–900.
12. Karavidas A, Lazaros G, Tsiachris D, Pyrgakis V. Aging and the cardiovascular system. Hellenic J Cardiol. 2010;51:421–42.
13. North BJ, Sinclair DA. The intersection between brain and cardiovascular disease. Circ Res. 2012;110:1097–108.
14. Nassimiha D, Aronow WS, Ahn C, Goldman ME. Association of coronary risk factors with progression of valvular aortic stenosis in older persons. Am J Cardiol. 2001;87:1313–4.
15. Lakatta EG, Yin FCP. Myocardial aging: functional alterations and related cellular mechanisms. Am J Physiol. 1982;242:H927.
16. Pugh KG, Wei JV. Clinical implications of physiological changes in the aging heart. Drugs Aging. 2001;18(4):263–73.

17. Virmani R, Avahu AP, Mergner WI, Robinourtz M, Mederik EE, Cornhill JF, et al. Effect of aging on aortic morphology in populations with high and low prevalence of hypertension, atherosclerosis: comparison between occidental and Chinese communities. Am J Pathol. 1991;139:1119–29.
18. Kovacic JC, Moreno P, Nabel EG, Hachinski V, Fuster V. Cellular senescence, vascular disease and aging. Circulation. 2011;123:1900–10.
19. Lim MA, Townsend RR. Arterial compliance in the elderly: its effect on blood pressure measurement in cardiovascular outcomes. Clin Geriatr Med. 2009;25:198–205.
20. Hafeez A. Age related changes in the cardiovascular system. http://www.physio-pedia.com/Age_related_changes_in_Cardiovascular_System. Accessed 27 Apr 2015.
21. Lakatta EG. Arterial and cardiac aging: major shareholders in cardiovascular disease enterprises, part an molecular clues to heart and arterial aging. Circulation. 2003;107:490–7.
22. Lakatta EG. Cardiovascular regulatory mechanisms in advanced age. Physiol Rev. 1993;73: 413–67.
23. Esler MD, Turner AG, Kaye DM, Thompson JM, Kingwell BA, Morris M, et al. Aging effects on human sympathetic neuronsal function. Am J Physiol. 1995;268(pt2):R278–85.
24. Taddei S, Virdis A, Mattee GL, Gennari A, Fesolo CB, et al. Aging and endothelial function in normotensive subjects and patients with essential hypertension. Circulation. 1995;91:1981–7.
25. Stamato N, Cahill J, Goodwin M, Winters G. Cardiac amyloidosis causing ventricular tachycardia: diagnosis mage by endomyocardial biopsy. Chest. 1989;96:1431–3.

Heart Failure

26. Mann DL, Bristow MR. Mechanisms and models in heart failure. Circulation. 2005;111: 2837–49.
27. Sowers JR, Lester M. Hypertension, hormones and ageing. J Lab Clin Med. 2000;135:379–86.
28. Luche RJ, Taffet GE. Tearsdale. Congestive heart failure in the elderly. J Am Geriatr Soc. 1991;39:810.
29. Beroni AG, Handley WG, Massing MW, Bonds DE, Burke GL, Gott Jr DC. Heart failure prevalence, incidence and mortality in the elderly with diabetes. Diabetes Care. 2004;27(3):699–703.
30. Burlew BS, Weber KT. Connective to issue and the heart. Functional significance and regulatory mechanisms. Cardiol Clin. 2000;18(3):435–42 (abstract).
31. Oxenham H, Sharpe N. Cardiovascular aging and heart failure. Eur J Heart Fail. 2003;5(4): 427–31.
32. Pugh KG, Wei JY. Clinical implications of physical changes in aging heart. Drugs Aging. 2001;18(4):263–76.
33. Olivetti G, Melissari M, Canasso I, Anversa P. Cardiomyopathy of the aging human heart. Myocyte loss and reactive cellular hypertrophy. Circ Res. 1991;68:1560–8.
34. Lakatta EG. Cardiovascular aging health. Clin Geriatr Med. 2000;16:419–44.
35. Morley IF, Reece SS. Clinical implications of aging heart. Am J Med. 1989;86:77–86.
36. Stratton IR, Levy WC, Cernueira MD, Schwartz RS, Abrass IB. Cardiovascular responses to exercise. Effects of ageing and exercise training in healthy men. Circulation. 1994;89: 1648–55.
37. Swine C. Aging of heart function in man. Presse Med. 1992;21(26):1216–21.
38. The American College of Cardiology and American Heart Association (ACC/AHA). Guidelines update; 2005.
39. Klabunde RE. The Pathophysiology of heart failure. http://cvpharmacology.com/clinical%20topics/heart%20failure-3.htm. Accessed 19 Apr 13.
40. Jackson G, Gibbs CR, Davies MK, Lip GYH. Pathophysiology of heart failure. BMJ. 2000;320(7228):167–70.

Cardiac Arrhythmias in the Elderly

41. Wit AL, Rosen MR. Pathophysiologic mechanisms of cardiac arrhythmias. Am Heart J. 1983;106(4Pt2):798–811 (abstract).
42. Fulberg CD, Psaty BM, Manolio TA, Gardin JM, Smith VE, Rautahanu PM. Prevalence of atrial fibrillation in elderly subjects (the Cardiovascular Health Study). Am J Cardiol. 1994;74:236–41.
43. Luria DM, Shen WK. Syncope in the elderly: new trends in diagnostic approach and non-pharmacologic management. Am J Geriatr Cardiol. 2001;10:91–6.
44. Roffe C. Ageing of the heart. Br J Biomed Sci. 1998;55(2):136–48 (abstract).
45. Klausner SC, Schwartz AB. The aging heart. Clin Geriatr Med. 1985;1(1):119–41 (abstract).
46. Fujino M, Okada R, Arakawa K. The relationship of aging to histopathological changes in the conducting system of the normal human heart. Jpn Heart J. 1983;24(1):13–20 (abstract).
47. Hatch F, Lancaster MK, Jones SA. Aging is a primary risk factor for cardiac arrhythmias: disruption of intracellular Ca2+ regulation as a key suspect. Expert Rev Cardiovasc Ther. 2011;9(8):1059–67 (abstract).
48. Sanchez-Quintana D, Yen HS. Anatomy of cardiac nodes and atrioventricular specialised conduction system. Rev Esp Cardiol. 2003;56(11):1085–92 (abstract).
49. Iaizzo PA, Laske TG. Chap 4. Anatomy and physiology of the cardiac conducting system. In: Cardiac electrocradiography methods and models. New York: Springer Science+Business MedLLc; 2010.
50. Schucht J. The cardiac conducting system: clinical electrophysiology and cardiac ablation. A senior thesis. Liberty University Fall 2011. Digitalcommon.liberty.edu. Accessed 1 Jan 2014.
51. Levy MN, Pappano AJ. Cardiovascular physiology. 9th ed. Philadelphia: Mosby Elsevier; 2007.
52. Ho S. Atrial structure and fibres: morphological basis of atrial fibrillation. Cardiovasc Res. 2002;54(2):325–36.
53. Mahadevan V. Anatomy of the heart. Surgery (Oxford). 2008;26(12):473–6.
54. Anderson RH, Ho SY. The architecture of the sinus node, the atrioventricular conduction axis, and the intermodal atrial myocardium. J Cardiovasc Electrophysiol. 1998;9(11):1233–48 (abstract).
55. Mohrman DE, Heller LJ. Cardiovascular physiology. 7th ed. New York: The McGraw Hill Companies; 2010.
56. Parks DS, Fishinan GI. Basic science for clinicians. The cardiac conductive system. Circulation. 2011;123:904–15.
57. Antoni H. Pathophysiology of cardiac arrhythmias. Z Kardiol. 1992;81 Suppl 4:111–7 (abstract).
58. Hoffman BF, Dangman KH. Mechanisms for cardiac arrhythmias. Experientia. 1987;43(10): 1049–56.

Infective Endocarditis in the Elderly

59. Gergoratos G. Infective endocarditis in the elderly: diagnosis and management. Am J Geriatr Cardiol. 2003;12:183–9.
60. Hill EE, Herijgers P, Herregods MC, Peetermans WE. Evolving trends in infective endocarditis. Clin Microbiol Infect. 2006;12:5–12.
61. Fernandez-Hidalgo N, Almirante B, Tornos P, Pigran C, Samola A, Iqual A, et al. Contemporay epidemiology and prognosis of health care-associated infective endocarditis. Clin Infect Dis. 2008;47:1287–97.
62. Benito N, Miro JM, de Lazzari E, Cabell CH, del Rio A, Altilas J, et al. Health care-associated native valve endocarditis: importance of non-noscomial acquisition. Ann Intern Med. 2009;150:586–94.
63. Kumar V, Cotran RS, Robbins SL. Basic pathology. 5th ed. Philadelphia: WB Saunders Company; 1992.

64. Durack DT, Karchmer AW. Infective endocarditis: clinical presentation. APC Medicine Online. 2006. www.medscape.com/viewarticle/534843.
65. Moreillon P, Que YA, Bayer AS. Pathogenesis of streptococcal and staphylococcal endocarditis. Infect Dis Clin North Am. 2002;16(2):297–318 (abstract).
66. Widmer E, Que YA, Entenza JM, Moreillon P. New concepts in the pathophysiology of infective endocarditis. Curr Infect Dis Rep. 2006;8(4):271–9 (abstract).
67. Gagliardi IP, Nettles RF, McCarty DF, Sanders LL, Corey GR, Sexton DJ. Native valve infective endocarditis in elderly and younger adult patients: comparison of clinical features and outcomes with use of the Duke criteria and duke Endocarditis Database. Clin Infect Dis. 1998;26:1165–8.
68. Dhawan VK. Infective endocarditis in elderly patients. Clin Infect Dis. 2002;34(6):806–12.
69. Brusch J. Infective endocarditis: management in the case of intravascular devices. New York: Informa Health Care; 2007.
70. Durante-Mangoni E, Bradley S, Selton-Suty C, Tripodi MF, Barsil B, Bonza E, et al. Current features of infective endocarditis in elderly patients. Arch Int Med. 2008;168(19):2095–103 (abstract).
71. Cunha RA, Gill MV, Lazar IM. Acute infective endocarditis. Diagnostic and therapeutic approach. Infect Dis Clin North Am. 1996;10:811–34.
72. Murdoch DR, Corey GR, Hoen B, Miro JM, Fowler VG, Bayer AS, et al. Clinical presentation etiology and outcome of infective endocarditis in the 21st century: the International Collsboration on Endocarditis-Prospective Cohort Study. Arch Intern Med. 2009;169: 463–73.
73. Fowler Jr VG, Miro JM, Hoen B, Cabell CH, Abrutyn E, Rubinstein E, et al. Staphylococcus aureus endocarditis: a consequence of medical progress. JAMA. 2005;293:3012–21.
74. Werner GS, Schulz R, Fuchs JB, Andreas S, Prange H, Ruschewski W, et al. Infective endocarditis in the elderly in the era of tranesophgeal echocardiography: clinical features and prognosis compared with younger patients. Am J Med. 1996;100:90–7.
75. Bayer A, Bolger AF, Taubert KA, Wilson W, Steckberg J, Karchmer AW, et al. Diagnosis and management of infective endocarditis and its complications. Circulation. 1998;98:2936–48.
76. Di Salvo G, Rosenberg V, Pergola V, Pergola V, Belhard O, Derumeaux G, et al. Endocarditis in the elderly: clinical, echocardiographic, and prognostic features. Eur Heart J. 2003;24: 1575–82.
77. Vahanian A. The growing burden of infective endocarditis in the elderly. Eur Heart J. 2003;24:1539–90.

Coronary Artery Disease in the Elderly

78. Australian Institiute of Health and Welfare. Coronary heart disease. 2006. http://www.aihw.gov.au/cvd/majordiseases/coronary.cfm. Accessed 23 Nov 2007.
79. Boyle Jr EM, Lille ST, Allaire E, Clowes AW, Verrier ED. Endothelial cell injury in cardiovascular surgery: atherosclerosis. Ann Thorac Surg. 1997;63:885–94 (abstract).
80. Kumar V, Cotran RS, Robbins SL. Basic pathology. 5th ed. Philadelphia: WB Saunders Company; 1992.
81. Reiner Z, Tedeschi-Reiner E. New information on the pathophysiology of atherosclerosis. Lijec Vjesn. 2001;123(1–2):26–31 (abstract).
82. Steinberg D, Witzum JL. Lipoproteins and atherogenesis: current concepts. JAMA. 1990;264:3047–52.
83. Tegos TJ, Kalodiki E, Sabetai MM, Nicholaides AN. The genesis of atherosclerosis and risk factors. A review. Angiology. 2001;52:89–94.
84. Libby P. Inflammation in atherosclerosis. Nature (London). 2002;420:868–74.
85. Moons AH, Levi M, Peiers RJ. Tissue factor and cotonary artery disease. Cardiovasc Res. 2002;53:313–5.
86. Rainer EW. PDGF and cardiovascular disease. Cytokine Growth Factor Rev. 2004;15:237–54 (abstract).

87. Davies MJ, Thomas AC. Plaque fissuring-the cause of acute myocardial infarction, sudden ischaemic death and crescendo angina. Brit Heart J. 1985;53(6):363–73.
88. Brass LF. Thrombin and platelet activation. Chest. 2003;124:195–255.
89. Savi P, Nurden P, Nurden AT, Levy-Tolando S, Herbert JM. Clopidergrol: a review of its mechanisms of action. Platelets. 1998;9(3–4):251–5.
90. Jansson HH, Nilsson TK, Johnson O. vonWillibrand factor in plasma: a novel risk factor for recurrent myocardial infarction and death. Br Heart J. 1991;66:351–5.
91. Mintz GS, Pichard AD, Pooma II, Kent KM, Satler LF, Bucher TA, et al. Determinants and correlates of target lesion calcium in coronary artery disease: a clinical angiographic and intravascular ultrasound study. J Am Coll Cardiol. 1997;29:268–74.
92. Kinlay S, Ganz P. Role of endothelial dysfunction in coronary artery disease and implications of therapy. Am J Cardiol. 1997;80(9A):11I–6 (abstract).
93. Michel JB, Virmani R, Arbustini E, Pasterkamp G. Intraplaque haemorrhages as the trigger of plaque vulnerability. Eur Heart J. 2011;32(16):1977–85.
94. Virmani R, Kolodgie FD, Burke AP, Finn AV, Gold HK, Tulentko TN, et al. Athersclerotic plaque progression and vulnerability to rupture: anfiogenesis as a source of intraplaque haemorrhage. Arterioscler Thromb Vasc Biol. 2005;25(10):205–11 (abstract).
95. De Stefano R, Felice F, Balbarini A. Angiogenesis as a risk factor for plaque vulnerability. Curr Pharm Des. 2009;15(10):1095–106 (abstract).
96. Falk E, Shah P, Fuster V. Pathogenesis of plaque rupture. In: Fuster V, Ross R, Topol E, editors. Atherosclerosis and coronary artery disease. Philadelphia/New York: Lippincott-Raven; 1996. p. 491–500.
97. Shah P. Pathophysiology of plaque rupture and the concept of plaque stabilization. Cardiol Clin. 1996;14:17–29.
98. Fuster V, Gotto AM, Libby P, Loscalzo J, McGill HC. 77th Bethseda Conference matching the intensity of risk factor management with the hazard for coronary artery disease events. Pathogenesis of coronary disease: the biologic role of risk factors. J Am Coll Cardiol. 1996;27:964–76.
99. Braunwald F, Jones RH, Mark DR, Brown J, Brown L, Cheitlin MD, et al. Diagnosing and managing unstable angina. Agency for Health Care Policy and Research. Circulation. 1994;90:613–22.
100. Braunwald E. Unstable angina. An etiologic approach to management. Circulation. 1998;98:2219–22.
101. Hirsh PD, Hillis LD, Campbell WB, Firth BG, Willerson JT. Release of protoglandins and thromboxane into coronary circulation in patients with ischaemic heart disease. N Engl J Med. 1981;304:685–91.
102. Kaski JC, Chester MR, Chen L, Katritsis D. Rapid angiographic progression of coronary artery disease in patients with angina pectoris: the role of complex stenosis morphology. Circulation. 1995;92:2058–65.
103. De Boer OJ, van der Wal AC, Becker AE. Atherosclerosis inflammation and infection. J Pathol. 2000;190(3):237–43 (abstract).
104. Gurfinkel E, Bozovich G. Chalmydia pneumonia: inflammation and instability of the atherosclerotic plaque. Atherosclerosis. 1998;14 Suppl 1:S31–5 (abstract).
105. Becker AE, de Boer OJ, van Der Wal AC. The role of inflammation in coronary artery disease. Annu Rev Med. 2001;52:289–97 (abstract).
106. Pasceri V, Cammarota G, Patti G, Cuoco L, Gasharrani A, Grillo RL, et al. Association of virulent *Helicobacter pylori* strains with ischaemic heart disease. Circulation. 1998;97:1675–9.
107. Mehta JL, Saldeen TGP, Rand K. Interactive role of infection inflammation and traditional risk factors in atherosclerosis and coronary artery disease. J Am Coll Cardiol. 1998;31:1217–25.
108. Nagaratnam N. Toxoplasmosis and heart disease. J Natl Sci Coun Sri Lanka. 1974;2(2):115–27.
109. Nagaratnam N, Siripala KA. Myocardial toxoplasmosis. Cardiology. 1970;55:272–80.
110. Nagaratnam N, Stephen SJ. Chronic constrictive pericarditis associated with toxoplasmosis. Br Heart J. 1973;35:868–70.

Valvular Heart Disease in the Elderly

111. Desai MY, Gerstinblith G. Valvular heart disease in the elderly. In: Cardiovascular disease in the elderly. Contemporary cardiology. Totowa: Humana Press Inc; 2005. p. 231–59.
112. Novaro GM, Tiong IY, Pearce GL, Lauer MS, Strecher DL, Griffin B. Effect of hydroxymethylglutaryl coenzyme a reductase inhibitors on the progression of calcific aortic stenosis. Circulation. 2001;104:2205–9.
113. McKilop GM, Stewart DA, Burns JM. Doppler echocardiography in elderly patients with ejection systolic murmurs. Postgrad Med J. 1991;67(794):1059–61.
114. Aronow WC, Kronzon I. Prevalence and severity of valvular aortic stenosis determined by Doppler echocardiography and its association with echocardiography and electrocardiographic left ventricular hypertrophy and physical signs of aortic stenosis in elderly patients. Am J Cardiol. 1991;67(8):776–7.
115. Stewart BF, Siscovick D, Lind BK, Gardin JM, Gottdiener JS, Smith VE, et al. Clinical factors associated with calcific aortic valve disease. Cardiovascular Health Study. J Am Coll Cardiol. 1997;29:630–4.
116. Rajamannan NM, Gersh B, Bonow RO. Calcific aortic stenosis: from bench to the bedside-emerging clinical and cellular concepts. Heart. 2003;89:801–5.
117. Freeman RV, Otto CM. Spectrum of calcific aortic valve disease. Circulation. 2005;111:3316–26.
118. Curtin RJ, Griffin BP. Valvular heart disease: etiology. ACP Medicine Online. website: www.medscape.com/viewarticle/535378.
119. Soler-Soler J, Galve E. Worldwide perspective of valve disease. Heart. 2000;83:724–5.
120. Roberts WC, Ko JM. Frequency by decades of unicuspid, bicuspid and tricuspid aortic valves in adults having isolated aortic valve replacement for aortic stenosis with or without associated aortic regurgitation. Circulation. 2005;111:120–5.
121. Enriquz-Sarano M, Tajik AJ. Aortic regurgitation. N Engl J Med. 2004;351:1539–46.
122. Bekeredjian R, Grayburn PA. Valvular heart disease. Aortic regurgitation. Circulation. 2005;112:125–34.
123. Singh JP, Evans JC, Levy D, et al. Prevalence and clinical determination of mitral, tricuspid and aortic regurgitation. (The Framingham Heart Study). Am J Cardiol. 1999;83:897–902.
124. Klein AL, Burstow DJ, Fujika AJ, Tajik AJ, Zacharian PK, Taliercio CP, et al. Age related prevalence of valvular regutrgitation in normal subjects. A comprehensive colour flow examination of 118 volunteers. J Am Soc Echocardiogr. 1990;3:54–63.
125. Waller BF, Howard J, Fess S. Pathology of aortic valve stenosis and pure aortic regurgitation. A clinical morphologic assessment.-part II. Clin Cardiol. 1994;17:150–6.
126. Nkomo VT, Gardin JM, Skelton TN, Gottdiener JS, Scott CG, Enriqiez-Sarano M. Burden of valvular heart diseass: a population – based study. Lancet. 2006;368:1005–11.
127. Sutton MG, Gorman LC. Surgery for asymptomatic severe aortic regurgitation in the elderly. Early surgery or wait and watch? Circulation. 2006;114:258–60.
128. Stout KK, Verrier ED. Acute valvular regurgitation. Circulation. 2009;119:3232–41.

Hypertension and Hypertensive Heart Disease in the Elderly

129. The sixth report of the Joint National Committee in prevention, detection, evaluation and treatment of high blood pressure. Ann Int Med. 1997;157:2413–46.
130. Levy D, Larson MG, Vasan RS, Kannel WB, Ho KK. The progression from hypertension to congestive failure. JAMA. 1996;275:1557–62.
131. Meeks WM. Pathophysiology of hypertension in the elderly. Semin Nephrol. 2002;22(1):65–70 (abstract).
132. Lidman D. Histopathology of human extremital arteries throughout life: including measurements of systolic pressures in ankle and arm. Acta Chir Scand. 1982;148:575–80.

133. Laurent S, Boutouyrie P, Benetos A. Pathophysiology of hypertension in the elderly. Am J Geriatr Cardiol. 2002;11(1):34–9 (abstract).
134. Cohen DL, Townsend RR. Update on pathophysiology and treatment of hypertension in the elderly. Curr Hypertens Rep. 2011;13:330–7 (abstract).
135. Gimbrone Jr MA. Vascular endothelium, hemodynamic forces and atherogenesis. Am J Pathol. 1999;155(1):1–5.
136. Avolio A. Genetic and environmental factors in the function and structure of the arterial wall. Hypertension. 1995;26:34–7.
137. McEmery CM, Yasmin IR, Qasem A, Wilkison IB, Cockcroft JR. Normal vascular aging: differential effects on wave reflection and aortic pulse wave velocity; the Anglo-Cardiff Collaborative Trial (ACCT). J Am Coll Cardiol. 2005;46:1753–60.
138. Walsh T, Donnelly T, Lyons D. Impaired endothelial nitric oxide bioavailability: a common link between aging, hypertension and atherogenesis? J Am Geriatr Soc. 2009;57:140–5.
139. Aslami OO, Fang TD, Song HM, Nacamuli RP. Physiological features of aging patients. Arch Surg. 2003;138:1068–76.
140. Millar JA, Lever AF. Implications of pulse pressure as a predictor of cardiac risk in patients with hypertension. Hypertension. 2000;36:907–11.
141. Sagie A, Larson MG, Levy D. The natural history of borderline isolated systolic hypertension. N Engl J Med. 1993;329:1912–7.
142. van Zwieten PA. Drug treatment of isolated hypertension. Nephrol Dial Transplant. 2001;16(6):1095–97.
143. Wallace SM et al. Isolated systolic hypertension is characterised by increased stiffness and endothelial dysfunction. Hypertension. 2007;50:228–33.

Peripheral Arterial Disease

144. Fowler B, Jamrozuk K, Allen Y, Norman P. Prevalence of peripheral arterial disease: persistence of excess risk in former smokers. Aust N Z J Public Health. 2002;26:219–24.
145. Meijer W, Hoes A, Rutgers D, Bots ML, Hofman A, Grobbee DE. Peripheral arterial disease in the elderly. The Rotterdam study. ArteriosclerThromb Vasc Biol. 1998;18:185–92.
146. Ouriel K. Peripheral arterial disease. Lancet. 2001;358(9289):1257–64 (abstract).

Carotid Artery Disease

147. Niesen WD, Sliwka U, Lingnan A, Noth J. Cerebral emboli in cryptogenic ischaemia: a reason to enforce diagnostic testing. J Stroke Cerebrovasc. 2001;10:44–8.
148. Graham AM, Moore WS, Baker W. Carotid artery disease. Website: http://updvs.vascular-webng/APDVS_contribution_PagesCurriculum/clinical/os-carotid. Accessed 20 Mar 2010.
149. Fusler V, Badimon L, Badimon JJ, Chesebro JH. The pathogenesis of coronary artery disease and the acute coronary syndromes. N Engl J Med. 1992;326:242–50.
150. Ogunrinade O, Kameya GT, Truskey GA. Effect of fluid sheer stress on permeability of the arterial endothelium. Ann Biomed Eng. 2002;30(4):430–46 (abstract).
151. Kumar V, Contran RS, Robbins SL. Basic pathology. 5th ed. Philadelphia: WR Saunders Co; 1992.
152. Wadsworth R. Oxidative stress and the endothelium. Exp Physiol. 2008;93:155–7 (abstract).
153. Hugashi Y, Noma K, Yoshimi M, Kihara Y. Endothelial function and oxidative stress in cardiovascular diseases. Circ J. 2009;73(3):411–8 (abstract).
154. Davies MJ. Arterial thrombosis and acute coronary syndromes in Acute Coronary Syndromes. Am Coll Cardiol. 1999.
155. Hogan N, Boenau I. Transient ishaemic attack. Emerg Med. 2006;38:41–6.

156. Craven TE, Ryu JE, Espeland MA, Kahl FR, McKinney WM, Toole JF. Evaluation of the associations between carotid artery atherosclerosis and coronary artery stenosis. A case–control study. Circulation. 1990;82:1230–42.
157. O'Leary DH, Polak JF, Kronmal RA, Manolio TA, Burke GJ, Wolfson Jr SK, et al. Coronary-artery intima and media thickness as a risk factor for myocardial infarction and stroke in older adults. N Engl J Med. 1999;340:14–22.
158. Selhub J, Jacques PF, Bostom AG, D'Agostino RB, Wilson PWF, Belager AJ, et al. Association between plasma homocysteine concentrations and extra carotid-artery stenosis. N Engl J Med. 1995;332:286–91.
159. Momjian-Mayor I, Baron J-C. The pathophysiology of watershed infarction in internal carotid artery disease. Stroke. 2005;36:567–77.

Related Disorders: Syncope

160. Forman DE, Lipsitz LA. Syncope in the elderly. Cardiol Clin. 1997;15(2):295–311.
161. Benditt DG, van Dijk JG, Sutton R, Wieling W, Lin JC, Sakaguchi S, et al. Syncope. Curr Probl Cardiol. 2004;29(4):152–229 (abstract).
162. Kapoor WN, Smith MA, Miller NL. Upright tilt testing in evaluation of syncope. A comprehensive literature review. Am J Med. 1994;97:78–88.
163. Lipsitz LA, Wei JY, Rowe JW. Syncope in an elderly institutionalised population: prevalence, incidence and associated risk. Q J Med. 1985;55:45–54.
164. Day SC, Cook EF, Funkenstein LI, Goldman L. Evaluation and outcome of emergency room patients with transient loss of consciousness. Am J Med. 1982;72:15–23.
165. Savage DD, Corwin L, McGee D, Kannel WB, Wolf PA. Epidemiologic features of isolated syncope: The Framingham Study. Stroke. 1985;10:626–8.
166. Kapoor W, Snustad D, Peterson J, Wieand HS, Cha R, Karpf K. Syncope in the elderly. Am J Med. 1986;80:419–28.
167. McIntosh S, Da Costa D, Kenny RA. Clinical characteristics of vasodepressor, cardioinhibitory and mixed carotid sinus syndrome in the elderly. Am J Med. 1993;95:203–8.
168. Miller TH, Kruse JE. Evaluation of syncope. Am Fam Physician. 2005;72(8):1492–5000 (abstract).
169. Kapoor WN, Karpf FM, Wieand S, Peterson JR, Levey GS. Appropriate evaluation and follow up of patients with syncope. N Engl J Med. 1983;309:197–204.
170. Hainsworth R. Syncope: what is the trigger? Heart. 2003;83:123–4.
171. Seger JJ. Syncope evaluation and management. Tex Heart Inst J. 2005;32(2):204–6.
172. Grubb BP, Kosinski D. Tilt table testing: concepts and limitaions. Pacing Clin Electrophysiol. 1997;20:781–7.
173. Davies AJ, Steen N, Kenny RA. Carotid sinus hypersensitivity is common in older patients presenting to an accident and emergency department with unexplained falls. Age Ageing. 2001;30(4):289–93.
174. Thomas JE. Hyperactive carotid sinus reflex in carotid sinus syncope. Mayo Clin Proc. 1967;44:127–39.
175. Strickberger SA, Benson W, Biaggioni I, Callans DJ, Cohen MI, Ellenbogen KA, et al. AHA/ACCF Scientific Statement on the evaluation of syncope. Circulation. 2006;113:316–27.
176. Kenny RA. Syncope in the elderly. J Cardiovasc Electrophysiol. 2003;14(9 Suppl):S74–7 (abstract).
177. Linzer M, Young EU, Ester MA, Wang P, Vorperian VR, Kapoor WN, et al. Clinical guide – diagnosing syncope. Ann Intern Med. 1997;127:78–86.
178. Wayne HH. Syncope. Physical considerations and an analysis of clinical characteristics in 510 patients. Am J Med. 1961;30:413–38.
179. Lipsitz LA, Pluchino FC, Wei JY, Rowe JW. Syncope in institutionalised elderly: the impact of multiple pathological conditions and situational stress. J Chronic Dis. 1986;39:619–30.

180. Vaitkevicius PV, Esserwwin DM, Maynard AK, O'Connor FC, Fleg JL. Frequency and importance of postprandial blood pressure reduction in elderly nursing-home patients. Ann Intern Med. 1991;115:865–70.
181. Kenny RA, Traynor G. Carotid sinus syndrome-clinical characteristics in elderly patients. Age Ageing. 1991;20:449–54.
182. Brignole M, Menozzi C, Gianfranchi L, Oddone D, Lotti G, Bertulla A, et al. Neurally mediated syncope detected by carotis sinus massage in older patients with syncope. Am J Cardiol. 1991;68:1032–6.
183. Munro NC, McIntosh S, Lawson J, Morley CA, Sutton R, Kenny RA. Incidence of complications after carotid sinus massage in older patients with syncope. J Am Geriatr Soc. 1994;42:1248–51.
184. Kapoor N. Current evaluation and management of syncope. Circulation 2002;106:1606–9.

Related Disorders: Leg and Foot Ulcers

185. Ebbesskog B. Lindh in South Stockholm, Sweden Scand. J Primary Care. 1996;14:238–47.
186. Andersson E, Hansson C, Swanbeck G. Leg and foot ulcer prevalence and investigation of the peripheral arterial and venous circulation in a randomized elderly population. A epidemiological survey and clinical investigation. Acta Derm Venereol. 1993;73:57–61.
187. Slagsvold CE, Stranden E. Venous leg ulcers. Tidsskr Nor Laegeforen. 2005;125(7):891–4 (abstract).
188. Trent JT, Falabella A, Eaglstein WH, Kirsner RS. Venous ulcers: pathophysiology and treatment options. Ostomy Wound Manage. 2005;51(5):38–54 (abstract).
189. Toporcer T, Lakyova L, Radonak J. Venous ulcer-present view on aetiology, diagnostics and therapy. Cas Lek Cesk. 2008;147(4):199–205 (abstract).
190. Gonsalves CF. Venous leg ulcers. Tech Vasc Interv Radiol. 2003;6:132–6.
191. Abbade LP, Lastoria S. Venous ulcer: epidemiology, diagnosis and treatment. Int J Dermatol. 2005;44(6):449–56 (abstract).
192. Boike A, Maier M. Prevention and treatment of leg and foot ulcers in diabetes mellitus. Disease Management Project. Cleveland Clinic. http://mm.clevelandclinic.med.ed.com/medicalpubs/diseasemanagement/endocrinology/prevention-treatment-diabetic-leg-and-foot-ulcers/. Accessed 12 Nov 2013.
193. Meehan M. Multisite pressure ulcer prevalence survey. Decubitus. 1990;3:14–7.
194. Brandeis AH, Morris JN, Nash DJ, Lipsitz VA. The epidemiology and natural history of pressure ulcers in elderly nursing home residents. JAMA. 1990;264:2905–9.
195. Anders J, Heinemann A, Leffmar C, Lentenegger M, Protener F, von Rentedn-Kruse W. Decubitus ulcers: pathophysiology and primary prevention. Dtsch Arztebl Int. 2010;107(21): 371–82 (abstract).
196. Agale SV. Chronic ulcers. Epidemiology, aetiopathology and management. Review article. Ulcers Vol 2013. Article ID413604. http://dxdoi.org/10.1155/2013/413604.
197. Singer AJ, Clark RAF. Cutaneous wound healing. N Engl J Med. 1999;341:738–46.
198. Sumpio BE. Foot ulcers. N Engl J Med. 2000;343:789–92.
199. Hopkins NFG, Wolfe JHN. Deep venous insufficiency and occlusion. ABS of Vascular disease. Br Med J. 1991;304:107–10.
200. Kahn SR, Ginsberg JS. Relationship between deep vein thrombosis and postthrombotic syndrome. Arch Intern Med. 2004;164:17–26.
201. Negus D. The post-thrombotic syndrome. Arris and Galle Lecture, 28th May 1970. Ann R Coll Surg Engl. 1970;47:92–105.
202. Valencia IC, Falabella A, Kirsner RS, Eaglstein WH. Chronic venous insufficiency and venous leg ulceration. J Am Acad Dermatol. 2001;44(3):401–21 (abstract).
203. Coleridge-Smith PD, Thomas I, Scurr JH, Dormandy JA. Causes of venous ulceration: a new hypothesis. Br Med J. 1988;296:1726–7.

204. Rudolph R, Shannon ML. The normal healing process. In: Eaglstein WH, editor. New directions in wound healing. Princeton: ER Squibb & Sons; 1990.
205. Falanga V, Eaglstein WH. The trap hypothesis of venous ulceration. Lancet. 1992;341: 1006–8.
206. Newton H. Leg ulcers: differences between venous and arterial wounds. Essentials. 2011;6(1): 20–8.
207. Levin ME. Preventing amputation in patients with diabetes. Diabetes Care. 1985;18: 1383–94.
208. Hutton W, Stokes I. The mechanism of the foot. In: Klenerman L, editor. The foot and its disorders. Oxford: Blackwell Scientific; 1991. p. 11–25.
209. Goode PS, Allman RM. The prevention amd management of pressure ulcers. Med Clin North Am. 1989;73(6):1511–24 (abstract).
210. Yarkony GM. Pressure ulcers. A review. Arch Phys Med Rehabil. 1994;76:908–17.
211. Overgaard C. Pressure ulcers: a review of pathophysiology, risk factors and management principles. www.healthplexus.net. Sept 2000 (abstract).
212. Spentzouris G, Labropoulos N. The evaluation of lower extremity ulcers. Semin Intervent Radiol. 2009;26(4):286–95.
213. Hart DIT. 5 differences between venous and arterial leg ulcers. www.nurses.for.nurses.com.au. 2012. Accessed 21 Feb 2014.

Respiratory Diseases in the Elderly 2

2.1 Anatomical and Physiological Changes with Ageing

The lungs continue to develop throughout life reaching their maximal functional status in the early third decade and thereafter a gradual decline [1]. Normal physiological and structural changes occur in the respiratory system with ageing [2]. Anatomical changes in both lungs and chest wall with multiple changes in structure and function [2] give rise to changes in pulmonary mechanics, respiratory muscle strength [3] and ventilation control. In spite of these changes, the gas exchange is adequately maintained [4]. Age-related changes in pulmonary function result in decrease in respiratory reserve during acute illness [3, 4]. Changes occur in the pulmonary vasculature resulting in increase in pulmonary vascular stiffness, vascular pressures and vascular resistance [5]. It is important therefore to have a clear understanding of the changes in respiratory structure and function associated with ageing as these changes may affect, for instance, the perioperative period of elderly patients [1].

Table 2.1 summarises the structural and physiological changes and the resultant effects of ageing on respiratory function.

Box 2.1. Key Points. Anatomical and Physiological Changes with Ageing

- Anatomical changes result in changes in pulmonary mechanics, respiratory muscle strength and ventilation control [2].
- Changes in pulmonary function result in decrease in respiratory reserve during acute illness [3, 4].
- Changes in pulmonary vasculature result in increase in pulmonary vascular stiffness, vascular pressures and vascular resistance [5].
- Thickening of the alveolar basement membrane results in decrease gas diffusing capabilities and increase in ventilation/perfusion heterogeneity (see Table 2.1).
- Decrease in small airway diameter gives an obstructive flow pattern (see Table 2.1).
- The conduction zone increases in size resulting in increased residual volume and functional residual capacity and decreased vital capacity (see Table 2.1).

N. Nagaratnam et al., *Diseases in the Elderly: Age-Related Changes and Pathophysiology*, DOI 10.1007/978-3-319-25787-7_2

Table 2.1 Fundamental changes in respiratory structure and function with ageing

Anatomical changes	Physiological changes	Effects in respiratory function
I. Changes in thoracic cage		
(i) Calcification of the intercostal cartilages; arthritis of the costo-vertebral joints	Rigidity and stiffness of the wall increases and chest wall compliance decreases	Expiratory flow movement decreases/shifts chest wall pressure-volume curve to the right
(ii) Gradual atrophy of intercostals muscles (loss of muscle mass)	Weakening of the intercostals muscles	Reduction in the muscle strength demands greater contribution from diaphragmatic and abdominal muscles and may lead to diaphragmatic fatigue
II. Airway changes		
(i) The cilia beat decreases with age and there is a reduction in number of cilia	Reduces clearance of debris and pathogens	Increases chance of infection
(ii) The conduction zone (the area between nose and bronchioles) increases in size of the larger airways – trachea, Iry and II ry bronchi	Increase in volume of anatomical dead space	Increased residual volume and functional residual capacity and decreased vital capacity
(iii) Bronchioles and alveolar ducts increase in size, grouping of the alveoli, widening and loss of depth and loss of supporting tissue ('senile emphysema')	Decreased state of elastic recoil	Increased ventilation/perfusion heterogeneity
(iv) Thickening of the alveolar basement membrane	Decrease gas-diffusing capabilities, increase in ventilation/perfusion heterogeneity	Arterial oxygenation declines, CO transfer decreases
(v) Decrease in small airways diameter	Decrease in maximal expiratory flow	Obstructive flow pattern
III. Ventilation control	Diminishes	Diminishes response to hypercapnia and hypoxia

Information sources: Janssens et al. [3]; Fowler et al. [6]; Knight and Nigamy [7]; Levitsky [8]; Niewoehner and Kleincman [9]; Tolep et al. [10]; Verbeken et al. [11]

2.2 Pneumonia in the Elderly

Introduction

Pneumonia is an infection or inflammation of one or both lungs. Pneumonia is one of the most common infections in the elderly. Approximately 20 % of nosocomial infections in the elderly are due to pneumonia which is only second in prevalence to urinary tract infections [12, 13].

Pathophysiology

In the elderly there is a greater susceptibility to infection because of the age-related decline in immune response. Invasion by bacteria, viruses and other pathogens evokes a systemic inflammation in response to the active immune system. Innate immunity mechanisms include physical barriers and phagocytic cells such as neutrophils and macrophages which destroy the pathogenic bacteria. Elimination of bacteria is by activation of the phagocytes locally in the lung brought about by the innate defence mechanism [14]. Structural changes occur with ageing [15], for instance, there is a decrease in the cilia beat and numbers [7] which reduces the clearance of debris and pathogens [16] resulting in increased chance of infection. In the aged there is also a reduction in the total number of phagocytes resulting in their reduced bactericidal activity [17]. During infection, antigen contact induces neutrophil activation and release of matrix metalloproteinases (MMPs) and possibly by setting off proinflammatory cytokines cause bacterial clearance. There is evidence that various levels of different MMPs have been detected in community-acquired and hospital-acquired pneumonias [18, 19]. Pulmonary inflammation may also be brought about by mechanical ventilation [14]. Neutrophil recruitment with MMP release and activation induced by cytokine release may result in lung injury in this setting [14, 20].

Box 2.2. Key Points. Pneumonia

- In the elderly there is age-related decline in immune response.
- Structural changes occur with ageing, for instance, a decrease in number of cilia [7].
- There is reduction in the number of phagocytes [17].
- Various levels of different MMPs have been detected in community- and hospital-acquired pneumonias [18, 19].

2.3 Chronic Obstructive Pulmonary Disease (COPD)

Introduction

According to the Global Initiative for Chronic Obstructive Lung Disease (GOLD) [21], COPD is a disease state characterised by airflow limitation usually progressive and is not fully reversible. The American Thoracic Society [22] defines COPD as a disease process involving progressive airflow obstruction due to chronic bronchitis, emphysema or both. The prevalence in those over 65 years is fourfold that in the 45–64-year-old group [23, 24]. The major causative factor is cigarette smoking, but inhalational exposure to other irritants and genetic factors are also important. Ageing of the population and past smoking are the major causes of the increase in COPD [25]. Air pollution and occupational exposures may be important and interact with cigarette smoking. Non-specific airway hyperresponsiveness may predispose smokers to the development of COPD [26]. Genetic factors may cause an accelerated decline in lung function which can lead to COPD in a susceptible population of individuals who smoke [27], and there are several inherited forms of antiproteinase deficiency which may predispose to the development of emphysema. Approximately 50 % of COPD is caused by cigarette smoking [28]. The common risk factors associated with non-smoking COPD are air pollution and occupational exposures to fumes and dust [29]. Little consideration has been given to the possibility of chronic adult diseases such as COPD to have their origins in early life [30]. There is considerable evidence that adverse maternal factors can interact with the environment of a susceptible host to promote altered lung growth and development in early childhood [30].

Pathophysiology

The alveolar walls play an important pathophysiological roles in obstructive pulmonary disease. Destruction of the alveolar walls is caused by an imbalance between alveolar proteases and anti-protease activity in the alveolar tissues [31]. Macrophages play an important role in the pathogenesis of emphysema [32]. Macrophages activated by cigarette smoke release neutrophilic chemotactic factors interleukins (IL-8) and leukotriene B4 (LTB4) [33] which in turn release proteases, metalloproteinases (MMPs), cathepsin [32] and Protein 3 [34]. The proteases are responsible for the breakdown of lung parenchyma resulting in emphysema and also stimulate mucous secretion and are counteracted by alpha-antitrypsin and tissue inhibitor of metalloproteinases (TIMP).

The airflow limitation is associated with an abnormal inflammatory response of the lungs to noxious particles and gases [35]. Neutrophil-derived elastase is an important protease which mediates elastolysis and stimulates mucous secretion, and alpha-antitrypsin is the prime anti-protease inhibitor [36]. Increased number of activated neutrophils are found in the sputum and bronchoalveolar lavage and air smooth muscle of patients with COPD [37]. In the smaller airways, bronchial biopsies have shown that smokers with or without obstruction had increased inflammation of the bronchial epithelium with increased numbers of mononuclear cells and CD4+ and CD8+ T lymphocytes [38]. The inflammatory cellular pattern changes during exacerbations with further increase of eosinophils and neutrophils and various inflammatory mediators, cytokines, chemokines and markers of oxidative stress [39].

COPD is further characterised not only by the inflammation but also by tissue remodelling which follows tissue destruction and repair [36]. 'Airway remodelling' embraces all the architectural changes which include bronchoconstriction, mucous plugging, bronchial wall oedema, inflammatory cell infiltration, airway smooth muscle hypertrophy and subepithelial fibrosis [40].

More recently another contributor to airway narrowing is oxidative stress which is increased in COPD [41]. Oxidative stress promotes inflammation by exacerbating the protease/anti-protease imbalance and by activating the former and deactivating the latter in patients with COPD. Oxidants are present in cigarette smoke and are also produced by activated inflammatory cells including neutrophils and macrophages [36]. They contribute to the pathophysiology of COPD by the potentiation of elastic activity, increase in mucous secretion and damage to serum protease inhibitors [36].

Ninety percent of COPD is caused by cigarette smoking; less than 20 % of smokers develop significant airway obstruction [42]; hence there may be other factors other than exposure to cigarette smoke which predispose an individual to smoking-related respiratory disease [43]. COPD tends to occur more frequently in individuals with a family history of asthma and COPD, low lung function in childhood and hyperresponsiveness, and a host of genetic factors may regulate the effects of cigarette smoking-induced airway inflammation [43]. Spontaneous changes in the lungs consistent with emphysema have been shown to be associated with ageing [44]. Airflow limitation is generally progressive with COPD; however, the rate of decline is highly variable. Ultimately COPD is complicated by chronic hypoxia and intimal and smooth muscle thickening causing pulmonary hypertension [45].

Box 2.3. Key Points. Chronic Obstructive Airway Disease

- Cigarette smoke activates macrophages which release neutrophilic chemotactic factors resulting in the release of proteases [33].
- Imbalance between alveolar proteases and anti-protease activity results in destruction of the alveolar walls [31].
- The proteases are counteracted by alpha-antitrypsin and tissue inhibitor metalloproteinases [36].
- Airflow limitation is associated with abnormal inflammatory response, tissue remodelling and oxidative stress [40, 41].
- Ultimately COPD is complicated by hypoxia and intimal and smooth muscle thickening causing pulmonary hypertension [45].

2.4 Asthma in the Elderly

Introduction

Bronchial asthma is characterised by periodic, reversible widespread narrowing of the airways. The prevalence of asthma in the elderly is between 4.5 and 8 % and is similar to that in the adult age group [46, 47] and affects more than 10 % in the over 60 years of age [48]. In at least half of the elderly patients, asthma is recently acquired. It is reported that 50 % of asthmatics older than 65 years had not been diagnosed, and only 30 % of the diagnosed are treated with inhaled corticosteroids [49].

Pathophysiology

The airflow obstruction in asthma is the result of bronchoconstriction which is the result of a complex interaction of inflammatory cells, mediators and cytokines [50]. Reversible air flow obstruction and bronchial hyperreactivity are the hallmarks of asthma. It is characterised by inflammation, hyperresponsiveness [51] and remodelling of the airways [52, 53]. There is sound evidence that both genetic and environmental factors influence the risk of developing asthma, and several studies have emphasised that specific genes are involved in the pathogenesis of asthma [54]. Genes including IL2RB on chromosome 22 and IL33 on chromosome 9 have been implicated [55]. Asthma can be categorised as allergic and non-allergic based on the presence of IgE antibodies to common environmental allergens [56]. There have been several attempts to define asthma subtypes, and cluster analyses had identified different adult-onset asthma phenotypes [57]. The early-onset allergic group is characterised by high levels of airway eosinophilia, mast cells, IgE and exhaled nitric oxide with prominent T helper type 2 (T_H2) cell pathway [58]. The second cluster group with adult-onset asthma has notable eosinophilia, notable patterns of interleukins (IL) and T_H2 pathway but generally absence of important allergic disease [59]. The remaining third are exercise induced with mast cells playing an important role, obesity and with minimal T_H2 response and sputum neutrophilia [58, 59].

Many inflammatory cells take part in the inflammatory process and mediate a complex display of mediators [60]. The inflammatory response is characterised by the infiltration of the airway by increased amounts of inflammatory cells which include mast cells, lymphocytes, eosinophils [61], macrophages, dendritic cells and T helper 2 (Th2) lymphocytes and are regulated by interacting cytokines [62]. The cytokines are of particular importance as mediators of chronic inflammation [60]. It has been advanced that CD4- T cells produce the Th2 pattern of cytokines [61] such as IL-4, IL-5 and IL-13 [56]. These cytokines stimulate mast cells, increase B-cell IgE production and cause eosinophilia and stimulate leucocytosis [56]. The smooth muscle also contributes to bronchial inflammation by secreting a number of inflammatory mediators mobilising and stimulating inflammatory cells such as mast cells or T lymphocytes [63].

Bronchial hyperresponsiveness is documented as decreased airflow after bronchoprovocation with histamine or methacholine [52], and other triggers include respiratory allergens, cold air, exercise, viral upper respiratory infection and cigarette smoke [52]. Recent data suggest that there is an interaction between mast cells and smooth muscle cells, and this can be a significant contribution to hyperresponsiveness [65]. Following the triggers of asthma, the activated mast cells and eosinophils generate their cytokines, and complex interplay of mediators may lead to chronic inflammation [66] resulting in long-term structural alterations of the airway 'remodelling' [52, 62]. Remodelling is associated with increased deposition of collagen and fibronectin together with smooth muscle hypertrophy [58], and structural changes such as epithelial injury, increased basement thickness, airway smooth muscle mass and goblet metaplasia [59].

Box 2.4. Key Points. Asthma

- Bronchoconstriction results in complex interaction of inflammatory cells, mediators and cytokines [50].
- Asthma is characterised by inflammation, hyperresponsiveness and remodelling of airways [51–53].
- Remodelling refers to structural changes – increased basement thickness, airway smooth muscle mass, epithelial injury and goblet metaplasia [52, 62].
- Inflammatory response increased inflammatory cells – mast cells, lymphocytes, eosinophils and macrophages [61].
- Bronchial hyperresponsiveness is documented as decreased airflow after bronchoprovocation [52].

2.5 Lung Cancer in the Elderly

Introduction

Lung cancer is characterised as cancerous growth in the lungs which may be primary, originating from the lung cells, or secondary, metastatic from another source. The mortality secondary to primary cancer has increased in those 65 years and older during the period 1980–1998 and decreased in those younger than 55 years reflecting generational patterns in smoking prevalence [67] and is not uncommon in persons older than 85 years [68]. In the United Kingdom, the peak incidence of lung cancer is between 75 and 80 years of age [69]. Between 30 and 45 % of all lung cancers are diagnosed in patients older than 70 years [70–72].

Pathophysiology and classification

Lung cancers, like all other cancers, are initiated by the accumulation of genetic changes resulting in the activation of oncogenes or inactivation of the tumour suppressor gene [73]. The pro-oncogenes when exposed to particular carcinogens turn into oncogenes [74]. Mutations of KRAS proto-oncogenes are responsible for 20–30 % of the non-small cell lung cancer (NSCLC) [75], and they are of particular relevance in adenocarcinoma as activation of these genes is associated with poor prognosis [76]. However, the role of KRAS oncogene in NSCLC is unclear, and recent studies have indicated that KRAS mutant could be predictive of lack of response to chemotherapy, but these results have not been confirmed [77]. Small cell lung cancer is associated with changes in several oncogenes and mutation of the *raf* gene. Smoking and other environmental insults are mainly responsible for the genetic changes that give rise to lung cancers. Nitrosamine, benzopyrene and radioisotopes from radon decay are among the several carcinogens found in cigarette smoke [78]. There is a strong epidemiologic relationship between smoking and lung cancer [79]. Genetic factors may play an important role in modifying an individual's risk for lung cancer [79].

Based on the histology bronchogenic carcinoma of the lung is classified as non-small cell lung carcinoma (NSCLC) and small cell lung carcinoma (SCLC). The NSCLC is subdivided into squamous cell carcinoma, adenocarcinoma and large cell carcinoma. Even though each has its own epidemiological, histological and clinical features, they have been grouped together because they share similar prognosis and management. NSCLC accounts for 80–85 % of the lung cancers [70], of which 25–30 % is squamous cell carcinoma, 30–35 % adenocarcinoma and 10–15 % large cell carcinoma [80]. The incidence of SCLC is between 15 and 20 % [70]. Squamous cell carcinoma arises in the central bronchi and extends to the hilum and mediastinum. Adenocarcinoma which is more frequently located peripherally is a large cell carcinoma. SCLC arises in the proximal airways and involves the hilum and mediastinum.

Box 2.5. Key Points. Lung Cancer

- Lung cancer is initiated by accumulation of genetic changes resulting in activation of oncogenes or inactivation of tissue suppression gene [73].
- Genetic factors may play an important role in modifying an individual's risk for lung cancer [79].
- Smoking and other environmental factors are responsible for the genetic changes which predispose the development of lung cancers [78, 79].
- Small cell lung cancer is associated with changes in several oncogenes and mutation of the *raf* gene.

2.6 Acute Pulmonary Embolism in the Elderly

Introduction

Acute pulmonary embolism is an abrupt lodgement of a clot in the pulmonary artery compromising the blood flow to the lung parenchyma. The incidence rate of acute pulmonary embolism (PE) is not known. PE incidence, prevalence and mortality increase steadily with age [81, 82]. PE is predominantly a disease of the elderly and is often underdiagnosed. Less than 30 % of the PE is diagnosed on the index visit in the elderly [83]. The incidence of thromboembolic events is greater in elderly men than women, whereas the incidence of PE is higher in women than in men younger than 55 years [84].

Pathophysiology

The effects of the embolic thrombus will depend on a number of factors, namely, the size of the clot, the size of the affected pulmonary artery and the cardiopulmonary status of the individual [84, 85]. Occlusion of the major pulmonary vessels of more than 60 % reduction of the pulmonary vasculature is considered a major factor in increasing the pulmonary arterial pressure giving rise to right ventricular decompensation and diminishing the cardiac output [84]. There is evidence to suggest that vasoconstriction, caused by vasoactive mediators, thromboxane A_2 and serotonin released mainly by activated platelets may also be another factor in the pathophysiology of pulmonary embolism [85, 86].

A number of factors give rise to arterial hypoxaemia which is seen in majority of patients with PE and is proportional to the size of the embolus and the degree of ventilation and perfusion mismatch [87]. Because of the decreased cardiac output, the diverted blood from the obstructed area may not attain normal oxygenation. Arterial hypoxaemia however may not always occur with PE owing to possible compensation resulting from hyperventilation. PE is a complication of deep vein thrombosis. The most common cause of the pulmonary embolus is the thrombus which has originated from the popliteal vein or the larger veins above it. More than two-thirds of the thromboemboli lodge in the large or intermediate pulmonary arteries.

Box 2.6. Key Points. Acute Pulmonary Embolism(PE)

- Less than one-third of PE is diagnosed on the index visit in the elderly [83].
- Effects of PE will depend on the size of the embolus, size of the affected artery and the cardiopulmonary status of the individual [84, 85].
- Arterial hypoxaemia is proportionate to the size of the embolus [87].
- PE is a complication of deep vein thrombosis.

Multiple Choice Questions (MCQs)

1. The following in COPD are true, EXCEPT:
   A. 90 % of COPD is caused by cigarette smoking; less than 30 % of smokers develop significant airway obstruction.
   B. In cigarette smokers susceptible to COPD, the rate of decline as measured by FEV_1 is three- to fivefold compared to age-related rate.
   C. Smokers with a family history of airway obstructive disease are more likely to develop COPD.
   D. Airway limitation is generally progressive and the rate of decline is variable.
2. The following are true of asthma in the elderly, EXCEPT:
   A. In at least half of the elderly patients, asthma is recently acquired.
   B. In one study 20 % of the elderly patients with asthma were wrongly diagnosed as COPD.
   C. Asthma in the elderly is often associated with allergic triggers.
   D. Asthma in the elderly results from effects of ageing on the airways.
3. The following in relation to lung cancer are true, EXCEPT:
   A. 65 % of lung cancer occurs in the 65 years and over.
   B. Mutations of KRAS proto oncogenes are responsible for 20–30 % of non-small cell lung cancer.
   C. Small cell lung cancer is associated with changes in several oncogenes and mutation of the *raf* gene.
   D. Small cell lung cancer is weakly associated with smoking.
4. The following are true in relation to pulmonary embolism, EXCEPT:
   A. More than two-thirds of the thromboemboli lodge in the large or intermediate pulmonary arteries.
   B. The most common cause of the pulmonary embolus is the thrombus which has originated from the popliteal vein or the larger veins below it.
   C. The effects of the embolic thrombus will depend on a number of factors, namely, the size of the clot, the size of the affected pulmonary artery and the cardiopulmonary status.
   D. Arterial hypoxaemia is proportional to the size of the embolus.

Answers to MCQs

1 = A; 2 = B; 3 = D; 4 = B.

References

Anatomical and Physiological Changes with Aging

1. Sprung J, Gajic O, Warner DO. Review article: age-related alterations in respiratory function-anaesthetic considerations. Can J Anaeth. 2006;53:1244–57.
2. Oyarzun GM. Pulmonary function in aging. Rev Med Chil. 2009;137(3):411–8 (abstract).
3. Janssens JP, Pache JC, Nicol NP. Physiological changes in respiratory function associated with aging. Eur Res J. 1999;13:197–205 (abstract).
4. Janssens JP. Aging of the respiratory system: impact on pulmonary function tests and adaptation to exertion. Clin Chest Med. 2005;26(3):469–84 (abstract).
5. Taylor BJ, Johnson BD. The pulmonary circulation and exercise responses in the elderly. Semin Respir Crit Care Med. 2010;31(5):528–38 (abstract).
6. Fowler RW, Pluck RA, Hetzel MR. Maximal expiratory flow-volume curves in Londoners aged 60 years and over. Thorax. 1987;42:173–82.
7. Knight J, Nigam Y. Exploring the anatomy and physiology of aging part 2-the respiratory system. Nurs Times. 2008;104:24–5.
8. Levitzky MG. Effects of aging on the respiratory system. Physiologist. 1984;27(2):102–7.
9. Niewoehner DE, Kleinerman J. Morphologic basis of pulmonary resistance in human lung and effects of aging. J Appl Physiol. 1974;36:412–8.
10. Tolep K, Higgins N, Muza S, Criner G, Kelsen SG. Comparison of diaphragm between healthy adult elderly and young men. Am J Respir Crit Care Med. 1995;152:677–82.
11. Verbeken EK, Canberghs M, Merteus K, Clement J, Lanweryns JM, Van de Woestijne KP. The senile lung: comparison with normal and emphysematous lungs 1. Structural aspects. Chest. 1992;101(3):793–9.

Pneumonia in the Elderly

12. Scheld WM, Mandell GI. Nosocomial pneumonia: pathogenesis and recent advances in diagnosis and therapy. Rev Infect Dis. 1991;13 Suppl 9:S743–51.
13. Emori TG, Banerjee SN, Culver DH, Gaynes RP, Horan TC, Edwards JR, et al. Nosocomial infections in the elderly patients in the United States. 1986–1990. Am J Med. 1991;91(S3B):289S–93.
14. Schaaf B, Liebau C, Kurowski V, Droemann D, Dalhoff CK. Hospital acquired pneumonia with high-risk bacteria is associated with increased pulmonary matrix metalloproteinase activity. BMC Pulm Med. 2008;8:12. doi:10.1186/1471-2466-8-12.
15. Miller MR. Structural and physiological age associated changes imaging lungs.Semin Respir Crit Care Med 2010;31(5):521–7.
16. Knight J, Nigam Y. Exploring the anatomy and physiology of aging part 2-the respiratory system. Nurs Times. 2008;104:24–5.
17. Strout RD, Suttles J. Immunosenescence and macrophage functional plasticity: dysregulation of macrophage function by age-associated microenvironmental changes. Immunol Rev. 2005;205:60–71.
18. Yang SF, Chu SC, Chiang IC, Kuo WF, Chiou HL, Chon FB, et al. Excessive matrix metalloproteinase-9 in the plasma of community-acquired pneumonia. Clin Chim Acta. 2005;352: 209–15.

19. Hartog CM, Wermelt JA, Sommerfield CO, Eichler W, Dalhoff K, Braun J. Pulmonary matrix metalloproteinase excess in hospital-acquired pneumonia. Am J Respir Crit Care Med. 2003;167:593–8 (abstract).
20. Halbertma FJ, Vanekar M, Scheffer GJ, van der Hoeven JG. Cytokines and biotrauma in ventilator-induced lung injury: a critical review of the literature. Neth J Med. 2005;63:382–92 (abstract).

Chronic Obstructive Pulmonary Disease (COPD)

21. Global initiative for COPD (GOLD) workshop summary. Am J Respir Crit Care Med. 2001;163:1256–76.
22. American Thoracic Society. Standards for the diagnosis and care of patients with Chronic obstructive pulmonary disease. Am J Respir Crit Care Med. 1995;152:S77–121.
23. Hurd S. The impact of COPD on lung health worldwide: epidemiology and incidence. Chest. 2000;117(suppl):1S–4.
24. Sullivan SD, Ramsey SD, Lee TA. The economic burden of COPD. Chest. 2000;117 suppl 2:5S–9.
25. Feenstra TL, van Genugten ML, Hoogenveen RT. The impact of aging and smoking on the future burden of chronic obstructive pulmonary disease: a model analysis in the Netherlands. Am J Respir Crit Care Med. 2001;154:590–6.
26. Willemse BW, Hacken NH, Rutgers B, Lesman-Leegte JG, Timens W, Postma DS. Smoking cessation improves both direct and indirect airway hyperresponsiveness in COPD. Eur Respir J. 2004;24(3):391–6.
27. Ohar J. New data in the pathophysiology of COPD. Website: http://www.medscape.com/view.article/540983.
28. Mannino DM, Buist AS, Petty TI, Enright PL, Redd SC. Lung function and mortality in the United States: data from the First National Health and National Examination Survey follow-up study. Thorax. 2003;58:388–93.
29. Salvi SS, Barnes PF. Chronic obstructive pulmonary disease in non-smokers. Lancet. 2009;374:733–43.
30. Narang I, Bush A. Early origins of chronic obstructive pulmonary disease. Semin Fetal Neonatal Med. 2012;17:112–8.
31. Ritcher D, Russi EW. Alpha 1-antiproteinase deficiency. Ther Umsch. 1999;56(3):142–6 (abstract).
32. Abboud RT, Vimanathan S. Pathogenesis of COPD. Part I. The role of protease-antiprotease imbalance in emphysema. Int J Tuberc Lung Dis. 2008;12(4):361–7 (abstract).
33. Keatings VM, Collins PD, Scott DM, Barnes PJ. Differences on interleukin-8 and tissue necrosis factor-alpha in induced sputum from patients with COPD or asthma. Am J Respir Crit Care Med. 1996;153:530–4.
34. Baraldo S, Bazzan S, Zanin ME, Turarato G, Garbisa S, Maestrelli P, et al. Matrix metalloproteinase-2 protein in lug periphery is released to COPD progression. Chest. 2007;132: 1733–40.
35. Pauwels RA, Brust AJ, Calverly PM, Jenkins CR, Hurd SS. GOLD Scientific Committee: Global strategy for diagnosis, management and prevention of chronic obstructive pulmonary disease: NHLBI/WHO. Global Initiative for Chronic Obstructive Lung Disease (GOLD).
36. Barnes PJ. Managing chronic obstructive – pulmonary disease. 2nd ed. London: sP. Science Press Ltd; 2001.
37. Thompson PB, Daughton D, Robbins GA, Ghafonki MA, Ochlerking M, Rennard SI. Intramural airway inflammation in chronic bronchitis. Characterization and correlation with clinical parameters. Am Rev Respir Dis. 1989;140:1527–37.
38. Lofdahal M, Blomberg A, Roos-Engstrand E, Skold M. Increased CD4+ T cell infiltration in bronchial epithelium of patients with COPD. Program and abstracts of the American Thoracic Society. 19–24 May 2006, San Diego.

39. Papi A, Luppi F, Franco F, Fabbri LM. Pathophysiology of exacerbations of chronic obstructive pulmonary disease. Proc Am Thorac Soc. 2006;3(3):245–51.
40. Braman SS. Asthma in the elderly. Clin Geriatr Med. 2003;19:57–75.
41. Repine JE, Bast A, Lankhorst I. Oxidative stress in chronic obstructive pulmonary disease. Oxidative Stress Study Group. Am J Respir Crit Care Med. 1997;156:341–57.
42. Mannino DM. COPD: epidemiology, prevalence, morbidity and mortality and disease heterogeneity. Chest. 2002;121:1215–65.
43. Ohar J. New data in the pathophysiology of COPD. Website: http://www.medscape.com/view.article/540983.
44. Biswal S, Huang K, Misra V, et al. Physiological genomics of emphysema in aging normal lungs. Program and abstracts of the ATS 2000. International Conference My 19–24, San Diego.
45. Giard A, Yanagisawa M, Langliben D, Michel RP, Levy R, Schennib H, et al. Expression of endothelium-I in the lungs of patients with pulmonary hypertension. N Engl J Med. 1993;328:1732–9.

Asthma in the Elderly

46. Parameswaran K. Asthma in the elderly: under recognised, underdiagnosed and undertreated: a community survey. Respir Med. 1998;92:573–7.
47. Radenne F, Verkinne C, Tonnel AS. Asthma in the elderly. Res Mal Respir. 2003;20:9S–10 (abstract).
48. Murtagh E, Heaney L, Gingles J, Shepherd R, Kee F, Patterson C, et al. The prevalence of obstructive lung disease in a general population sample: the NICECOPD study. Eur J Epidemiol. 2005;20(3):443–53.
49. Enright PL, McClelland RL, Newman AB, Gottlieb DJ, Lebowitz MD. Underdiagnosis and undertreatment of asthma in the elderly. Chest. 1999;116:603–13.
50. Bouquet J, Jeffery PK, Busse WW. Asthma: from bronchoconstriction to airways inflammation and remodeling. Am J Respir Crit Care Med. 2000;161:1720–45.
51. Currie GP, Lee DK, Lipworth BJ. Long-acting beta-2 agonists in asthma: not so smart. Drug Saf. 2006;29(8):647–56 (abstract).
52. Fireman P. Understanding asthma pathophysiology. Allergy Asthma Proc. 2003;24(2):79–83 (abstract).
53. Page S, Ammit AJ, Black JL, Armour CL. Human mast cell and airway smooth muscle cell interactions: implications for asthma. Am J Physiol Lung Cell Mol Physiol. 2001;281(6):L1313–23 (abstract).
54. Melen E, Pershagen G. Pathophysiology of asthma: lessons from genetic research with particular focus on severe asthma. J In Med. 2012;272:108–20. doi: 10.1111/J1365_2796.2012.02555x. (abstract).
55. Moffat MF, Gut IG, Demenais F, Strachan DP, Bonzigon E, Heath S, et al. A large-scale consortium-based genomewide association study of asthma. N Engl J Med. 2010;363:1211–21.
56. Murphy DM, O'Byme PM. Recent advances in the pathophysiology of asthma. Chest. 2010;137(6):1417–26. doi:10.1378/chest.09-1895.
57. de Nijs SB, Venekamp LN, Bel EH. Adult-onset asthma: is it really different? Eur Respir Rev. 2013;22(127):44–52.
58. Wenzel SE. Asthma phenotypes: the evolution from clinical to molecular approaches. Nat Med. 2012;18:716–25.
59. Olin JT, Wechsler ME. Asthma: pathogenesis and novel drug treatment. BMJ. 2014;349:g5517.
60. Barnes PJ. Managing chronic obstructive – pulmonary disease. 2nd ed. London: sP. Science Press Ltd; 2001.
61. Wills-Karp M. Immunologic basis of antigen-induced airway hyperresponsiveness. Annu Rev Immunol. 1999;17:255–81 (abstract).

62. Kips JC. The relation between morphologic and functional airway changes in bronchial asthma. Verh K Acad Geneeskd Belg. 2003;65(4):247–65 (abstract).
63. Bara I, Ozier A, Tunon de Lara JM, Marthan R, Berger P. Pathophysiology of bronchial smooth muscle remodelling in asthma. Eur Respir J. 2010;26(5):1174–84 (abstract).
64. Armour C, Johnson P, Anticeviel S, Ammit A, McKay K, Hughes M. Mediators on human airway smooth muscle. Clin Exp Pharmacol Physiol. 1997;24(3–4):269–72 (abstract).
65. Robinson DS. The role of mast cells in asthma: induction of airway hyperresponsiveness by interaction with smooth muscle. J Allergy Clin Immunol. 2004;114(1):58–65 (abstract).
66. Elsassar S, Perruchoud AP. Pathophysiology of bronchial asthma. Schweiz Rundsch Med Prax. 1992;81(45):1346–9 (abstract).

Lung Cancer in the Elderly

67. Wingo PA, Cardinez CJ, Landes SH, Greenlee RT, Ries LA, Anderson RN, et al. Long term trends in cancer mortality in the United States. Cancer. 2003;97 suppl 12:3133–275.
68. Balducci L. Lung cancer in the elderly. CA Cancer J Clin. 2003;53:322. doi:10.3322/canjclin.53.6.322.
69. Brown JS, Eraut D, Trask C, Davison AG. Age and the treatment of lung cancer. Thorax. 1996;51:564–8.
70. Maione P, Rossi A, Sacco PC, Bareschino MA, Schettino C. Treating advanced non-small cell lung cancer in the elderly. Ther Adv Med Oncol. 2010;2(4):251–60.
71. Bunn PA, Lilenbaum R. Chemotherapy for elderly patients with advanced non-small cell lung cancer. J Natl Cancer Inst. 2003;95:341–3.
72. De Cos JS, Miravet L, Abal J, Nunez A, Munoz FJ, Gercia L, et al. The EpicliCP-2003 Study: a Multicenter epidemiological and clinical study of lung cancer in Spain. Arch Bronconeumol. 2006;42:446–52.
73. Fong KM, Sekido Y, Gazdar AF, Minna JD. Lung cancer: molecular biology of lung cancer: clinical implications. Thorax. 2003;58:892–900.
74. Salgia R, Skarin AT. Molecular abnormalities in lung cancer. J Clin Oncol. 1998;16.1207–17.
75. Aviel-Ronen S, Blackhall FH, Shepherd FA, Tsao MS. K-ras mutations in non-small cell lung carcinoma: a review. Clin Lung Cancer. 2006;8:30–8.
76. D'Arcangelo M, Capuzzo F. K-RAS mutations in non-small cell lung cancer: prognostic and predictive value. ISRN Mol Biol. 2012; doi:10.5402/2012/837306
77. Martin P, Leigh NB, Tsao MS, Shepherd FA. KRAS mutations as prognostic and predictive markers in non-small cell lung cancer. J Thorac Oncol. 2013;8(5):530–42 (abstract).
78. Hecht S. Tobacco carcinogens, their biomarkers and tobacco-induced cancer. Nat Rev Cancer. 2003;3:733–44.
79. Billelo KS, Murin S, Matthay RA. Epidemiology, etiology and prevalence of lung cancer. Clin Chest Med. 2002;23:1–25.
80. Kumar V, Cotran RS, Robbins SL. Basic pathology. 5th ed. Philadelphia: WB Saunders Company; 1992.

Acute Pulmonary Embolism in the Elderly

81. Kniffer Jr WD, Baron JA, Barrett J, Birkmeyer JD, Anderson Jr FA. The epidemiology of diagnosed pulmonary embolism and deep vein thrombosis in the elderly. Arch Intern Med. 1994;154:861–6.
82. White RH. Four topics of venous thromboembolism. Circulation. 2003;107:1-4-1-8. doi:10.1161/01.CIR.0000078468.11849.66.
83. Barrit W, Jordan SE. Anticoagulant drugs in the treatment of pulmonary embolism: a controlled trial. Lancet. 1960;1:1309–12.

84. Garg K. Acute pulmonary embolism (Helical CT). eMedicine. http://www.emedicine.com/radio/byname/Acute-Pulmonary-Embolism-(Helical-CT).htm. Accessed 28 Sep 2008.
85. Kostadima E, Zakynthinos E. Pulmonary embolism: pathophysiology diagnosis and treatment. Hellenic J Cardiol. 2007;48(2):94–107.
86. Smulders YM. Pathophysiology and treatment of haemodynamic instability in acute pulmonary embolism: the pivotal role of pulmonary vasoconstriction. Cardiovasc Res. 2000;48:23–33 (abstract).
87. Dantzker DR, Bower JS. Alterations in gas exchange following pulmonary thromboembolism. Chest. 1982;81(4):495–501.

3 Gastrointestinal System

3.1 Anatomical and Physiological Changes with Ageing Gastrointestinal Tract

The oesophagus

Alterations in function with ageing are primarily related to neuromuscular degeneration giving rise to alterations in the ability to coordinate the complex reflexes that lead to swallowing and propulsion of food bolus along the oesophagus [1]. Age-related loss of enteron neurons in the oesophagus has been demonstrated by morphological studies [2]. When objective criteria are assessed, actual age-related changes in the function of the oesophagus are minimal [3]. There is however evidence of reduced peristaltic contractions in the lower oesophagus in the elderly [4]. The oesophageal peristaltic contractions are reduced both in amplitude and duration in the over 90 age group [5].

Stomach and intestines

The main functions of the bowel are (i) storage, (ii) absorption, (iii) secretion, (iv) synthesis and (v) elimination. The changes that occur with ageing can basically be attributed to three areas, namely, changes in neuromuscular function, changes in the structure of the gastrointestinal tract and changes in the absorptive and secretory functions of the bowel [1]. The exact effect of ageing due to altered neuromuscular function of the stomach is unclear. Studies involving gastric emptying have provided data to indicate that homeostatic mechanisms regulating gastric emptying in elderly persons may be disrupted [6], but the small bowel has shown no alteration in transit rate [7].

In the small intestine the primary structures affected by age are the intestinal villi with loss in height resulting in a decreased area available for absorption [8]. Motility declines in the seventh and eighth decade of life [9]. In the large intestine with increasing age and more so after the age of 60 years, there is thickening of the muscle layers of the colon. The teniae coli are more affected than the circular

N. Nagaratnam et al., *Diseases in the Elderly: Age-Related Changes and Pathophysiology*, DOI 10.1007/978-3-319-25787-7_3

muscle layers and its contraction in the longitudinal direction and contribute to constipation, hard stool and faecal impaction [1]. There are mucosal changes which do not affect the absorptive capabilities of the colon. There is reduced tonic activity of the external anal sphincter at a smaller volume due to reduction in rectal wall elasticity [10]. Structural changes also occur in the internal anal sphincter and have been shown by endosonography to be thicker in older people [11]. There is evidence to suggest an age-dependent increase in rectal pressure threshold to produce initial sensation of rectal filling [12]. The difference between maximum resting anal pressure and rectal pressure falls in old age [7]. Decreased rectal compliance and an increase in the sensory threshold for an urge to defaecate are the more consistent findings. However, whether these changes are the result of physiological changes associated with ageing or are related to chronic bowel habits requires further clarification. Table 3.1 summarises the fundamental changes with ageing.

The enteric nervous system (ENS) is the division of the autonomic nervous system that regulates gastrointestinal function. Even though a large number of enteric neurons may be lost with age, the gastrointestinal tract remains functional [13]. However, neuronal loss can contribute to disturbing normal responsiveness, and this may be the reason for the higher frequency of gastrointestinal diseases in the elderly [14]. In the elderly the sensitivity of the gastrointestinal tract for usual concentration

Table 3.1 Changes in the gastrointestinal structure and function with ageing

Anatomical changes	Physiological changes	Effects in gastrointestinal function
I. Oesophagus		
Neuromuscular degeneration of enteron neurons	Inability to coordinate the complex reflexes of swallowing	Changes in function, reduced peristaltic contractions in lower oesophagus
II. Stomach		
Structural changes	Changes in neuromuscular, absorption and secretory functions	Gastric emptying may be disrupted
III. Small intestine		
Loss of enteric neurons	Disturbed normal responsiveness	High frequency of GI diseases
Intestinal villi loose height	Decreased area of absorption	Decrease GI reserves
IV. Large intestine rectum and anus		
Thickening of muscle layers teniae coli, circular muscles reduced tonic activity of external anal sphincter, thickening of internal anal sphincter	Contraction along longitudinal direction declines Rectal pressure increased	Faecal impaction

Information Sources: Aalami et al. [1]; Shaker and Lang [5]; Kupper et al. [6]; Haadem et al. [7]; Ibre [10]; Burnett and Barham [11]; Abelo et al. [14]; Atkins et al. [18]

of drugs is increased and may in part be the reason for the increased frequency of adverse drug reactions [15].

Few gastrointestinal functions decline to any significant level as a result of old age. Nevertheless, in older people there is a decrease in the gastrointestinal reserves which make them extremely vulnerable to minor insults and decompensation can occur rapidly. In ill and bedridden elderly patients, the colonic transit time is prolonged, but in the normal elderly, there is no conclusive evidence that the colonic transit time is altered compared with the younger adults [16]. Interestingly strength training shortens bowel transit but this is entirely limited to the colon [17].

Box 3.1. Key Points. Anatomical and Physiological GIT Changes with Age

- Age-related loss of enteron neurons in the oesophagus has been demonstrated by morphological studies, and there are reduced peristaltic contractions in the very old [2, 5].
- Gastric emptying in elderly persons may be disrupted [6].
- In the small intestine, loss of height of intestinal villi may result in disturbed normal responsiveness and decreased area of absorption [8].
- Structural changes within the large intestine result in decline in the contractions in the longitudinal direction, and the rectal pressure is increased [1, 12].

3.2 The Oesophageal Disorders

Introduction

Oesophageal disorders are a variety of pathological disorders that affect the oesophagus and alter the oesophageal function causing symptoms of dysphagia, heartburn and noncardiac chest pain. With advancing age there is an increase in the prevalence of swallowing impairment [19–21].

Pathophysiology

Although functional and structural changes in the oesophagus have been demonstrated with ageing, it does not cause clinically relevant oesophageal dysphagia in the elderly. Oral abnormalities including difficulty ingesting, controlling and delivering bolus relative to swallowing initiation were seen in 63 % [22]. Pharyngeal dysfunction consisting of bolus retention and lingual propulsion or pharyngeal constrictor paralysis was seen in 29 %. 39 % showed pharyngoesophageal segment abnormalities, mostly cricopharyngeal muscle dysfunction and minor abnormalities of oesophageal function were seen in 36 % [22]. Deficits in neurological function caused by true central nervous system degenerative processes and stroke and their differentiation from age-related changes [23] can be difficult.

A variety of pathological conditions seen in the elderly affect the oesophagus and can alter oesophageal function and cause symptoms. Organic abnormalities of swallowing can be related to the initiation of the swallowing reflex in the oropharynx or to propulsion of the food bolus through the oesophagus. Any pathology that interferes with the normal swallowing reflex may result in difficulty in swallowing and termed dysphagia. There are two main subcategories of dysphagia, namely, oropharyngeal dysphagia and oesophageal dysphagia, [24, 25] involving different phases of swallowing [25]. Oropharyngeal dysphagia results from disturbances in the oropharyngeal physiology such as poor tongue movement in chewing, reduced peristalsis in the pharynx, reduced laryngeal elevation or closure and cricopharyngeal dysfunction [26]. Oesophageal dysphagia is caused by disordered motility or a result of obstruction to the passage of the food bolus through the oesophagus to the stomach [24]. Oropharyngeal dysphagia and oesophageal dysphagia often present as a symptom of a systemic disease process and are a secondary diagnosis.

3.2.1 Gastro-oesophageal Reflux Disease (GORD)

Gastro-oesophageal reflux disease (GORD) is a chronic disorder that affects the lower oesophageal sphincter allowing gastric acids to reflux into the oesophagus. The prevalence and severity of GORD increases with age. And the elderly are more likely to develop severe disease.

Pathophysiology
GORD is caused by failure of the lower oesophageal sphincter (LES). There are several factors which may contribute to the competence of the gastro-oesophageal junction. These include:

(i) The intrinsic sphincter pressure. In recent years attention has shifted from sustained hypotension to transient lower oesophageal relaxation [27].
(ii) The angle at which the oesophagus enters the stomach creates a valve preventing gastric contents transiting back into the oesophagus.
(iii) Permeability as a pathogenic factor in GORD. Psychological stress may induce a permeability defect on the stratified epithelia and oesophagus [28].
(iv) The action of the diaphragm that functions as an external sphincter [29].

Some of the factors that contribute or predispose to the development of GORD include gastric acid, delayed gastric emptying, oesophageal clearance mechanisms, ingested irritants, mucosal integrity and genetic factors [29]. Factors that lead to the oesophagitis are the corrosiveness and increase in the number of long-lasting refluxate, prolonged oesophageal clearance time [30], the resistance of the oesophageal mucosa and the volume of the gastric contents. In the elderly age-related changes such as decreased salivary secretions, reduced or loss of lower oesophageal sphincter tone, diminished oesophageal motility and gastric acid hypersecretion may lead to GORD. The 'classical' GORD is referred to as erosive GORD. A non-erosive or negative endoscopy reflux disease (NERD) is now recognised and constitutes about 60 % of all GORD [31].

Box 3.2. Key Points. Oesophageal Disorders

- Oropharyngeal dysphagia results from disturbances in the oropharyngeal physiology such as poor tongue movement in chewing, reduced peristalsis in the pharynx, reduced laryngeal elevation or closure and cricopharyngeal dysfunction [26].
- Oesophageal dysphagia is caused by disordered motility or a result of obstruction to the passage of food [24].
- In the elderly age-related changes such as decreased salivary secretion, reduced or loss of lower oesophageal sphincter tone, diminished oesophageal motility and gastric acid hypersecretion may lead to gastro-oesophageal reflux disease [29].

3.3 Peptic Ulcer Disease in the Elderly

Introduction

A peptic ulcer is a breach in the mucosal lining of the stomach (gastric ulcer) or in the first part of duodenum (duodenal ulcer) caused by an imbalance between gastroduodenal mucosal protective factors that normally limit injury and inimical factors. The main causes of peptic ulcers are *Helicobacter pylori* infection and the use of non-steroidal anti-inflammatory drugs (NSAIDs) [32]. The prevalence of *H. pylori* increases with age [33], and the prevalence of *H. pylori* infection in patients with peptic ulcer has been reported to range from 58 to 78 % in patients aged over 65 years [34]. In the age group 20–30 years, the prevalence of the infection was 18 % and this rose to 53 % in those aged over 70 [35]. About 65–70 % of patients with gastric ulcer and 95 % with duodenal ulcer are *H. pylori* positive [36]. NSAID use in the elderly is increasing steadily and about half of such all medications are used by the elderly aged over 60 years and approximately 15 % of persons over the age of 60 take NSAIDs [37]. Almost 40 % of gastric ulcers and 25 % of duodenal ulcers in the elderly are associated with the use of NSAIDs [38]. There is three to four times increase in risk with the use of NSAIDs for gastric ulcer. Although the prevalence of *H. pylori* is falling, the elderly remain at risk for peptic ulcer because of the widespread use of NSAIDs [39].

Physiology

The production of gastric juice in the stomach is tightly regulated by positive and negative feedback mechanisms, neural and hormonal. Four types of cells are involved – parietal cells, G cells, D cells and enterochromaffin-like cells (ECLs). Endings of the vagus nerve and intramural nervous plexus in the digestive tract influence secretion significantly. The nerve endings in the stomach secrete stimulating neurotransmitters. Acetylcholine (ACh), gastrin and histamine have physiological roles in regulating gastric acid secretion [40]. ACh is the neurotransmitter released by muscarine nerve endings of the parasympathetic nerve in the gastric mucosa. Gastrin a hormone is released by peptides in the stomach [40]. The release of histamine is the most important positive regulatory mechanism of secretion of gastric acid in the stomach and is the final common chemical mediator at the oxyntic cell [41]. Its release is stimulated by ACh and gastrin and inhibited by somatostatin. There are three phases of secretion of gastric acid: (1) cephalic phase (30 % of total stimulated by anticipation of eating, smell and taste), (2) gastric phase (60 % by distension of the stomach with food) and (3) intestinal phase (10 %) [42]. There is also a small continuous basal secretion of gastric acid between meals. Gastric acid production is regulated by autonomic nervous system and several hormones. The parasympathetic nervous system (via the vagus) and hormone gastrin stimulate parietal cell to produce acid and directly and indirectly through the stimulation of the secretion of hormone histamine from enterochromaffin-like cells. Vasoactive intestinal peptide cholecystokinin and secretin inhibit production. The acidity in the stomach is maintained by the gastric H^+ K^+-ATPase (proton pump). This enzyme is the ultimate common step of acid secretion [43] on which all stimulating pathways merge [44].

Pathophysiology

Peptic ulcer disease is associated with hyperfunction of the G cell, increased gastric secretion and pepsinogen, impaired bicarbonate secretion and the presence of inflammatory indicators [45]. The main cause of peptic ulcers is *Helicobacter pylori* infection. *H. pylori* infection is highly associated with peptic ulcer disease [46], gastric carcinoma [47] and gastric lymphoma [48]. In duodenal ulcer *H. pylori* is common up to 90–100 % of patients and in gastric ulcer 60–70 % [49]. It is still unclear how *H. pylori* is transmitted from person to person and it is generally believed that it is by faecal-oral route. On reaching the stomach, it adheres to the mucosal lining of the stomach and is found in the inner surface of the epithelial cell and also within the cell [50]. The bacterial colonisation patterns will depend on the amount of acid in the stomach. In persons producing large amount of acid, *H. pylori* will colonise in the pyloric antrum [51]. *H. pylori* evokes an inflammatory response which induces the secretion of gastrin. Gastrin acts on the parietal cells to increase acid production. The increased amounts of acid damage the duodenum resulting in the formation of duodenal ulcers [51]. Gastric ulcers on the other hand are associated with normal or low levels of acid production. This would suggest that in these individuals the mechanisms that protect the gastric mucosa are impaired [52].

H. pylori produces urease in large amounts which is necessary for the pathogenesis and survival of the organism [53]. The urease breaks down urea into carbon dioxide and ammonia. It also produces other enzymes, proteases (break down glycoproteins in the gastric mucous) and phospholipases (hydrolyse phospholipids into fatty acids) [54]. Ammonia is produced by urease activity; the protease and lipase degrade the gastric mucous and by disrupting the phospholipid-rich layer at the epithelial cell layer cause cell injury suggesting that *H. pylori* contributes to gastric mucosal injury by direct pathogenic mechanisms [55]. *H. pylori* triggers an inflammatory response; the bacterial polysaccharides attract inflammatory cells to the mucosa and cause high levels of TNF-α and/or interleukin-6 [51]. A platelet-activating factor promotes thrombotic occlusion of the surface capillaries [56].

Apart from *H. pylori* infection, other causes of peptic ulcers are the use of non-steroidal anti-inflammatory drugs (NSAIDs) and aspirin, Zollinger-Ellison syndrome and those related to other forms of gastritis [45]. Corticosteroids, smoking and heavy intake of alcohol also increase the risk of peptic ulcer disease. High level of prostaglandins enhances mucosal resistance to injury perhaps by increasing blood flow and stimulating the secretion of mucous [57]. Age is a risk factor and is associated with low prostaglandin concentration. The precursor of prostaglandins, arachidonic acid, is catalysed by two enzymes – cyclooxygenase coenzymes 1 and 2. The anti-inflammatory properties of NSAIDs are mediated through inhibition of cyclooxygenase coenzyme 2. Peptic ulcers result from the effects of cyclooxygenase 1. No anti-inflammatory drug is completely safe including cyclooxygenase (COX)-2 inhibitors [58], and switching to selective COX-2 inhibitors in patients with previous bleeding is not without risk and the addition of PPI is needed [58]. The role of *H. pylori* infection in NSAID-related peptic ulcer is unclear, nor is there clear evidence for testing and treating *H. pylori* infection in elderly patients on NSAID or aspirin for prevention of drug-related peptic ulcer [34].

Box 3.3. Key Points. Peptic Ulcer Disease

- It is associated with hyperfunction of the G cells, increased gastric secretion and pepsinogen level, impaired bicarbonate secretion and presence of inflammatory marker [45].
- The main cause is *Helicobacter pylori* infection [46].
- *H. pylori* triggers an inflammatory response; the bacterial polysaccharides attract inflammatory cells to the mucosa and cause high levels of TNF-α and/or interleukin-6 [51].
- Gastric ulcers are associated with normal or low levels of acid production [52].

3.4 Colorectal Cancer

Introduction

Colorectal cancer is a malignant tumour arising from the mucosa of the colon or rectum. Colorectal cancer is the fourth common cancer in men and the third in women worldwide [59, 60]. Australia has one of the highest rates of colorectal cancer in the world and is the second leading cause of death.

Pathophysiology

The cause of colorectal cancer is not understood and appears to involve interactions between inherited susceptibility and environmental factors. Colorectal cancers evolve from colonic polyps, mostly from the conventional adenomas and from mutation of the APC gene through a multistep process involving mutations of the DCC, k-ras and p53 genes. The basic genetic defect in the latter is not known [61]. Large polyps (>1 cm) at villous adenomas have a high risk of cancer [62].

Genetic factors are important. Familial risk of colon cancer is common [67]. Family history of colorectal cancer or adenomas in the first-degree relatives, hereditary non-polyposis colorectal cancer (HNPCC) and familial adenomatous polyposis (FAP) and the presence of high-risk mutation in the adenomatous polyposis coli (APC) place the individual at potentially high risk of developing colorectal cancer. The genes that give rise to HNPCC and FAP have been identified [63]. About 2 % of patients with colorectal cancer suffer from genetic syndromes associated with an exceptionally high risk, and another 15–20 % have a family history of colorectal cancer without genetic predisposition [64].

Environmental factors play an important role and can increase the risk of colon cancer [61]. Western diet (particularly one rich in red meat, high fat and low vegetables) is a predisposition [65]. It has been shown that intake of energy, fat and protein had a greater impact on risk among older men and women than among the young. The data suggested that age at diagnosis may interact with other factors to alter the risk of colon cancer [66]. Nutritional intervention (fresh fruit and vegetables) and controlling energy balance have been identified as an important part in its prevention [65]. Changing dietary and physical activity habits is considered an important factor in the development of the disease [67].

Box 3.4. Key Points. Colorectal Cancer

- It involves interaction between inherited susceptibility and environmental factors.
- Genetic factors are important and familial risk of colon cancer is common [67].
- Environmental factors play an important role [61].
- Changing dietary and physical activity habits is considered an important factor in the development of the disease [67].

3.5 Inflammatory Bowel Disease in the Elderly

Introduction

Inflammatory bowel disease (IBD) embraces two diseases, Crohn's disease (CD) and ulcerative colitis (UC), which are immunologically mediated, chronic, relapsing, inflammatory conditions of unknown aetiology [68]. With ageing of the population, IBD has become a growing problem in the elderly [69]. 10–30 % of the IBD population are above the age of 60 years, and 10–15 % of the cases of IBD are diagnosed in patients 60 years and over [69]. Crohn's disease has its peak onset in early life and a second peak among the elderly [70], and a third of newly diagnosed occurs in the elderly with prevalence in females twice that of males [71, 72].

Pathophysiology

The aetiology and pathogenesis are unclear. It is generally accepted that the patho-aetiology involves complicated multifactorial interactions among various genetic, environmental and microbial factors and immune responses [73, 74] and their secreted mediators (cytokines and chemokines) [74]. Multiple genes contribute to disease susceptibility and studies have indicated that genetic factors are integrally involved. One-quarter of patients with IBD has an affected family member [75], and a genetic background is responsible for at least 50 % of the risk or susceptibility to develop CD [76]. Twin studies have demonstrated the increased incidence in IBD in first-degree relatives of probands with either disease [68]. About 163 susceptibility gene foci have been ascertained for IBD [73]. A genetic susceptibility to CD has been proven with the identification of variations as a risk factor CARD15 (caspase recruitment domain family member 15) formerly known as NOD2 [76, 77]. Genetic factors seem to have a stronger influence in CD than in UC [75]. Environmental risk factors both protective and inciting have been investigated among them being gastrointestinal infections, breastfeeding, stress, smoking and diet [78].

The innate lymphoid cells (macrophages, monocytes, neutrophils) and adaptive (T cells and B cells) immune system are activated with loss of tolerance to enteric commensal bacteria and in patients with UC and CD [68, 79]. In genetically susceptible hosts, environmental factors transiently break the mucosal barrier [68], and alterations in the gut microbiome stimulate an inflammatory response [78], and the microbial antigen exposure results in the onset and perpetuation of the disease [68, 80]. In UC the T-cell response is either Th2 (interleukin (IL)-4, IL-13) or mediated by a subset of natural killer (NK) T cells (IL-13) which are cytotoxic for epithelial cells [80, 81]. The Th2 immune responses lead to B-cell hyperactivity and the production of autoantibodies. In CD the T-cell response is T helper (Th) 1 dominant [80]. Various types of autoantibodies including pANCA and antibodies against goblet cells are present [81]. Antibodies to *Saccharomyces cerevisiae* do not commonly occur with UC but have been strongly associated with Crohn's disease. The presence of anti-*Saccharomyces cerevisiae* antibody (ASCA) increases the possibility of Crohn's disease.

Box 3.5. Key Points. Inflammatory Bowel Diseases in the Elderly

- Pathophysiology involves multifunctional interactions among various genetic, environmental and microbial factors, immune responses and their secreted mediators [73, 74].
- Genetic factors seem to be stronger in Crohn's disease (CD) than in ulcerative colitis (UC) [75].
- In genetically susceptible hosts, environmental factors transiently break the mucosal barrier, and alterations in the gut microbiome stimulate inflammatory response [68, 78].
- Various types of autoantibodies including pANCA and antibodies against the goblet cells are present [81].
- The presence of anti-*Saccharomyces cerevisiae* antibody (ASCA) increases the possibility of Crohn's disease.

3.6 Related Disorders

3.6.1 Diarrhoea in the Elderly

Introduction

Diarrhoea is usually defined as an increase in stool frequency (three or more stools per day [82]), fluid content (>150–200 ml/24 h) [83] and volume or weight. The exact incidence rate of diarrhoeas in the elderly is not available but it is greater than in young adults. Diarrhoea can be mild or severe in the elderly and severe diarrhoea in the elderly can be life-threatening. It is an important cause of morbidity worldwide and is the second leading cause of morbidity [84] and mortality in the elderly [85, 86]. Deaths due to diarrhoeal illnesses occur in the elderly living in the community and in nursing homes but more so in the latter, and outbreaks have been associated with more deaths from nursing home residents [87]. Fifty per cent of deaths due to diarrhoea occur in individuals over the age of 75 years.

Pathophysiology

Mechanisms of diarrhoea. The main function from the midgut to the transverse colon is the absorption of fluids and electrolytes by nonpropulsive contractions resulting in the formation of solid faeces. In the remaining colon, the faecal mass is propelled forwards to the rectum and lubricated by mucous secreted by the goblet cells. The elderly are at increased risk of dying from dehydration and electrolyte abnormalities and impaired mobility and are frequently institutionalised. It is likely that deficits in both immune and non-immune defences may play a role in gastrointestinal infections in the elderly [88]. Basically diarrhoea develops from the following mechanisms:

(i) Mucosal injury – disruption of the absorptive and secretory mechanisms both in the large and small intestine. Decreased absorption and increased secretion result in diarrhoea [89]. It is largely caused by infection or inflammation. Infection causes diarrhoea by mucosal adherence and invasion or by toxin production [83]. The causative agent, for example, bacteria, may adhere to specific receptors on the mucosa causing a watery diarrhoea [90] or invade the mucosa and damage the epithelial cells and vascular endothelium causing a bloody diarrhoea or by producing toxins, enterotoxin and cytotoxin [83]. The former gives rise to a watery diarrhoea and the latter a bloody diarrhoea.

(ii) Secretory – due to disorder of sodium chloride transport. There are two mechanisms. The first is by affecting the exchange pump, the energy for which is provided by the Na^+ K^+ ATPase-mediated breakdown of ATP, thereby disrupting the transintestinal movement of water and electrolytes. The second mechanism is through activation of the adenylate cyclase within the intestinal enterocyte which increases the level of cyclic AMP resulting in secretion of Na and Cl ions together with water into the bowel lumen [91–93]. This leads to loss of water and salts from the body as watery stools. Secretory diarrhoea can result from bacterial toxins [94]. The enteropathogens, e.g. *Vibrio cholerae*, *E.*

coli and viruses such rotavirus, and therapeutic and humoral agents give rise to secretory diarrhoea [94].

(iii) Osmotic – due to ingestion of non-absorbable solutes. Osmotic agents, for example, sorbitol and lactulose, draw fluid across the membranes into the lumen. The absorption of carbohydrate depends on the presence of disaccaridases in the brush border of the intestine. Lack of these enzymes will lead to attraction of water by the unabsorbed disaccharides in the gut lumen [95].

(iv) Increase in intestinal motility – by making the bowel overactive. The increase in intestinal motility results in reduction of the contact time and therefore increases the volume and liquid in the stool. This can be due to diabetic neuropathy, hyperthyroidism, and postvagotomy (Fig. 3.1) [96].

Box 3.6. Key Points. Diarrhoea in the Elderly

- Results from the following mechanisms:
- Mucosal injury results in disruption of absorption and secretory mechanisms in both large and small intestines.
- Secretory – interfering with fluid and electrolyte transport [91–93].
- Osmotic – due to ingestion of non-adsorbable solutes.
- Increased intestinal motility results in reduction of the contact time and increases the volume of the liquid in the stool [96].

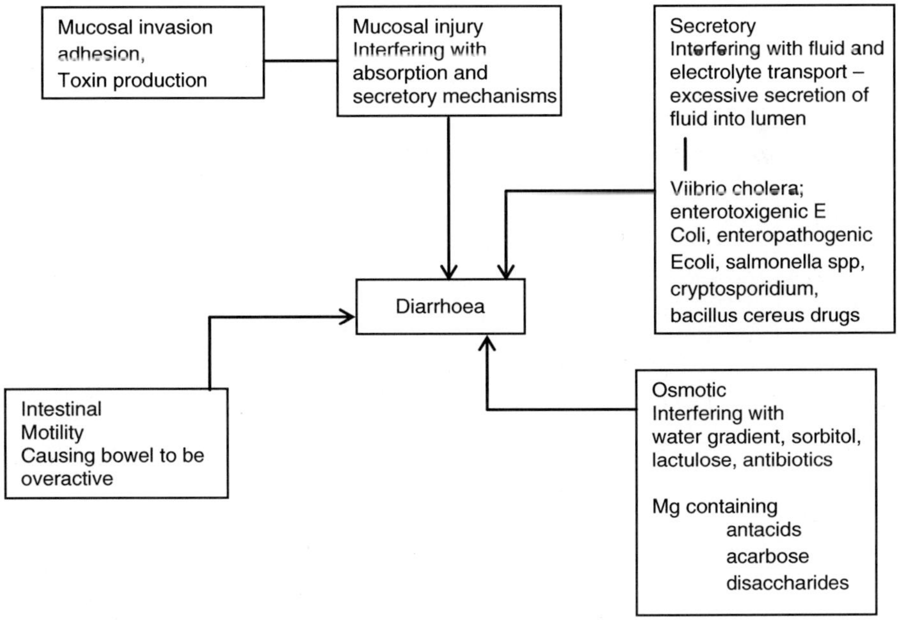

Fig. 3.1 Pathophysiology underlying diarrhoeas (Information sources: Binder [83]; Ratnaike and Jones [91]; Cutting [92]; Ewe and Wanitscke [93])

3.6.2 Malabsorption in the Elderly

Introduction

Malabsorption is the impairment of either absorption and uptake of nutrients or impaired digestion (maldigestion). Malabsorption may occur for several nutrients or for specific nutrients and can lead to severe nutritional problems. Malabsorption is present in the elderly more often than is realised, and symptoms resulting from malabsorption tend to be muted in the elderly [97]. In a study of 490 patients admitted to an acute geriatric ward, presented with non-gastrointestinal symptoms, 24 patients with previously unrecognised malabsorption was detected [98].

Pathophysiology

The extraction of nutrients requires both digestion and absorption. Normal absorption involves three steps, intraluminal phase (premucosal), mucosal phase and post-absorptive processing (postmucosal) [99]. Defect in the intraluminal phase gives rise to maldigestion and defect in the mucosal phase to malabsorption [100]. Malabsorption can be caused by gastric hypochlorhydria with small bowel bacterial overgrowth [101]. There is little evidence that ageing causes significant malnutrition in the normal elderly, but decrease in the gastrointestinal reserve makes the elderly more susceptible to small insults [101]. There may be altered absorption of calcium and possibly zinc and magnesium as a result of physiological changes with ageing [102].

3.6.2.1 Intraluminal Phase

Although digestion begins in the mouth, the greater part of digestion occurs in the stomach. Protein, an essential nutritional component, undergoes a series of degradation processes elicited by hydrolytic enzymes from the stomach, pancreas and small intestine resulting in a mixture of amino acids and small peptides which are absorbed by the enterocytes [103]. Hydrochloric acid and pepsin facilitate digestion by hydrolytic actions and in the small intestine through the pancreatic enzymes, namely, amylase, lipase and trypsin. In the mouth the salivary enzyme amylase breaks down the starch and glycogen into disaccharides. The major part of the digestion however is in the lumen of the small intestine by pancreatic alpha-amylase [104]. The digestion of carbohydrate is in two phases, luminal phase involving the pancreatic alpha-amylase and the membrane phase involving the enzymes disaccharidases (sucrase, maltase and lactase) [104] in the epithelial cells of the villi. Disaccharides are broken down into monosaccharides and are absorbed. Maldigestion occurs as a result of enzyme deficiency, inactivation or inadequate mixing.

Digestion of dietary triacylglycerols begins in the stomach and continues in the duodenum with the synergistic action of gastric and colipase-dependent pancreatic lipases [105]. The products formed are transported into structures made of bile salts and phospholipids. Fat solubilisation occurs with bile salts to form lamellar vesicles and mixed micelles and is then absorbed by the enterocytes [105]. Fat digestion could be interfered by diminished bile salt secretion, synthesis or increased loss.

Luminal availability of nutrients, for example, vitamin B_{12}, is converted into forms capable of being absorbed or bound to cofactors necessary for absorption. The absorption process of vitamin B_{12}, for instance, involves five stages. The vitamin B_{12} in the food is bound to proteins. (i) In the stomach the gastric acid and pepsin release the cobalamin from the protein complex, (ii) the released cobalamin binds to the salivary R-protein, (iii) the cobalamin-protein complexes are then degraded by pancreatic enzymes [106], (iv) the released cobalamin combines in the duodenum with the intrinsic factor (IF) [106] and (v) the IF-cobalamin complex then attaches itself to the brush border membrane of the terminal ileum and is absorbed [107]. Any interruption of the necessary steps in the sequence will lead to vitamin B_{12} deficiency. Luminal availability of vitamin B_{12} may also be affected by bacterial overgrowth.

3.6.2.2 Mucosal Phase

Mucosal phase involves brush border hydrolysis and epithelial transport. At the brush border further hydrolysis, for example, of the carbohydrates occurs, and deficiency of lactase in the brush border of the small intestinal epithelial cells impairs the breakdown of the unabsorbable disaccharide such as lactose into its absorbable components, glucose and galactose [108].

3.6.2.3 Post-absorptive Processing

The nutrients after absorption enter the systemic circulation via the portal vein to the liver or via the lymphatic or thoracic duct.

Box 3.7. Key Points. Malabsorption in the Elderly

- There is little evidence that ageing causes symptomatic malnutrition in the elderly, but decrease in the gastrointestinal reserve makes the elderly more susceptible to small insults [105].
- Maldigestion occurs as a result of enzyme deficiency, inactivation or inadequate mixing.
- Defect in the intraluminal phase gives rise to maldigestion and defect in the mucosal phase to malabsorption
- Fat absorption could be interfered by diminished bile salt secretion, synthesis or increased loss.
- Luminal availability, for instance, of vitamin B_{12} may be affected by bacterial overgrowth.
- Deficiency of lactase in the brush border of the small intestinal epithelial cells impaired the breakdown of unabsorbable disaccharides, lactose into absorbable glucose and galactose [108].

3.6.3 Malnutrition in the Elderly

Introduction

Malnutrition can be defined as nutritional inadequacy resulting from an imbalance in food intake and body needs; the outcome is loss of lean body mass and/or deficiency of one or more micronutrients. Malnutrition is not uncommon in the elderly and is a problem of immense concern. It has a high prevalence among hospitalised patients ranging from 12 to 50 % and from 23 to 60 % among institutionalised elderly patients [109, 110]. In one study 78.3 % were found to be malnourished on admission [111]. In other studies the prevalence among institutionalised patients ranged from 23 to 85 % [112–114]. The differences in the variation are due to variation in the diagnostic criteria and screening tools used which make comparison difficult.

Pathophysiology Age-related physiological changes together with other factors place the elderly at a high risk of developing malnutrition. Many age-related changes are not completely understood. Nutritional inadequacy could be due to physiological, pathological, functional and socio-economic causes [115, 116] (Box 3.10). With ageing there is decreased food intake often referred to as *anorexia of ageing* and is related to several factors (Box 3.11). In more than 75 % of the adults aged 89 years or older, the sense of smell and taste is depressed [117]. There is degeneration of the taste buds together with a reduction in the number of tastes buds. The taste detection threshold varies across different taste modalities, the sweet taste is least affected in the elderly [117]. There is also a marked decline in the ability to smell with ageing due to a regression of olfactory receptors on the roof of the nasal cavity and a decline in the olfactory nuclei in the brain. Alterations in the neurotransmitters and hormones affect the central feeding system and the peripheral satiety system [118, 119]. There is a decline in gastric emptying of large meals associated with satiation [120]. The reduced food intake and appetite could also be attributed to the loss of lean body mass and decreased basal metabolic rate (BMR) seen with advancing age.

Box 3.8. Key Points. Malnutrition in the Elderly

- Age-related changes with other factors place the elderly at high risk of developing malnutrition [115, 116].
- With ageing there is decreased food intake referred to as anorexia of ageing.
- Similar to several factors such as smell, taste is depressed [117].
- Alterations in the neurotransmitters and hormones affect central feeding sites and peripheral satiety system [118, 119].
- There is decline in gastric emptying of large meals associated with satiation [120].
- Decrease in food intake is also due to decrease in fat intake.

Box 3.9. Anorexia of Ageing
Decreased sense of smell [117]
Decreased sense of taste [117]
Decreased fat intake
Alterations to central feeding system
Alterations to peripheral satiety system [118, 119]
Decline in gastric emptying [120]
Loss of lean body mass
Decreased basal metabolic rate

3.6.4 Constipation and Faecal Incontinence

Physiology of defaecation
It is mandatory for those treating constipation and faecal incontinence to have a clear understanding of the physiological mechanisms of defaecation and continence [121]. Both conditions are of diverse aetiology and many mechanisms may be involved in their pathophysiology. The rectum serves as a reservoir for faecal contents, whereas the anal canal regulates continence and defaecation [122]. Normal defaecation begins with the passage of faecal bolus into the rectum. The rectum distends and there is transient relaxation of the internal anal sphincter. The nature of the rectal contents (solid, liquid or gas) is recognised by the sensory epithelium of the proximal anal canal. Continence is preserved by the contraction of the external anal sphincter which allows time for impulses to attain conscious awareness as to the nature of the material and decide the course of action. This is associated with an urge to defaecate. Voluntary deferring of evacuation until an appropriate moment is by voluntary control of the external anal sphincter [123]. If the individual complies and adopts a squatting position, the anorectal angle becomes straightened. Valsalva manoeuvre increases the intra-abdominal pressure and overcomes the resistance of the external anal sphincter. The pelvic floor descends and pressure on the faecal mass increases the intra-rectal pressure. The internal anal sphincter, the external anal sphincter and the puborectalis muscle relax synchronously and the faecal mass is discharged. Once the mass is expelled and defaecation is over, the anal canal sphincters and the pelvic muscles regain their resting activity and the anal canal closed. The entire train of events is regulated by the interplay between sympathetic and parasympathetic nerves, striated and smooth muscles and environmental factors [121, 124] and initiated by higher cortical function [125].

Nerve pathways
The anal function is controlled by the smooth and striated sphincter muscles which are innervated with the autonomic and somatic nerves. The sympathetic pathway to the

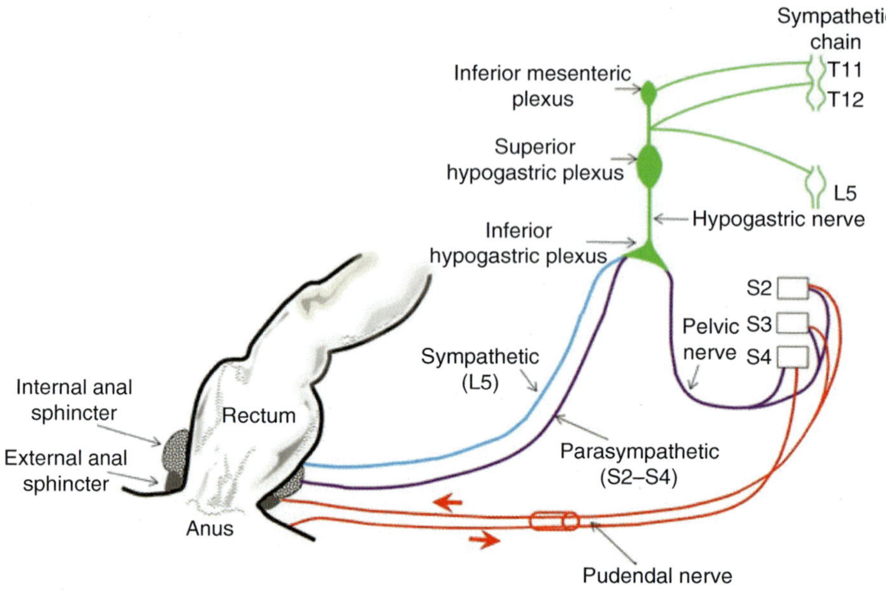

Fig. 3.2 Segmental and peripheral innervation of the rectum

IAS emerges from the 5th lumbar segment. The IAS is also supplied by the preganglionic parasympathetic fibres that emerge from 2nd, 3rd and 4th sacral segments. The EAS is supplied by the inferior rectal nerves and by the perianal branch of the 4th sacral nerve, and the reflex has its afferent and efferent pathway in the pudendal nerve. The fibres in the pelvic splanchnic nerves reach the intestines by way of plexuses (Fig 3.2). Defaecation involves integrated sensorimotor functions including the ultimate common path, the pelvic floor and anal sphincters [124] (Fig. 3.3).

3.6.4.1 Constipation

Introduction

There is no satisfactory definition of constipation, but generally in clinical practice, it is fewer than three bowel movements per week and has both functional and organic causes. Constipation is a common condition in the elderly and the prevalence increases with age [126]. The estimated prevalence of constipation is highly variable from 2 % [127] to 28 % [128]. Older men and women are equally affected and are often related to multiple age-related problems which may account for the increased prevalence in older people. About three-quarters of the elderly hospitalised patients and nursing home residents use laxatives for bowel regulation [129]. About half the number in nursing homes and 15–20 % of the community dwelling elderly suffer from constipation [130]. Chronic constipation is often a cause of great discomfort and often affects the quality of life negatively [131]. It may be a sign of a more serious underlying problem such as mass lesions or colonic dysmotility [132].

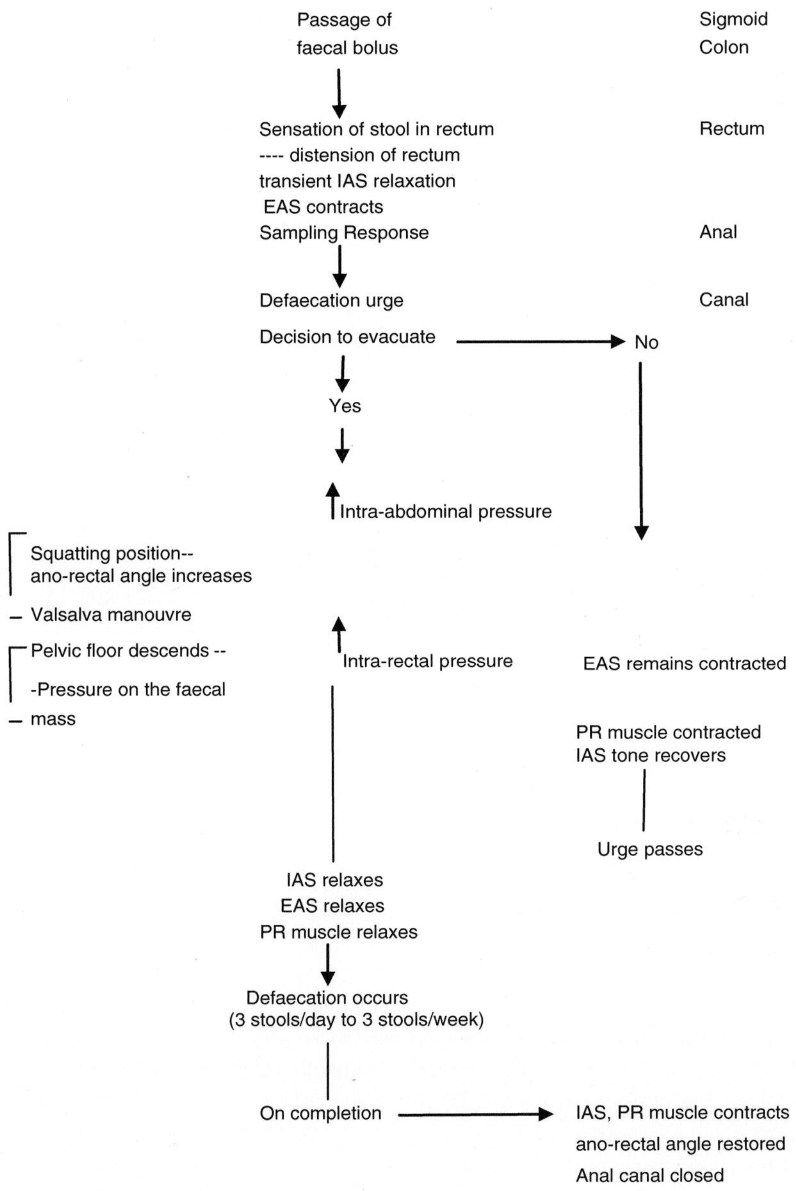

Fig. 3.3 Physiology of defaecation. *IAS internal anal sphincter, *EAS* external anal sphincter, *PR* muscle puborectal muscle

Pathophysiology

The pathophysiology of constipation in the elderly is complex [126]. Slow colon transit, irritable bowel syndrome and pelvic floor dysfunction are three distinct pathophysiologies which can contribute to constipation [133]. In older people the increased prevalence of constipation can be attributed to the many age-related problems such as multiple medical conditions, increased use of medications with a side effect profile that includes constipation, decreased mobility and dietary changes. The last is especially due to reduced fibre intake as the result of their poor chewing ability. Frailty and bedriddeness and weak straining ability contribute to the increased prevalence of constipation in this group [134]. Drug-induced constipation is the use of medications that affect the central nervous system, nerve conduction and smooth muscle fibres. Drugs that are associated with constipation are the anticholinergics and dopaminergics (used in Parkinson's disease [134]. Other causes of secondary constipation are the (i) neurological diseases (stroke, autonomic neuropathy, Parkinson's disease, spinal cord injury and Hirschsprung disease), (ii) endocrine and metabolic diseases (diabetes mellitus, hypercalcaemia, hypothyroidism, hyperparathyroidism and uraemia), (iii) psychological conditions (anxiety, depression) and (iv) structural abnormalities (haemorrhoids, strictures, anal fissure, rectal prolapse, rectocele and obstruction of the colon) [135].

Box 3.10. Key Points. Constipation

- The pathophysiology of constipation is complex [126].
- Three distinct pathophysiologies can contribute to the development of constipation are slow transit time, pelvic floor dysfunction and irritable bowel syndrome [133].
- Increased in prevalence can be attributed to the many age-related problems [134].
- Multiple medical problems and medications, decreased mobility and dietary changes contribute to constipation [134].

3.6.4.2 Faecal Incontinence

Physiology of continence

The puborectalis and the other pelvic floor muscles have sensory and motor function, the rectum and anal sphincters are essential to continence [123] as is the continuous tonic activity of the puborectalis muscle. The presence of a compliant rectum together with the above augments sphincter activity and allows continence to be preserved since the relationship of lower pressures in the rectum and higher pressures in the anal canal is maintained.

Introduction

Faecal incontinence is defined as inability to control voluntarily the internal anal sphincter with passage of faeces and flatus. True prevalence of faecal incontinence is not known but could be as high as 2.2 % in the general population [136]. In institutionalised patients the prevalence had been estimated between 30 and 60 % [137]. Almost one in ten residents in 30 residential homes for the elderly had faecal incontinence at least once weekly [138]. In 73 % of the patients, faecal incontinence had been present for over a year, and yet only 4 % had been referred to the general practitioner [138]. Estimates of the prevalence of incontinence in older adult population vary widely, but clearly it is significantly more common in older adults [139].

Pathophysiology

Several mechanisms may be involved in its pathophysiology. The rectum acts as a storage reservoir [122] until the contents can be disposed. The pelvic floor muscles including the puborectalis muscle and the anal sphincters are essential for defaecatory process and to maintain continence [136]. There are broad categories of faecal incontinence among the elderly, namely, (i) overflow incontinence, (ii) reservoir incontinence and (iii) rectosphincteric incontinence [140, 141]. Altered stool consistency and delivery of contents to the rectum, abnormal rectal capacity and compliance, decreased anorectal sensation and pelvic floor or anal sphincter dysfunction may result in incontinence [142]. Table 3.2 shows the pathophysiology of faecal incontinence.

In the female vaginal delivery is the most common cause of structural damage to the anal sphincter [144]. Other conditions associated with faecal incontinence are faecal impaction which is an important factor in the elderly, diarrhoeal states, connective tissue disorders and neurological impairment related to stroke, diabetes and multiple sclerosis [136].

Table 3.2 Pathophysiology of faecal incontinence

Physiological function	Dysfunction	Cause	Result
Rectal capacity/compliance	Abnormal, rigid rectum, reduced compliance	Inflammatory bowel disease, radiation altered stool consistency and delivery to the rectum	Increased frequency, urgency, faecal incontinence
Rectal sensitivity and co-ordination	Decreased	Neurological diseases	Faecal incontinence
Pelvic floor muscles puborectalis and mucosal seal	Reduced tonic activity		Faecal incontinence
Motility	?Failure to keep the rectum and anal canal empty	Infection, radiation, emotions	Faecal incontinence
Sphincters			
IAS	Structural damage	Iatrogenic damage surgical, obstetric injury, degeneration	Passive soiling urge incontinence
EAS			

Information sources; Rasmussen [145]

Box 3.11. Key Points. Faecal Incontinence

- Several mechanisms are involved in the pathophysiology.
- Physiology: (i) The rectum acts a storage reservoir. (ii) The pelvic floor muscles including the puborectalis muscle and the anal sphincters are essential for defaecatory process and to maintain continence [122, 136].
- There are broad categories of faecal incontinence among the elderly, namely, (i) overflow incontinence, (ii) reservoir incontinence and (iii) rectosphincteric incontinence [140, 141].
- Altered stool consistency and delivery of contents to the rectum, abnormal rectal capacity and compliance, decreased anorectal sensation and pelvic floor or anal sphincter dysfunction may result in incontinence [142].
- In the female vaginal delivery is the most common cause of structural damage to the anal sphincter; other conditions associated with faecal incontinence are faecal impaction which is an important factor in the elderly, diarrhoeal states, connective tissue disorders and neurological impairment related to stroke, diabetes and multiple sclerosis [136, 144].

Multiple Choice Questions

1. The following are true of peptic ulcer EXCEPT:
   A. Duodenal ulcer is more common with blood group O.
   B. The male/female ratio is 4:1.
   C. Duodenal ulcer is three times more common in first-degree relatives.
   D. Gastric ulcer is more related to *H. pylori* than duodenal ulcer.
2. The following are true of peptic ulcer EXCEPT:
   A. The increased amounts of acid damage the duodenum resulting in the formation of duodenal ulcers.
   B. Cigarette smoking and *H. pylori* are cofactors for the formation of peptic ulcer disease.
   C. The prevalence of peptic ulcer is unrelated to the socio-economic status.
   D. The lifetime prevalence of developing ulcer disease in first-degree relatives of ulcer patients is three times greater than in the general population.
3. The following are true in relation to absorption and digestion, EXCEPT:
   A. Luminal availability of vitamin B_{12} is not affected by bacterial overgrowth.
   B. The fats are broken down to triglycerides and fatty acids in assumable forms.
   C. Deficiency of lactase in the brush border of the small intestine impairs the breakdown of the unabsorbable disaccharides.
   D. After absorption the nutrients enter the systemic circulation via the portal vein and via the thoracic duct.
4. The following are true of *H. pylori* infection, EXCEPT:
   A. *H. pylori* produces urease in large amounts which is necessary for its survival.
   B. *H. pylori* evokes an inflammatory response which induces secretion of gastrin.

C. *H. pylori* contributes to gastric mucosal injury by direct pathogenic mechanisms.
D. *H. pylori* infection is present in 60 % of patients with duodenal and 90–100 % in patients with gastric ulcer.

5. The following are true in inflammatory bowel disease(IBD) in the elderly, EXCEPT:
   A. Genetic factors seem to be stronger in Crohn's disease than in ulcerative colitis.
   B. One-quarter of IBD has an affected family member.
   C. Antibodies to *Saccharomyces cerevisiae* do not commonly occur in Crohn's disease but have been strongly associated with ulcerative colitis.
   D. Environmental factors including gastrointestinal infections, breastfeeding, stress, smoking and diet have inciting or protective roles.
6. The following are true in the pathophysiology of colon cancer, EXCEPT:
   A. Environmental factors play an important role and can increase the risk of colon cancer.
   B. Intake of energy, fat and proteins has a greater impact on risk among the young than among older men and women.
   C. Familial risk of colon risk is common.
   D. Large polyps (>1 cm) or villous adenomas have a high risk of cancer.
7. The following statements in relation to faecal incontinence are TRUE, EXCEPT:
   A. Neurological diseases cause decreased rectal sensitivity and co-ordination resulting in faecal incontinence.
   B. Obstetric injury causes structural damage to the sphincters resulting in passive soiling and urge incontinence
   C. Sphincter integrity, bowel motility, stool consistency and psychological factors among others are requisites for conserving continence.
   D. Many old people seek help early because of the great discomfort.

Answers to MCQs

1 = B; 2 = C; 3 = A; 4 = D; 5 = C; 6 = B; 7 = D.

References

Anatomical and Physiological Changes with Ageing-Gastro-Intestinal Tract

1. Aalami OO, Fong TD, Song HM, Nacamali RP. Physiological features of aging persons. Arch Surg. 2002;138:1068–76.
2. Meccano FJ, Carvalho VC, de Souza RR. Nerve cell loss in the myenteric plexus of the human oesophagus in relation to age: a preliminary investigation. Gerontology. 1995;41:18–21.
3. Tack J, Vantrappen G. The aging oesophagus. Gut. 1977;41:422–4.
4. Nishimura N, Hongo M, Yamada M, Kawakami H, Ueno M, Okuno Y, et al. Effect of aging on the oesophageal motor functions. J Smooth Muscles Res. 1996;32:43–52.

5. Shaker R, Lang IM. Effect of aging on the deglutitive oral, pharyngeal, and oesophageal motor function. Dysphagia. 1994;9(4):221–8 (abstract).
6. Kupper RM, Hepell M, Haggith TW, Bateman DN. Gastric emptying rate and small bowel transit rate in the elderly. Geriatr Soc. 1985;331:340–3.
7. Haadem K, Dahlstrom HA, Ling I. Anal sphincter competence in healthy women: clinical implications of age and other factors. Obstet Gynecol. 1991;78:823–7.
8. Adkins RB, Marshall BA. Anatomic and physiologic aspects of aging. In: Adkins RB, Scott HW, editors. Surgery in the elderly. 2nd ed. Philadelphia: Lipincott-Raven Publishers; 1998, xxi, 531.
9. Hanson GJ. Malabsorption in the elderly. A Clinician's approach. Mayo Clinic EAMA VI.-Jan 2005.
10. Ibre T. Studies on anal function in continent and incontinent patients. Scand J Gastroenterol. 1974;25:1–64.
11. Burnett SJ, Barham CI. Endosonographic variations in the normal internal anal sphincter. Int J Colorectal Dis. 1991;6:2–4.
12. Akerrvalil S, Nordgren S, Fasth S, Oresland T, Pettersson K, Hulten L. The effects of age, gender and parity on rectoanal functions in adults. Scand J Gastroenterol. 1990;25:1247–56.
13. Wade PR, Hornby PJ. Age-related neurodegenerative changes and how they affect the gut. Sci Aging Knowl Environ. 2005;2005:12pc8.
14. Abelo R, Vera R, Rivera AJ, Martin MI. Age-related changes in the gastrointestinal tract: a functional and immunohistochemical study in guinea pig ileum. Life Sci. 2007;80:2436–45.
15. Iber FL, Murphy PA, Connor ES. Age-related changes in the gastrointestinal system. Effects of drug therapy. Drugs Aging. 1994;5:34–48.
16. Melkersson M, Anderson H, Boeaeus I, Falkedn T. Intestinal transit time in constipated and non-constipated patients. Scand J Gastroenterol. 1983;18:593–7.
17. Koffler KH, Menties A, Ridmond RA, Whitehead WE, Pratley RE, Hurley BF. Strength training accelerates gastrointestinal transit in middle aged and older men. Med Sci Sports Exerc. 1992;24:415–9.
18. Atkins RB, Marshall BA. Anatomic and physiologic aspects of aging. In: Atkins RB, Scott HW, editors. Surgery in the elderly. 2nd ed. Philadelphia: Lipincott H-Raven Publishers; 1998. p. 37. XXXI.

The Oesophageal Disorders

19. Sheth N, Diner WC. Swallowing problems in the elderly. Dysphagia. 1982(2):209–15.
20. Groher ME, Bukatman R. The prevalence of swallowing disorders in two teaching hospitals. Dysphagia. 1986;1:3–6.
21. Donner MW, Jones B. Editorial. Gastrointest Radiol. 1985;10:194–5.
22. Ekberg O, Feinberg MJ. Altered swallowing function in elderly patients without dysphagia: radiologic findings in 56 cases. AJR Am J Roentgenol. 1991;156:1181–4 (abstract).
23. Khan TA, Shragge BW, Crispin JS, Lind JF. Esophageal motility in the elderly. Am J Dig Dis. 1977;22:10–4.
24. Mujica VR, Conklin J. When it's hard to swallow. What to look for in patients with dysphagia. Postgrad Med. 1999;105(7):131–4, 141-2,145 (abstract).
25. Marshall JB. Dysphagia, pathophysiology, causes and evaluation. Postgrad Med. 1985;77(5):58–63, 67–8 (abstract).
26. Longemann JA. Swallowing physiology and pathophysiology. Otolaryngol Clin North Am. 1988;21(4):613–23 (abstract).
27. Quigley EM. New development in the pathophysiology of gastro-oesophageal reflux disease (GERD): implications for patient management. Aliment Pharmacol Ther. 2003;17 suppl 2:43–51.
28. Soderholm JD. Stress related changes in oesophageal permeability filling the gaps of GORD? Gut. 2007;56(9):1177–80.

29. Diamont NE. Pathophysiology of gastro-oesophageal reflux disease. GI motility on line. 2006. doi: 10.1038/gimo21.
30. Cibor D, Clicko-Michalska I, Szulewski P, Mach T. Etiopathogenetic factors in patients with gastro-oesophageal reflux disease. Przegl Lek. 2007;64(1):1–4 (abstract).
31. Kennedy T, Jones R. The prevalence of gastro-oesophageal reflux disease symptoms in a UK population and the consultation behaviour of patients with these symptoms. Aliment Pharmacol Ther. 2000;14(12):1589–94.

Peptic Ulcer Disease in the Elderly

32. Burum ML. Peptic ulcer in the elderly. Clin Geriatr Med. 1999;15(3):457–71.
33. Pillotto A, Salles N. Helicobacter pylori infection in geriatrics. Helicobacter. 2002;7Suppl 1:56–62 (abstract).
34. Pillotto A. Helicobacter pylori-associated peptic ulcer disease in older patients: current management strategies. Drugs Aging. 2001;18(7):487–94.
35. Lockery GJ. Management of peptic ulcer disease in elder people. Aust J Hos Pharm. 1999;29:45–50.
36. Tytgat GN, Rauws EA. Campylobacter pylori and its role in ulcer disease. Gastroenterol Clin North Am. 1990;19:183–96.
37. Petersen AM. Bleeding peptic ulcer. Epidemiology and non-surgical management. Gastroenterol Clin North Am. 1990;19:155–70.
38. Pillotto A. Aging and upper gastrointestinal disorders. Best Pract Res Clin Gastronterol. 2004;18 Suppl:73–81 (abstract).
39. Linder JD, Wilcox CM. Acid peptic disease in the elderly. Gastroenterol Clin North Am. 2001;30(2):363–76.
40. Soll AH, Walsh JH. Regulation of gastric acid secretion. Annu Rev Physiol. 1979;41:35–53.
41. Cabano GCA. Histamine and gastric acid secretion. Acta Gastrenterol Latinoam. 1980;10(1):77–84.
42. Wikipedia, Regulation of gastric function. http://en.wikiedia.org/wiki/Regulation_of_gastric_function.retreived. 9 Jan 2015.
43. Lindberg P, Keeling D, Fryklund J, Andersson T, Lundborg P, Carlsson E. Review article-esomeprazole- enhanced bioavailability specificity for the proton pump and inhibition of acid secretion. Aliment Pharmacol Ther. 2003;17:481–8.
44. Sachs G. Proton pump inhibitors and acid related disease. Pharmacotherapy. 1997;17:22–7.
45. Lin SK, Lambert TJR. *H pylori* in ulcer genesis. Scand J Gasteroenterol Suppl. 1995;210:64–99 (abstract).
46. Blaser MJ. Hypothesis on the pathogenesis and natural history of *Helicobacter pylori*-induced inflammation. Gastroenterology. 1992;102:720–7.
47. Forman D, Newell DG, Fullerton F, Yarnell JWG, Stacey AR, Wald N, et al. Association between infection with *Helicobacter pylori* and risk of gastric cancer: evidence from a prospective investigation. Br Med J. 1991;302:1302–5.
48. Parsonnet J, Hansen S, Rodriquez L, Gelb AB, Warnke RA, Jellum E, et al. Helicobacter pylori infection and gastric lymphoma. N Engl J Med. 1994;330:1127–31.
49. Knipers EJ, Thys JC, Fester HP. The prevalence of H pylori in peptic ulcer disease. Aliment Pharmacol Ther. 1995;9(Supp 2):59–69.
50. Petersen AM, Krogfelt KA. Helicobacter pylori: an invading microorganism? A review. FEMS Immunol Med Microbiol. 2003;36(3):117–26.
51. Microbewiki. Gastritis and peptic ulcer disease caused by Helicobacter pylori. http://microbewiki.kenyon.edu/index.php/Gastritis_and_Peptic_Ulcer_Disease_Cause. Accessed 21 Nov 2012.
52. Schubert ML, Peura DA. Control of gastric acid secretion in health and disease. Gastroenterology. 2008;134(7):1842–60.

53. Krishmurthy P, Parlow M, Zitzer JB, Vakel NB, Mobley HT, Levy M, et al. Helicobacter pylori containing cytoplasmic urease is susceptible to acid. Infect Immun. 1998;66(11):5060–6.
54. Ruiz C, Falcocchio S, Pastor FI, Saso L, Diaz P. Helicobacter pylori EstV: identification cloning characteristics of the first isolated fraction in Epsilon- Proteobacterium. Appl Environ Microbiol. 2007;73(8):2423–31.
55. Smoot DT. How does Helicobacter pylori cause mucosal damage? Direct mechanisms. Gastroenterology. 1997;113:S31–4 (abstract).
56. Roy S. Pathology and pathogenesis of peptic ulcer. www.sosgastro.org.pc.biblioteen/ulcrapeptic/ulcera320008.ppt. 18 Nov 2012.
57. Flier JS, Underhill LH. Prostaglandins of peptic ulcer and implications for therapy. N Engl J Med. 1990;322:909–16.
58. Zullo A, Hassan C, Campo SM, Morini S. Bleeding peptic ulcer in the elderly: risk factors and prevention strategies. Drugs Aging. 2007;24(10):815–28 (abstract).

Colorectal Cancer

59. Parkin DM. International variation. Oncogene. 2004;23:6329–40.
60. Parkin DM, Forag F, Ferlay J, Pisani I. Global cancer statistics. 2002. CA Cancer J Clin. 2005;56:74108.
61. Sharma S, O'Keefe SJ. Environmental influences on the high mortality from colorectal cancer in African Americans. Postgrad Med J. 2007;83(983):583–9 (abstract).
62. Burt RW. Familial risk and colorectal cancer. Gastroenterol Clin North Am. 1996;25(4):793–803 (abstract).
63. NHMRC Guidelines for the prevention, early detection and management, A guide for general practitioners. ISBN. 1864960914. Cat No. 9925182.
64. Cappell MS. From colonic polyps to colon cancer: pathophysiology clinical presentation screening and colonoscopic therapy. Minerva Gastroenterol Dietol. 2007;53(4):351–73 (abstract).
65. Slattery et al. Clinical Practice: Guidelines for the prevention early detection and management of colorectal cancer. ISBN 18649609.14. Cat No.9925182.NHMRC 8 December 2005.
66. Slattery ML, Potter JD, Sorenson AW. Age and risk factors for colon cancer (United States and Australia): are there implications for understanding differences in case-control and cohort studies? Cancer Causes and Control. 1994;5(6):557–63 (abstract).
67. Center MM, Jemal A, Ward E. International trends in Colorectal cancer. Incidence rates. Cancer Epidemic Biomarkers Prev. 2009;18:1685.

Inflammatory Bowel Disease in the Elderly

68. Sartor RB. Mechanisms of disease: pathogenesis of Crohn's disease and ulcerative colitis. Nat Clin Pract Gastroenterol Hepatol. 2006;3:390–407.
69. Gisbert JP, Chaparro M. Inflammatory bowel disease in the elderly. Aliment Pharmcol Ther. 2014;39(5):459–77 (abstract).
70. Sandler RS, Golden AL. Epidemiology of Crohn's disease. J Clin Gastroenterol. 1986;8(2):160–5 (abstract).
71. Jones HW, Hoare A. Does ulcerative colitis behave differently in the elderly? Age Aging. 1988;17:410–4.
72. Robertson DJ, Grimm IS. Inflammatory bowel disease in the elderly. Gastroenterol Clinic of North America. 2001;30:409–26.
73. Zhang YZ, Li YY. Inflammatory bowel disease: pathogenesis. World J Gastroenterol. 2014;20(1):91–9 (abstract).
74. Wallace KL, Zheng LB, Kanazawa Y, Shih DQ. Immunopathology of inflammatory bowel disease. World J Gastroenterol. 2014;20(1):6–21 (abstract).

75. Karlinger K, Gyorke T, Mako E, Mester A, Tarjan Z. The epidemiology and the pathogenesis of inflammatory bowel disease. Eur J Radiol. 2000;35(3):154–67 (abstract).
76. Vavricka SR, Rogler G. New insights into the pathogenesis of Crohn's disease: are they relevant for therapeutic options? Swiss Med Wkly. 2009;139(37–38):527–34.
77. Ogura Y, Bonen DK, Inohara N, Nicholae DL, Chen FF, Ramos R, et al. A frameshift mutation in NOD2 associated with susceptibility to Crohn's disease. Nature. 2001;411:603–6.
78. Ponder A, Long MD. A clinical review of recent findings in the epidemiology of inflammatory bowel disease. Clin Epidemiol. 2013;5:237–47.
79. Duchmann R, Kaiser I, Hernmann E, Mayet W, Ewe K, Meyer Zum Buschenfelde KH, et al. Tolerance exists towards resident intestinal flora but is broken in active inflammatory bowel disease (IBD). Clin Exp Immunol. 1995;102:448–55.
80. Targan SR, Karp LC. Defects in mucosal immunity leading to ulcerative colitis. Immunol Rev. 2005;206:296–305 (abstract).
81. Fries VV, Comunale S. Ulcerative colitis. Curr Drug Targets. 2011;12(10):1373–82 (abstract).

Diarrhoea in the Elderly

82. Gerok W. Pathophysiology of chronic diarrhoea. Praxis (Bern 1994). 2000;89(41):1635–41 (abstract).
83. Binder HJ. Pathophysiology of acute diarrhoea. Am J Med. 1990;88(6A):25–45.
84. Faruque ASG, Malik RI, Kahu AI, Huq S, Salam MA, Sack DA, et al. Diarrhoea in elderly population: aetiology and clinical characteristics. Scand J Infect Dis. 2004;36:204–8.
85. Lew JF, Glass RI, Gangarosa RE, Cohen IP, Bern C, Moe CL. Diarrhoeal deaths in the United States. 1979 through 1987. A special problem for the elderly. JAMA. 1991;265:3280–4.
86. Hoffman J, Zeitz M. Small bowel disease in the elderly: diarrhoea and malabsorption. Best Pract Res Clin Gastroenterol. 16(1):17–36 (abstract) Website: http://benkinghub.elsevier.com.retrieve/pii/S152169180.2902635.
87. Bennett RG, Greenough WB. Approach to acute diarrhoea in the elderly. Gastrenterol Clin North Am. 1993;22:517–33.
88. Ratnaike RN. Diarrhoea in the elderly. Epidemiological and aetiological features. J Gastrenterol Hepatol. 1990;5(4):449–58.
89. Whyte LA, Jenkins HR. Pathophysiology of diarrhoea. Paediatr Child Health. 2012;22:443–7 (abstract).
90. Website. Pathology of diarrhoea. http://www.vivo.colostate.edu/hbooks/pathphys/digestion/smallgut/diarrhoea.html. Accessed 9 Jan 2015.
91. Ratnaike RN, Jones TE. Mechanisms of drug-induced diarrhoea in the elderly. Drugs Aging. 1998;13:245–53.
92. Cutting WA. Mechanisms of diarrhoea and why they do matter. Dialogue Diarrhoea. 1988;35:45.
93. Ewe K, Wanitscke R. Current concepts in the pathophysiology of diarrhoea. Leber Magen Dam. 1977;7(1):1–2 (abstract).
94. Schiller LR. Secretory diarrhoea. Curr Gastroenterol Rep. 1999;1(5):389–97 (abstract).
95. Low-Bier TS, Read AE. Progress report: diarrhoea: mechanisms and treatment. Gut. 1971;72:1021–36.
96. Shan S. Evaluation of diarrhoea. The challenge continues. Part 1. Ind J Med Sci. 2004;58:75–8.

Malabsorption in the Elderly

97. Holt PR. Diarrhoea and malabsorption in the elderly. Gastroenterol Clin North Am. 2009;30:427–44 (abstract).

98. McEvoy A, Dutton J, James OF. Bacterial contamination of the small intestine is an important cause of occult malabsorption in the elderly. Br Med J (Clin Res Ed). 1983;287 (abstract).
99. Owens SR, Greenon JK. The pathology of malabsorption: current concepts. Histopathology. 2007;50:64–82.
100. Blaauw R. Malabsorption: causes, consequences diagnosis and treatment. Afr J Clin Med. 2011;24(3):125–7.
101. Lovat LB. Age related changers in gut physiology and nutritional status. Gut. 1996;38(3):306–9 (abstract).
102. Holt PR. Intestinal malabsorption in the elderly. Dig Dis. 2007;25(2):144–50 (abstract).
103. Erickson RH, Kim YS. Digestion and absorption of dietary protein. Annu Rev Med. 1990;41:133–9.
104. Holmes R. Carbohydrate digestion and absorption. J Clin Pathol. 1991;5:10–3.
105. Armand M, Pasquier B, Andre M, Borel P, Senft M, Peyrot J, et al. Digestion and absorption of 2 fat emulsions with different droplet sizes in the human digestive tract. Am J Clin Nutr. 1999;70(6):1096–106.
106. Felsen H. Intrinsic factor secretion and cobalamin absorption. Physiology and pathophysiology in the gastrointestinal tract. Scand J Gastroenterol Suppl. 1991;188:1–7.
107. Schjonsby H. Vitamin B_{12} absorption and malabsorption. Gut. 1989;30:1686–91.
108. Ingram CJE, Swallow DM. Lactose malabsorption. In: Advanced dairy chemistry. Springer; 2009, p. 203–29.

Malnutrition in the Elderly

109. Wallace JI. Malnutrition and enteral/parenteral alimentation. In: Hazzard WR, Blass JP, Ettinger WH, Halter JB, Ouslander JG, editors. Principles of geriatric medicine and gerontology. 4th ed. New York: McGraw –Hill; 1999. p. 1455–69.
110. Ennis BW, Saffel-Shrier S, Verson H. Diagnosing malnutrition in the elderly. Nurse Pract. 2001;26(3):52–6,61–2, 65.
111. Pablo AMR, Izaja MA, Aldey LA. Assessment of nutritional status on hospital admission: nutritional scores. Eur J Clin Nutr. 2003;57:824–31.
112. Silver AJ, Morley JE, Strome LS. Nutritional status in an academic nursing home. J Am Geriatr Soc. 1988;36:487–91.
113. Shaver HJ, Loper JA, Lutes RA. Nutritional status of nursing home patients. J Parenter Enteral Nutr. 1980;4:367–70.
114. Muncie HJ, Carbonetto C. Prevalence of protein-calorie malnutrition in an extended care family. J Fam Pract. 1982;14:1061–4.
115. Evans C. Malnutrition in the elderly: a multifactorial failure to thrive. Http://xnet.kp.org/permanente/sum05/elderly.html,2008
116. Hajjar RR, Kamel HK, Denson K. Malnutrition in aging. Int J Geriatr Gerontol. 2004;191:1–5.
117. Dudrik SJ. Eating disorders' prevalence increases. Todays Geriatr Med. 2013;6(4):18.
118. Endoy MP. Anorexia among older adults. Am L Nurse Pract. 2005;9:31–8.
119. Morley JE. Pathophysiology of anorexia. Clin Geriatr Med. 2002;18:661–73.
120. Morley JE, Keimar VB, Mattammal MB. Inhibition of feeding by nitric oxide synthase inhibitor effect of aging. Eur Pharmacol. 1996;15:311–5.

Constipation and Fecal Incontinence

121. Wald A. Constipation and faecal incontinence in the elderly. Gastroenterol Clin North Am. 1990;19(2):405–18.

122. Barieben A, Mills A. Anorectal anatomy and physiology. Surg Clin North Am. 2010;90(1):1–15 (abstract).
123. Bajwa A, Emmanuel A. The physiology of continence and evacuation. Best Pract Res Clin Gastrenterol. 2009;23(4):477–85 (abstract).
124. Palit S, Luniss M, Scott AM. The physiology of human defecation. Dig Dis Sci. 2012;57(6):1445–64 (abstract).
125. Gurjar SV, Jones OM. Physiology: evacuation, pelvic floor and continence mechanisms. Surgery. 2011;29(8):358–61.
126. Gallagher P, O'Mahony D. Constipation in old age. Best Pract Res Clin Gastroenterol. 2009; 23(875–87). doi. 10.1016()bpg.2009.09.001 (abstract).
127. Sonnenberg A, Koch T. Epidemiology of constipation in United States. Dis Colon Rectum. 1989;32:1–8.
128. Stewart WF, Liberman JN, Sandler RS, Woods MS, Stemhagen A, Chee E, et al. Epidemiology of constipation (EPOC) in the United States: relation of clinical subtypes to sociodemographic features. Am J Gastroenterol. 1999;94:530–40.
129. Primrose WL, Caperwell HE, Simpson GK, Smith RG. Prescribed patterns observed in registered nursing homes and long stay geriatric wards. Age Aging. 1987;16:25–8.
130. Bosshard W, Dreher R, Schnegg J-F, Bula CJ. The treatment of chronic constipation in elderly people: an update. Drugs Aging. 2004;21:911–30 (abstract).
131. Talley NJ, O'Keefe EA, Zinsmeister AR, 3rd Melton LJ. Prevalence of gastrointestinal symptoms in the elderly: a population based study. Gastroenterology. 1992;102:895–901.
132. Scheffer DC, Cheskin LJ. Constipation in the elderly. Am Fam Physician. 5 Sept 1998. Website: www.aafip.org/alp/980915ap/schaefer.html
133. Mertz H, Naliboff B, Mager E. Physiology of refractory chronic constipation. Am J Gastroenterol. 1998;94(3):608–15.
134. Miller-Lissner S. General geriatrics and gastroenterology: constipation and faecal incontinence. Best Pract Res Clin Gastroenterol. 2002;16:115–33. Website Science Direct (abstract).
135. Gallegos-Orozco JF, Foxx-Orenstein AE, Sterler SM, Stor JM. Chronic constipation in the elderly. Am J Gastroenterol. 2012;197:18–25.
136. Cooper ZR, Rose S. Faecal incontinence: a clinical approach. Mt Sinai J Med. 2000;67:96–105.
137. Roberts RO, Jacobson SJ, Reilly WT, Pemberton JH, Lieber MM, Talley NJ, et al. Prevalence of combined faecal and urinary incontinence: a community-based study. J Am Cleveland Soc. 1999;47:837–41.
138. Tobin GW, Brocklehurst JC. Faecal incontinence in residential homes for the elderly: prevalence, aetiology and management. Age Aging. 1988;15:41–6.
139. Johnson JF, Lafforty J. Epidemiology of faecal incontinence: the silent affliction. J Gastroenterol. 1996;91:33–6.
140. Wald A. Faecal incontinence in the elderly: epidemiology and management. Drugs Aging. 2005;22:132–9 (abstract).
141. Gordon PH, Nivatrongs S. Principles and practice of surgery for the colon, rectum and anus. 3rd ed. New York: Information Health Care; 2007.
142. Jorge JM, Wexner SD. Etiology and management of faecal incontinence. Dis Colon Rectum. 1993;36(1):77–97.
143. Snooks SJ, Swash M, Setchell M. Injury to innervation of pelvic floor sphincter musculature in child birth. Lancet. 1984;2:546.
144. Kalantar JS, Howell S, Tallet NJ. Prevalence of faecal incontinence and associated risk factors: an underdiagnosed problem in the Australian Community. Med J Aust. 2001;176:54–7.
145. Rasmussen O. Fecal incontinence. Studies on physiology, pathophysiology and surgical treatment. Dan Med Bull. 2003;50(3):262–82 (abstract).

Disorders of the Hepato-Biliary System in the Elderly

4

4.1 Anatomical and Physiological Changes with Ageing

Several physiological changes occur in ageing both functional and structural. Liver volume decreases with age as does the hepatic blood flow [1–3]. Although there is a decrease in the total number of hepatocytes, the remaining hepatocytes increase in size due to the increased biological demand of the remaining cells [4]. Apart from the increased hepatocyte size, there have been reports of an increase in number of binucleated cells, altered mitochondria and endoplasmic reticulum [5]. More recently, it has been shown that pseudocapillarisation occurs in the liver sinusoidal endothelial cells [3] resulting in thickening and reduction in the number of fenestrations [6]. The reduction in the fenestrations have significant impact on the hepatic lipoprotein metabolism [6].

Many theories assume that there is a decrease in the cellular functions with ageing but appear to be based on erroneous assumptions [7]. A decline in the intrinsic metabolic activity of hepatic parenchyma [3], hepato-biliary function, shifts in the expression of a variety of proteins and moderate decline in phase 1 metabolism of certain drugs have been documented [5]. The elderly exhibits a decline in the hepatic clearance of certain drugs with an increased frequency of adverse drug reactions, and this has been attributed to a decline in liver volume and blood flow [8] rather than to reduction in phase 1 metabolism [5]. There is a decline in the intracellular activity of cytochrome P450 enzyme which hinders the clearance of drugs from the system [9]. Hepatic synthesis of several proteins including the clotting factors can be reduced, but does not impact the baseline function.

The liver function in the elderly is well maintained even though the livers of the elderly are characterised by reduced capacity and adaptive responsiveness [5]. When challenged, however, it may not be able to increase significantly beyond the baseline [10]. The serum bilirubin, aminotransferase and fractionated alkaline phosphatase levels are not altered with age [11–13].

N. Nagaratnam et al., *Diseases in the Elderly: Age-Related Changes and Pathophysiology*, DOI 10.1007/978-3-319-25787-7_4

Box 4.1. Key Points. Anatomical and Physiological Changes in the Hepato-Biliary System with Ageing

- Liver volume decreases with age [1–3].
- Decrease in the hepatocytes with increase in size of remaining hepatocytes [4].
- Pseudocapillarisation occur with reduction in number of fenestrations which has an impact in hepatic lipoprotein metabolism [3, 6].
- The elderly exhibit a decline in hepatic clearance of drugs [8].
- Serum bilirubin, aminotransferase and fractionated alkaline phosphatase levels are not altered with age [11–13].

4.2 Viral Hepatitis in the Elderly

It is well known that viruses which do not normally produce liver damage with jaundice may occasionally display increased hepatotropism, producing a clinical picture similar to hepatitis [14], among them being the cytomegalovirus, herpes simplex, Coxsackie, yellow fever and others. By common usage, viral hepatitis is an acute inflammation caused by six viruses called hepatitis A, B,C, D, E and G. In countries with high standards of sanitation, HAV antibodies are found in 50 % or more in the elderly over the age of 50 years as compared to children [15]. The prevailing HAV antibodies were 40 %, 60 % and 80 % at ages 60,70 and 80 years, respectively, in a serological survey in the United States [16]. The elderly are at greater risk of severe effects of the illness, and the fatality rate increases with age [17]. The median length of stay was longer for those 50–60 years and over than for the younger age groups [18]. Although acute hepatitis B and C are more commonly recognised in younger adults, acute infection can occur in the elderly [19]. Chronic infection is prevalent in elderly patients and may be more symptomatic and severe than in younger adults. Hepatocellular carcinoma is a serious complication of chronic HBV infection. Hepatitis C has been the most frequent cause of acute hepatitis in older people [18, 20]. Hepatitis D virus (HDV) may occur as a co-infection with the hepatitis B virus or as a superinfection in individuals with existing chronic HBV infection. HEV has been described in a number of countries. In a study of 77 patients in New Zealand, the HEV IgG seroprevalence was 4 %[21], and data suggest that subclinical and unrecognised infection is common. One of the cases was misdiagnosed initially as a drug reaction. All cases were in elderly patients, and the NZ-acquired cases were more similar to HEV from Japan. It has been suggested all patients with unexplained hepatitis whatever their age or travel history be tested for HEV [21]. Hepatitis G (HGV) has been identified between 1 and 2 % of blood donors in the United States (Health A to Z) [22] and has been associated with liver disease in older people [23].

4.3 Chronic Liver Disease in the Elderly

Introduction

Viral infections are the commonest cause of chronic liver disease. Alcoholic liver disease, non-alcoholic fatty liver disease (NAFLD), autoimmune hepatitis, drug-induced hepatitis and metabolic diseases such as alpha-antitrypsin deficiency are the other causes. The prevalence of chronic liver disease is increasing in the elderly [24]. There are no age-related liver diseases, but the clinical course in the elderly differs in several aspects from those of younger adults [25].

Pathophysiology

With ageing, there is a decrease in the regenerative capacity, and this may partly account for the poor recovery after severe viral and toxic injury in the elderly [26]. Furthermore, ageing influences the pharmacokinetic and pharmacodynamic properties [27]. Acetaldehyde, the reactive metabolite from metabolism of ethanol together with ethanol, has a deleterious effect on the hepatocytes. Other factors which accelerate alcohol-related liver lesions are certain drugs, diet, infection, genetic factors and high-fat diet [28] and may be responsible for the variation in individual susceptibility to ALD [29].

4.3.1 Alcoholic Liver Disease (ALD)

ALD is a spectrum of conditions resulting ranging from alcoholic fatty liver, acute alcoholic hepatitis, alcoholic cirrhosis and liver failure from excessive drinking. The incidence of alcoholic liver disease in the last decade has increased [30] and is increasing in the elderly. This is largely due to increase in the consumption of alcohol in individuals over the age of 65 years [31]. There are three types of elderly drinkers, early onset, intermediate and late onset. Late-onset alcohol abuse can be due to a number of reasons, namely, increased longevity, loneliness, loss of life partner and depression [32], insomnia and retirement.

Pathophysiology and pathogenesis

Alcoholic fatty liver, acute alcoholic hepatitis and alcoholic cirrhosis are the three most widely recognised forms of ALD [33]. The exact pathogenesis of alcoholic liver disease is complex and implicates alcholol metabolism and secondary mechanisms involving immune-mediated and free radical hepatic injury, genetic, gender, nutritional, metabolic, environmental factors and cytokines [34, 35]. A genetic susceptibility as predisposing factor for ALD has emerged [36], and studies in gene polymorphism suggest that gene encoding for enzymes that metabolise both ethanol and acetaldehyde influences the predisposition to ALD development [37–39]. These genes include those encoding alcohol dehydrogenase (ADH), aldehyde dehydrogenase (ALDH) and cytochrome CYP2E1 [40]. Ethanol toxicity is linked to its metabolism by alcohol dehydrogenase and cytochrome P4502E1(CYP2E1) pathways resulting in production of toxic acetaldehyde [41]. The acetaldehyde is toxic to the mitochondria, aggravates their oxidative stress and together with cellular injury promotes inflammation via the proinflammatory cytokine tumour necrosis factor –alpha in the Kupffer cells [42]. Oxidative stress also has a vital role in the development of ALD [43, 44], and it promotes hepatocyte necrosis and apoptosis. Methionine-activated S-adenosylmethionine (SAMe) opposes oxidative stress resulting from cytochrome P4502E1 (CYP2E1) induction by alcohol, ketones and fatty acids [42]. The reduced form of nicotinamide adenine dinucleotide (NADH) generated by the alcohol dehydrogenase-mediated ethanol metabolism promotes steatosis by stimulating the synthesis of fatty acids and opposing their oxidation [41].

Following hepatocellular injury, the non-parenchymal cells release vasoactive compounds such as cytokines which take part in the modulation of extracellular matrix that is characteristic of fibrosis [45]. Depending on the cause of the liver disease and environmental and host factors, the fibrosis progresses at variable rate [46]. Cirrhosis is characterised by tissue fibrosis leading to destruction of the normal liver architecture into structural abnormal nodules [46].

With advancing age, the activity of enzymes such as alcohol dehydrogenase (ADH), acetaldehyde dehydrogenase (ALDH) and cytochrome CYP2E1 diminishes leading to increased blood concentrations of ethanol [31]. Thus, elderly people are more susceptible to the toxic effects of ethanol [32]. Chronic ethanol consumption has an extreme stimulating effect on microsomal enzymes and in particular cytochrome CYP2E [47]. The earliest change in alcoholic hepatitis is located mainly around the central vein [48], and alcohol is known to cause an exaggerated gradient from portal vein to the central vein which suggest that chronic alcohol use-induced hypoxia may contribute to hepatic damage [49].

4.3.2 Non-alcoholic Fatty Liver Disease (NAFLD)

NAFLD is a syndrome with a spectrum ranging from mild liver steatosis to non-alcoholic steatohepatitis (NASH) where the liver becomes inflamed and fibrous tissue begins to infiltrate the liver [50] to cirrhosis [51, 52] and liver cancer [50, 53–55]. It is one of the most common liver disorders seen by the primary care physician [56]. Its prevalence ranges from 3 to 24 % in the general population and increases with age and after menopause [57]. NAFLD affects mainly the middle aged and the elderly [58] for the prevalence of its risk factors increases with age [59].

Pathophysiology

What triggers the early stage is not known. Most cases occur in patients with obesity, often females with or without type 2 diabetes [60] but may occur in nonobese patients [61] and in a wide range of patients including children and nonobese males [62]. Older age, obesity, diabetes, hypertension, high triglycerides and insulin resistance are associated with more advanced stages of NAFLD [56]. Kagansky et al. [63] however found no such association. A sedentary life style and rapid weight loss are known to cause NASH [64]. Pathogenic concepts of NAFLD include overnutrition, insulin resistance and genetic factor [53, 65]. Symptoms are non-specific [66] and insulin resistance patients with obesity, hypertension and hypertriglyceridaemia are suggestive but not specific of diagnosis [67] and interestingly features of NAFLD are indistinguishable from ALD [68].

4.3.3 Autoimmune Hepatitis (AIH)

There are certain liver syndromes which can be classified as a group in which immunological abnormalities are commonly found, such as immune serum markers and association with other autoimmune diseases [69]. Several different names have been extended to this condition, namely, 'plasma cell hepatitis' and 'lupoid hepatitis' [70, 71]. Several systems may be involved, and it occurs in males and females of all ages. It occurs uncommonly in the elderly; nevertheless, there have been several studies of AIH in the elderly [72–76]. One reason for the low rate of diagnosis in the elderly is because AIH was incorrectly considered to be a disease of young age [74].

Pathophysiology
Autoimmune pathogenesis includes the occurrence of autoantibodies, the hepatic histopathology often composed of cytotoxic T cells and plasma cells, hypergammaglobinaemia and rheumatoid factor, association with other autoimmune disorders and response to steroids or immunosuppressive therapy [77]. Overlapping presentation with primary biliary cirrhosis and primary sclerosing cirrhosis has been observed [78]. There is a genetic predisposition and includes few risk factors such as presence of HLADR3 and HLADR4 and deletion of C4A alleles [79]. Between 40 and 80 % of the AIH patients will ultimately progress to cirrhosis [80–82].

4.3.4 Drug-Induced Liver Injury (DILI)

DILI embraces a spectrum of clinical diseases ranging from asymptomatic, liver function test abnormalities to acute liver failure [83] and to a lesser extent chronicity [84, 85].

Pathophysiology
There is an age-related reduction in blood flow and liver mass resulting in impaired drug metabolism which may be reduced by 40–50 % in old age [86]. Most drugs are lipophilic (fat soluble) and are easily absorbed across cell membranes and in the liver cell, It is rendered hydrophilic (water soluble) to facilitate excretion [87, 88]. Metabolism of drugs occur in two phases. In phase 1 reaction the drug is made polar by oxidation and hydroxylation [87]. Some drugs may undergo the phase 2 reaction directly. The cytochrome P450 [89] catalyses the phase 1 reactions, and several enzymes have been identified and are located in the endoplasmic reticulum of the liver. Some of the metabolites are highly reactive and are more toxic [90] than the parent substance and may result in liver injury [87]. Phase 2 reaction involves conjugation to a glucuronide or a sulphate or glutathione. The kidney excretes the drugs with a low molecular weight and the bile those with high molecular weight [91]. DILI can be either dose related or idiosyncratic. Idiosyncratic susceptibility has been attributed to interindividual variability in initial drug metabolism, the body's ability to curb the toxicity and the efficiency of

the immune system [90]. The susceptibility of older adults to idiosyncratic or hypersensitivity reactions cannot be reliably predicted because of the limited involvement of this group in clinical trials [92]. Genetic, environmental risk and immunological factors have a role in the pathogenesis of drug-induced hepatotoxicity [93–95]. Genetic polymorphisms of drug-metabolising enzymes such as P450 together with age and gender are risk factors for DILI [83].

4.3.5 Primary Biliary Cirrhosis (PBC)

PBC is a chronic progressive cholestatic disease with autoimmune features ultimately leading to cirrhosis and liver failure. PBC is now recognised more frequently than previously because of the increased awareness of the condition and the availability of diagnostic tools leading to earlier diagnosis [96]. The median age of onset is 50 years and varies between 20 and 90 years [97]. At the time of diagnosis, the affected persons are often in their 5 to 7th decades of life [98].

Pathophysiology
It was thought to be immune mediated, but more recently this view has been challenged [99] and another aetiological model involving retroviral infection has been put forward [100]. Clinical observations support a combination of genetic susceptibility [98, 101, 102] and environmental triggers such as infection, chemicals and smoking [98] to have a causative role [103, 104].

4.3.6 Hereditary Haemochromatosis

Hereditary haemochromatosis is a genetically inherited disorder where there is an increase absorption of dietary iron in excess of physiological need resulting in the accumulation of iron in the body iron stores. Symptoms occur at 40–60 years [105].

Pathophysiology
Iron in the ferrous state is absorbed in the proximal part of the duodenum. The ferrous ions are actively transported across the enterocyte apical membrane by the protein divalent metal transporter-I (DTM-I) [106, 107] after being reduced by ferric reductase Dcytb [108]. The amount of DTM-I regulates the iron absorption according to the body needs – the need for haematopoiesis and the amount of iron in the body stores. From within the enterocyte, the ferrous ions either enter the body by the basolateral transporter ferroportin [109] or bind to ferritin within the cell and is lost to the body when the cell ages and degrades. The iron that binds to the ferroportin is oxidised by a membrane bound ferroxidase hephaestin [108] into ferric ions and leaves the cell and is transported by transferrin iron binding for distribution around the body.

Hepcidin, a hormone formed in the liver, plays an important role in the regulation of iron absorption. Hepcidin binds to ferroportin causing it to degrade, and the iron remains within the cell [110]. This stimulates ferritin synthesis so that the iron that enters and binds to the ferritin is lost when the cell dies. The hepcidin is decreased when the body iron is low [111] and thus increases ferroportin activity and iron intake in the duodenum. When the body stores of iron are high, hepcidin is increased suppressing ferroportin and decreasing iron uptake. The expression of hepcidin is influenced by plasma transferrin saturation mediated by the proteins HFE, transferrin receptor 2 and hemojuvelin [108, 112].

In patients with hereditary haemochromatosis who are homozygous for the mutant HFE, there is a deficiency of hepcidin [111] so that iron absorption by the duodenal enterocyte continues even when the body iron stores are full. The normal level of body iron in the body for man is 4 g and for women 3 g, and in haemochromatosis the level may rise fivefold. The transferrin saturation is increased, and it determines if an individual has excessive load of iron in the body. Decades of iron deposition in the organs causes tissues damage. In the liver it gives rise to cirrhosis, in the pancreas diabetes, heart cardiomyopathy and the pituitary gland manifesting as loss of libido or impotence and joints.

4.3.7 Genetics

The HFE gene has two alleles C282Y and H63D. The most common genetic defect is the replacement of a amino acid cysteine with tyrosine in the position 282 (C282Y) in the HFE gene [113]. Homozygosity for the C282Y is the most common genotype and found in 52–100 % on clinically diagnosed probands [114]. Heterozygotes for either C282Y and H63D may not manifest clinical iron overload, and heterozygosity for C282Y/H63D results in clinically evident iron overload [115, 116]. Homozygous females delay the accumulation as the result of menstruation. An estimated 40–70 % of persons with C282Y homozygous genotype will develop clinical evidence of iron overload [114]. 41,038 individuals attending an appraisal clinic in the United States were screened, and the average age of 152 C282Y homozygotes was 57 years [116], and only one of the 152 homozygotes had signs and symptoms suggestive of haemochromatosis [117]. Large population studies had shown that the penetrance of the C282Y/C282Y genotype is very low. This indicates that C282Y homozygosity is necessary, but not adequate enough to cause the disease [118]. This discriminative expression of C282Y homozygosity is being studied bearing on other genetic and environmental factors including alcohol [118]. A recent study showed that there is a high clinical penetrance of HH in the Australian population [119]. Homozygous H63D mutation is not as penetrant as C282Y, and there are few reports of cases of haemochromatosis [114, 120].

Box 4.2. Key Points. Chronic Liver Disease in the Elderly

- With ageing, there is a decrease in regenerative capacity [26].
- The pathogenesis of alcoholic liver disease is complex and implicates alcohol metabolism and secondary mechanisms involving immune mediators and free radical hepatic injury, genetic, gender, nutritional, metabolic, environment and cytokines [34, 35].
- Most cases of NAFLD have underlying insulin resistance, and NAFLD is an important facet of metabolic syndrome [56].
- AIH is associated with autoantibodies, typical histopathology, hypergammaglobulinaemia and rheumatoid factor and other autoimmune disorders and response to steroids [77].
- Genetic polymorphism of drug-metabolising enzymes such as P450 together with age and gender is a risk factor for DILI [83].
- Primary biliary cirrhosis was thought to be immune-related, but now other aetiology model involving retroviral infection has been put forward [99, 100].
- In adult hereditary haemochromatosis who are homozygous for the mutant HFE, there is a deficiency of hepcidin which regulates iron absorption [11].

Multiple Choice Questions

1. The following physiological changes in the liver with ageing are true, EXCEPT:
   A. There is a decline in the number of hepatocytes, but the mean cell volume is increased.
   B. Pseudocapillarisation occurs in the liver sinusoidal endothelial cells resulting in the reduction in the number of fenestrations.
   C. The elderly exhibit a decline in hepatic clearance of certain drugs.
   D. Hepatic synthesis of several proteins can be reduced and has an impact on the baseline function.
2. The following are true of viral hepatitis in the elderly, EXCEPT:
   A. The elderly are at greater risk of severe effect with an increase in mortality.
   B. Chronic infection is present in the elderly, but they are asymptomatic and less severe.
   C. Hepatitis C has been the most frequent cause of acute hepatitis in the elderly.
   D. Patients with unexplained hepatitis whatever their age should be tested for HEV hepatitis.
3. The following are true in relation to chronic liver disease, EXCEPT:
   A. Non-alcoholic fatty liver disease is an important facet of metabolic syndrome.
   B. Primary biliary cirrhosis thought to be immune mediated, but recently this view has been challenged.
   C. Genetic polymorphism of drug-metabolising enzymes such as P450 together with age are risk factors for drug-induced liver injury.
   D. With advancing age, enzymes alcohol dehydrogenase and acetaldehyde dehydrogenase increase leading to increased concentration of ethanol.

4. The following relating to genotyping in haemochromatosis are true EXCEPT:
   A. Homozygosity for C282Y causes excessive iron absorption and overload.
   B. Heterozygosity for C282Y/H63D may not manifest iron overload.
   C. Heterozygosity for C282Y/H63D may not manifest iron overload.
   D. First-degree relatives of the individual with HH should be screened by transferrin saturation and genetic testing.

Answers to MCQs

1 = D; 2 = B; 3 = D; 4 = B

References

Anatomical and Physiological Changes with Aging

1. Koff RS, Garvey AJ, Burney SW, Bell B. Absence of an effect on sulfobromophtalein retention in healthy men. Gastroenterology. 1973;65:300–2.
2. Wynne HA. Age related changes in liver, gall bladder and pancreas. Rev Clin Gerontol. 2002;12(1):12–20.
3. Serste T, Bourgeois N. Aging and the liver. Acta Gastrenterol Belg. 2006;69:296–8.
4. Adkins RB, Marshall BA. Anatomic and physiological aspects of aging. In: Adkins RB, Scott HW, editors. Surgery for the elderly. 2nd ed. Philadelphia: Lippincott-Raven Publishers; 1998. xx1, 531.
5. Schumucker DL. Aging and the liver: an update. J Gerontol A Biol Sci Med Sci. 1998;53:B315–20 (abstract).
6. Le Couteur DG, Cogger VC, McCuskey RS, Cabo R, Smewdsred D, Sorensen KK, et al. Age related changes in the liver sinusoidal endothelium. Ann N Y Acad Sci. 2007;113:79–87 (abstract).
7. Kitani K. Aging of the liver: facts and theories. Arch Gerontol Geriatr. 1991;12:133–54.
8. le Couteur DG, McLean AJ. The aging liver: drug clearance and an oxygen diffusion barrier hypothesis'. Clin Pharmocokinet. 1998;34:359–73.
9. Gridelli C, Macone P, Comuncle D, Rossi A. Adjunct chemotherapy in elderly patients with non small cell lung cancer. Medscape Today. http://www.mediscape.co.viewarticle/553783_2. Accessed 19 May 2013.
10. Salem SA, Rajjayabun P, Shepherd AM, Stevenson H. Reduced induction of drug metabolism in the elderly. Age Ageing. 1978;7:68–73.
11. James OF. Parenchymal liver disease in the elderly. Gut. 1997;41:430–2.
12. Hodkinson HM, MacPherson CK. Alkaline phosphatase in geriatric in-patient population. Age Ageing. 1973;2:28–31.
13. Kamponann JP, Sinding J, Jorgeson IM. Effect of age on liver function. Geriatrics. 1975;20:91.

Viral Hepatitis in the Elderly

14. Zuckerman AJ. Virus diseases of the liver. London: Butterworth; 1969. p. p120.
15. Wikipedia. Viral hepatitis. http://enwikipedia.org/wiki/viral_hepatitis. Retrieved 3 Mar 2–14.
16. Bader TF. Hepatitis A, vaccine vaccine. Am J Gastroenterol. 1996;91:217–22.
17. Brown GR, Parsely K. Hepatitis epidemic in the elderly. Southern Med J. (abstract). http://www.medscope.com/viewarticle/444318.

18. Communicable Diseases Intelligence vol 34. Supplement. December 2010. Australian Government. Department of Health.
19. Carrion AF, Martin P. Viral hepatitis in the elderly. Am J Gastroenterol. 2012;107:691–7.
20. Laverdant C, Algayres JP, Daly JP, Molinie C, Flechaire A, Valmary J, et al. Viral hepatitis in patients over 60 years of age. Clinical, etiologic and developmental aspects. Gastroenterol Clin Biol. 1989;13:499–504.
21. Dalton HR, Fellows HJ, Gane E, et al. Hepatitis E in New Zealand. J Gastroenterol Hepatol. 2007;22:1236–40 (abstract).
22. Health A to Z. Hepatitis G. http://www.healthatoz.com/healthoz.Atoz/common/standard/transform.jsp?request URI=/h.
23. Marcus EL, Tur-Kaspa R. Viral hepatitis in older adults. J Am Geriatr Soc. 1997;45(6):755–63 (abstract).

Chronic Liver Disease in the Elderly

24. Frith J, Jones D, Newton J. The prevalence of chronic liver disease is increasing in the elderly. Age Ageing. 2009;38(1):11–8.
25. Floreani A. Liver damage in the elderly with an update. Dig Dis. 2007;25(2):138–43 (abstract).
26. Reger A, Schiff ER. Liver disease in the elderly. Gastroenterol Clin North Am. 2001;30(2):647–63 (abstract).
27. Hopf U. The elder patient with advanced liver disease. Praxis (Bern 1994). 2005;94(18):743–50.
28. Watuga M, Hartleb M. Alcoholic liver disease. Wiad Lek. 2003;56(1–2):61–70 (abstract).
29. Sherman DI, Williams R. Liver damage : mechanisms and management. Br Med Bull. 1994;50(1):724–38.

Alcoholic Liver Disease

30. Mandayam S, Jamal MM, Morgan TR. Epidemiology of alcoholic liver disease. Semin Liver Dis. 2004;24:217–32.
31. Meier P, Seitz HK. Age, alcohol metabolism and liver disease. Curr Opin Clin Nutrition Metab Care. 2008;11(1):21–0 (abstract).
32. Seitz HK, Tickel F. Alcoholic liver disease in the elderly. Clin Geriatr Med. 2007;23(4):105–21.
33. Walsh K, Alexander G. Alcoholic liver disease. Postgrad Med J. 2000;76(895):280–6 (abstract).
34. Mihas AA, Hung PD, Hueman DM. Alcoholic hepatitis. e-medicine updated June 30, 2008.
35. Seth D, Haber PS, Syn WK, Diehl AM, Day CP. Pathogenesis of alcohol induced liver disease: classical concepts and recent advances. J Gastroenterol Hepatol. 2011;26(7):1089–105.
36. Reubin A. Alcohol and the liver. Curr Opin Gastroenterol. 2006;22(3):263–7.
37. Yoshida A, Hsu LC, Yasinami M. Genetics alcohol-metabolising enzyme. Prog Nucleic Acid Res Col Biol. 1991;40:255–87.
38. Day DE, Bashir R, James OF, Bassendne MF, Crabb DW, Thomasson HR, et al. Investigation of the role of polymorphism at the alcohol and aldehyde dehydrogenase loci in genetic predisposition to acohol-related end organ damage. Hepatology. 1991;14:798–801.
39. Lee HC, Lee HS, Jung SH, Yi SY, Jung HK, Yoon JH, et al. Association between polymorphism of ethanol enzyme and susceptibility to alcoholic cirrhosis in a Korean male population. J Korean Med Sci. 2001;16:745–50.
40. Gramenzi A, Caputo F, Baselli M, Kuria F, Loggi E, Andreone P, et al. Review article: alcoholic liver disease: pathophysiological aspects and risk factors. Aliment Pharmacol Ther. 2006;24:1151–61.

41. Lieber CS. Alcoholic fatty liver: its pathogenesis and mechanism of progression to inflammation and fibrosis. Alcohol. 2004;34(1):9–19.
42. Lieber CS. New concepts of the pathogenesis of alcoholic liver disease lead to novel treatments. Curr Gastrenterol Rep. 2004;6(1):60–5.
43. Wu D, Cederbaum AI. Alcohol, oxidative stress and free radical damage. Alcohol Res Health. 2003;27:277–84.
44. Reinke LA, Lai EK, Dubose CM, McCay PB. Reactive free radical generation in the heart and liver of ethanol –fed rats: correlation in vitro radical formation. Proc Natl Acad Sci U S A. 1987;84:9223–7 (abstract).
45. Scholmerich J, Holstege A. Aetiology and pathophysiology of chronic liver disorders. Drugs. 1990;40 suppl 3:3–22 (abstract).
46. Pinzani M, Roselli M, Zuckermann M. Liver cirrhosis. Best Pract Res Clin Gastroenterol. 2011;25(2):281–90 (abstract).
47. Watuga M, Hartleb M. Alcoholic liver disease. Wiad Lek. 2003;56(1–2):61–70 (abstract).
48. Fairbanks K. Alcoholic liver disease. Cleveland Clinic. 2004. http://www.clevelandclinicmeded.com/medicalpubs/diseasemanagement/gastro/ald/ald.htm.
49. Stewart S, Jones D, Day CP. Alcoholic liver disease: new insights into maechanisms and preventative strategies. Trends Mol Med. 2001;7:408–13.

NAFLD

50. Brunt EM. Nonalcoholic steatohepatitis. Semin Liver Dis. 2004;24(1):3–20 (abstract).
51. Kichian K, McLean R, Gramlich LM, Bailey RJ, Bain VG. Non-alcoholic fatty disease in patients investigated for elevated liver enzymes 2003;17(1):38–42.
52. Saadeh S. Non alcoholic fatty liver disease and obesity. Natr Clin Pract. 2007;22(1):1–10 (abstract).
53. Raszeja-Wyszomirska J, Lawniczal M, Marlisz W, Miezynska-Kurtez J, Milkiewicz P. Non-alcoholic fatty liver disease –new review. Pol Merkur Lekarski. 2008;24(144):568–71 (abstract).
54. Yu AS, Keeffe ED. Non-alcoholic fatty liver disease. Rev Gastroenterol Disord. 2002;2(1):11–9.
55. Nugent C, Younossi ZZ. Evaluation and management of obesity –related non alcoholic fatty liver disease. Nat Clin Pract Gastroenterol Hepatol. 2007;4(8):432–41.
56. Bergquest CJ, SR H, Clouston AD, Jonsson JR, Powell EE, et al. Awareness and experiences of non-alcoholic fatty liver disease by hospital patients in France. J Hepatol. 2012;57:376–83.
57. Clark JM. The epidemiology of non-alcoholic fatty liver disease in adults. J Clin Gastroenterol. 2006;40(suppl-1):S5–10. abstract.
58. Koehler EM, Schonten JN, Hanser BE, van Rooij FJ, Hofman A, Stricker BH, et al. Prevalence and risk factors of non alcoholic fatty liver disease in the elderly: results from the Rotterdam study. J Hepatol. 2012;51(6):1305–11 (abstract).
59. Frith J, Day CO, Alstair AD, Newton JL. Non-alcoholic fatty liver disease in older people. Gerontology. 2009;55:607–15.
60. Youssef WI, McCullough AJ. Steatohepatitis in obese individuals. Best Pract Res Clin Gastroenterol. 2002;16:733–47.
61. Pinto HC, Baptista A, Camilo ME, Valente A, Saragosa A, de Moura MC. Nonalcoholic steatohepatitis. Clinicopathological comparison with alcoholic hepatitis in ambulatory and hospitalized patients. Dig Dis Sci. 1996;41:172–9.
62. Younossi ZM, Diehl AM, Ong JP. Nonalcoholic fatty liver disease: an agenda for clinical research. Hepatology. 2002;33:497–9.
63. Kagansky N, Levy S, Keter D, Rimon E, Taiba Z, Fridman Z, et al. Non-alcoholic fatty liver disease –a common and benign findings in octogenaian patients. Liver Int. 2004;24:588–94.
64. Clouston AD, Powell EE. Nonalcoholic fatty liver disease: is all the fat bad? Intern Med J. 2004;34:187–91.

65. Farrell GC, Larker CZ. Non-alcoholic fatty liver disease from steatosis to cirrhosis. Hepatology. 2006;43(2 supp 11):S99–112.
66. Powell EE, Cooksley WG, Hanson R, Searle J, Halliday JW, Powell LW. The natural history of nonalcoholic steatohepatitis: a follow-up study of forty-two patients for up to 21 years. Hepatology. 1990;11:74–80.
67. Adams LA, Talwahar JA. Diagnostic evaluation of non-alcoholic fatty liver disease. J Clin Gastroenterol. 2006;40(sup 1):S34–6.
68. Arrospide MT. Non-alcoholic fatty liver disease. Rev Gastroenterol Peru. 2013;23(1):49–57 (abstract).

Auto-immune Hepatitis

69. Nagaratnam N, Ambepitiya G, Rajaratnam RG. Lupoid hepatitis, Rendu-Osler-Weber syndrome, clubbing, cyanosis and hypertrophic osteoarthropathy. J Med. 1975;3&4:291–301.
70. Kunkel HG, Ahrens EH, Eisenmenger A, Bongiovanni AM, Slater RT. Extreme hypergammaglobulnaemia in young women with liver disease of unknown etiology. J Clin Invest. 1951;30:654–9.
71. Mackay TL, Cowley DC. Lupoid hepatitis'. Lancet. 1956;268:1323–6.
72. Newton JL, Burt AD, Park JB, Mathew J, Bassendine MF, James OF, et al. Autoimmune hepatitis in older patients. Age Ageing. 1997;21:441–4.
73. Selby CD, Toghill PJ. Chronic active hepatitis in the elderly. Age Ageing. 1986;15:350–6.
74. Schramm C, Kanzler S, zum Buschenfelde KH, et al. Auotimmune hepatitis in the elderly. Am J Gastroenterol. 2001;96(5):1587–91 (abstract).
75. Parker DR, Kingham JGC. Type1 auto-immune hepatitis in patients in later life. Q J Med. 1997;90:289–96.
76. Al-Chatabi T, Boccato S, Portmann DC, McFarlane IG, Heneghan M. Autoimmune hepatitis (AIH) in the elderly: a systematic retrospective analysis of a large group of consecutive patients with definite AIH followed at a tertiary referral centre. J Hepatol. 2006;45(4):575–83.
77. Wolf DC, Raghuraman UV. Autoimmune hepatitis. e-medicine update July 24, 2007.
78. Washington ML. Advance liver disease. Mod Pathol. 2007;20(Suppl):S15–30.
79. Obermayer-Straub P, Strassburg CP, Manns MP. Autoimmune hepatitis. J Hepatol. 2000;32(1):181–97 (abstract).
80. Oo YH, Hubsher SG, Adams DH. Autoimmune hepatitis: new paradigms in the pathogenesis, diagnosis and management. Hepatol Int. 2010;4(2):475–93.
81. Werner M, Prytz H, Ohlsson B, Almer S, Bjornsson E, Bergquist A, et al. Epidemiology and initial presentation of auto immune hepatitis in Sweden: nation wide study. Scand J Gastroenterol. 2008;43(15):1230–40.
82. Szabo Z. The risk of liver biopsy in the diagnosis of autoimmune hepatitis. Orv Hetil. 2006;147(35):1697–702 (abstract).

Drug Induced Liver Injury

83. Hussaini SH, Farrington EA. Idiosyncratic drug-induced liver injury: an overview. Expert Opin Drug Saf. 2007;6(6):673–84 (abstract).
84. Andrade RJ, Lucena MI, Kaplowitz N, Garcia-Munoz B, Bowax Y, Pachkona K, et al. Outcome of acute idiosyncratic drug-induced liver injury: Long-term follow-up ina hepatotoxicity registry. Hepatology. 2006;44(6):1581–8 (abstract).
85. Ghabril M, Chalasani N, Bjornsson E. Drug-induced liver injury: a clinical update. Curr Opin Gastroenterol. 2010;26(3):222–6.
86. le Couteur DG, McLean AJ. The aging liver: drug clearance and an oxygen diffusion barrier hypothesis. Clin Pharmacokinet. 1998;34(5):359–73.

87. Remmel MDH. The role of the liver in drug metabolism. Am J Med. 1970;49(5):617–29 (abstract).
88. Weinshilboum R. Inheritance and drug response. N Engl J Med. 2003;348:529–37.
89. Guengerich FP. Common and uncommon cytochrome P450 related to metabolism and chemical toxicity. Chem Res Toxicol. 2001;14:611–50.
90. Park KB, Kitteringham NR, Kenny JR, Pirmohamed M. Drug metabolism and drug toxicity. Infammopharmacol. 2001;9(1, 2):183–99. abstract.
91. Mehta N, Ozick L, Gbadehan E. Drug induced hepatitis. e-medicine updated 28, 2008.
92. Mitchell SJ, Hilmer SN. Drug induced liver injury in older adults. Ther Adv Drug Saf. 2010;1(2):65–77 (abstract).
93. Kaplowitz N. Drug-induced liver injury. Clin Infect Dis. 2004;38 Suppl 2:S44–8 (abstract).
94. Abboud G, Kaplowitz N. Drug-induced liver injury. Drug Saf. 2007;30(4):277–94 (abstract).
95. Rangnekar AS, Fontana RJ. An update on drug induced liver injury. Minerva Gastroenterol Dietol. 2011;57(2):213–29 (abstract).

Primary Biliary Cirrhosis

96. Prince MI, Jones DEJ. Primary biliary cirrhosis: new perspective in diagnosis and treatment. Postgrad Med J. 2010;76:199–206.
97. Talwalkar JA, Lindor K. Primary biliary cirrhosis. Lancet. 2003;362:53–61.
98. Kumagi T, Heathcote EJ. Primary biliary cirrhosis. Orphanet J Rare Dis. 2008;3:1. doi:10.1186/1756-1179-3-1. abstract.
99. Jones DEJ. Pathogenesis of primary biliary cirrhosis. J Hepatol. 2003;39:639–45.
100. Xu L, Shen S, Guo L, Fodera B, Keogh A, Joplin E, et al. Does a beta retrovirus infection trigger primary biliary cirrhosis. Proc Natl Heart Sci U S A. 2003;1000:8454–9.
101. Mehal WZ, Gregory WL, Lo YMD, Cross SJ, Fleming KA, Bassedine MF, et al. Defining the immunogenetic susceptibility to primary biliary cirrhosis. Hepatology. 1994;20(3):1213–9 (abstract).
102. Chon CY, Park JY. Primary biliary cirrhosis. Korean J Hepatol. 2006;12(3):364–72 (abstract).
103. Selmi C, Ichiki Y, Invermizzi P, Podda M, Gershwin ME. The enigma of primary biliary cirrhosis. Clin Rev Allergy Immunol. 2005;28(2):73–81 (abstract).
104. Invernizzi P, Selmi C, Gershwin ME. Update on primary biliary cirrhosis. Dig Liver Dis. 2010;42(6):401–8 (abstract).

Hereditary Haemochromatosis

105. Limdi JK, Crampton JR. Hereditary haemochromatosis. QJM. doi.http://dx.doi.org/10.1093/qjmed/hch065.315-324.
106. Kuhn LC. Iron overload: molecular clues to its cause. Trends Biochem Sci. 1999;24:164–6.
107. Zoller H, Pietrangelo A, Vogel W, Weiss G. Duodenal metal-transporter (DMT-1, NRAMP-2) expression in patients with hereditary haemochromatosis. Lancet. 1999;353:2120–3.
108. Anderson GJ, Frazer DM. Recent advances in intestinal iron transport. Curr Gastroenterol Rep. 2005;7(5):365–72.
109. Donovan A, Brownlie A, Zhou Y, Shepard J, Pratt SJ, Moynihan J, et al. Positional cloning of zebra fish ferroportin 1 identifies a conserved vertebrate iron exporter. Nature. 2000;403:776–81.
110. Vyrol D, Petrak J. Hepcidin: a direct link between iron metabolism and immunity. Int J Biochem Cell Biol. 2005;37(5):1768–73.
111. Nemeth E, Ganz T. Regulation of iron metabolism by hepcidin. Annu Rev Nutr. 2006;26:323–42.
112. Steele TM, Frazer DM, Anderson GJ. Systemic regulation of intestinal absorption. IUBMB Life. 2005;57(7):499–503.

113. JN F, Gnirke A, Thomas W, Tsuchihashi Z, Ruddy DA, Basava A, et al. A novel MHC class l-like gene is mutated in patients with hereditary haemochromatosis. Nat Genet. 1996;13:399–408.
114. Hanson EH, Imperatore G, Burke W. HFE Gene and hereditary hemochromatosis: a HUGE review. Am J Epidemol. 2001;154(3):193–206.
115. Bacon BR, Powell LW, Adams PC, Kresina TF, Hofnagle JH. Molecular medicine and haemochromatosis: at the cross roads. Gastroenterology. 1999;116:193–207.
116. Crawford DH, Jazwinska EC, Cullen LM, Powell LW. Expression of HLA-linked haemochromatosis in subjects homozygous or heterozygous for the C282Y mutation. Gastroenterology. 1998;114:1003–8.
117. Beutler E, Feliti VJ, Ho NJ, Koziol JA, Getbart T, et al. Penetrance of 845-A(C282Y) HFE hereditary haemochromatosis mutation in the USA. Lancet. 2002;359:211–8.
118. Waalen J, Nordestgaard BG, Beutler E. The penetrance of hereditary hemochromatosis. Best Pract Res Clin Haematol. 2005;18(2):203–20.
119. Powel LW, Dixon JL, Ramm GA, Purdie DM, Lincoln DJ, Anderson GJ, et al. Screening for haemochromatosis in asymptomatic subjects with or without family history. Arch Intern Med. 2006;166:294–301.
120. Bauder F, Scribans C, Renoux M, Borot N. Genetic haemochromatosis is a rare disease entity among French Basques: a center-based study from the general hospital of Basque. Trends Biochem Sci. 1999;24:164–6.

Blood Disorders in the Elderly

5

5.1 Haematopoiesis: Blood Cell Formation and Age-Related Changes

Haematopoietic stem cells (HSCs) are responsible for the production and replenishment of blood cells of all types throughout life. The lifelong homeostatic maintenance of tissues and organs is due to the dual ability for self-renewal and multilineage differentiation [1]. HSCs reside in the bone marrow in a physical niche with a specific microenvironment [2] which control their fate. The stem cell niches which are composed of stromal cells are vital for adult haematopoiesis [3] and there is evidence that stem cell niche is important for the regulation of cellular ageing in adult stem cells [2]. The stem cell niche maintains typical features of stem cells, mainly stem cell quiescence, maintenance or expansion [4], protects from radicals and toxic compounds and modulates gene expression [2]. Recently, it has been found that long-term bone marrow repopulating HSCs exist in the bone marrow trabecular bone surface and the osteoblasts are a vital component for sustaining HSCs [3]. Other studies have suggested that HSCs are associated with the sinusoidal epithelium ('vascular niche') and/or mesenchymal cells [5].

The glycoprotein hormones known as growth factors regulate the blood cell production. Growth factors are proteins that bind receptors on the cell surface with the primary result of activating cellular proliferation and/or differentiation. Many are able to stimulate cellular division in numerous different cell types, while others are specific to a particular cell type. Cytokines are a unique family of growth factors, secreted primarily from leucocytes. Cytokines stimulate both humoral and cellular immune responses and also activate the phagocytic cells. The haematopoietic cytokines maintain a firm control over the production of haematopoietic cells [6]. The cytokines of the haematopoietic system include colony-stimulating factors (CSFs), interleukins (ILs), interferons, erythropoietin (EPO) and thrombopoietin (TPO) [7]. Each cytokine binds to the cytokine receptors which contains specialised regions to initiate various responses [7] such as proliferation, survival, differentiation, maturation and functional activities [6].

N. Nagaratnam et al., *Diseases in the Elderly: Age-Related Changes and Pathophysiology*, DOI 10.1007/978-3-319-25787-7_5

The colony-stimulating factors (CSFs) are the cytokines that stimulate the proliferation of specific pluripotent stem cells of the bone marrow in adults. Granulocyte-CSF (G-CSF) is a glycoprotein specific for the proliferative effects on cells of the granulocyte lineage, differentiation and formation of granulocyte progenitor cells [8]. Macrophage CSF (M-CSF) is specific for cells of the macrophage range. Both G-CSF and M-CSF regulate myeloid cell the production, activation and differentiation [9]. Granulocyte-macrophage CSF (GM-CSF) has proliferative effects on both granulocytic and macrophage cells. It has more recently been shown that its major role is its ability to control properties of the more mature myeloid cells of the granulocyte and macrophage lineages [10, 11]. Erythropoietin is also considered a CSF as well as a growth factor since it stimulates the proliferation of erythrocyte colony-forming units. About 80 % of erythropoietin (EPO) is synthesised by the kidney and 20 % produced by the hepatic stellate cells [9] and is the primary regulator of erythropoiesis. Erythropoietin binds to the erythropoietin receptors (EPOR), stimulates the growth and induces the differentiation of the erythroid progenitors to increase the red mass [12] and differentiation of erythrocyte colony-forming units into proerythroblasts. Growth factor/cytokine IL-3 a multi-CSF supports the proliferation of a broad range of haematopoietic stem cells and is involved in a number of other activities [9]. Stem cell factor (SCF) is a cytokine which functions by binding to c-Kit, a tyrosine kinase receptor expressed on all HSCs [13]. Thrombopoietin is a primary cytokine that regulates megakaryocyte and platelet development [13].

Cytokines that are secreted by the lymphocytes are called lymphokines, whereas those secreted by monocytes or macrophages – monokines. Combined action of several cytokines and other hormones is required for the regulation of several fates of haematopoietic stem cells [13]. Many of the lymphokines are also called interleukins (ILs) since they are not only secreted by the leucocytes, but they are able to affect cellular response of leucocytes. Specifically interleukins are growth factors targeting cells of the haematopoietic organ.

The blood contains three primary cellular elements, the red cell, the white cell and the platelets. These blood cells have varying life span ranging from a few hours (neutrophils) to a few months (red cells). There is therefore a need for a continued blood cell production requiring a perpetual regeneration of blood cells throughout life. This continued production of blood cells is referred to as *haematopoiesis* which involves proliferation, commitment, differentiation of the early progenitor cells to mature cells and their release into the peripheral blood. The *pluripotent haematopoietic stem cell* has the capacity for self-renewal as well as a productive capacity and is capable of giving rise to all lymphoid and non-lymphoid haematopoietic cell lines. The non-lymphoid stem cell has the potential to differentiate into the different *progenitor cells* and which in turn gives rise to the *precursor cells* of the three cell series, the red cell, the white cell and the platelet. The erythroid progenitor cells give rise to the erythroid precursors (Fig. 5.1).

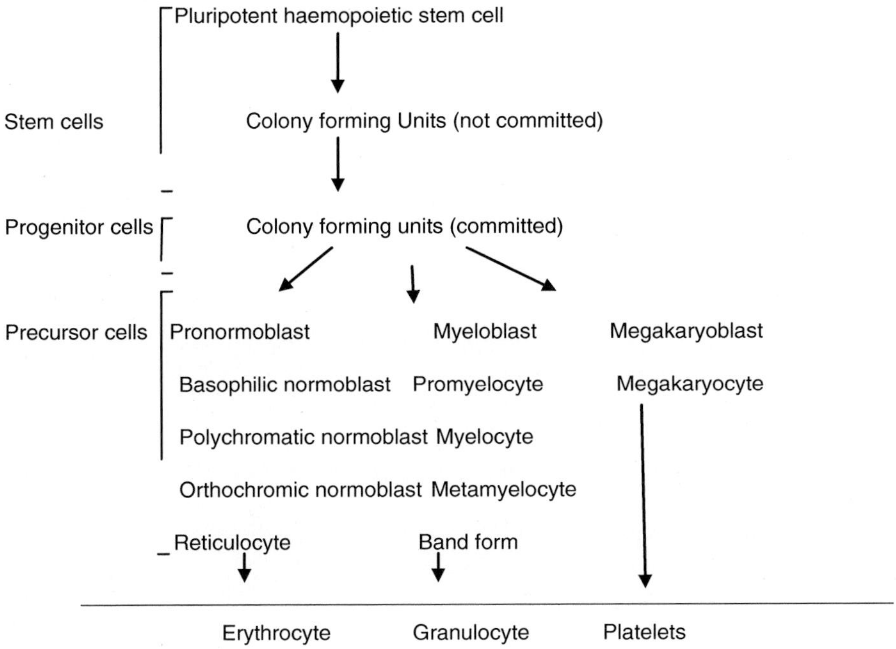

Fig. 5.1 Stages of development in normal haematopoiesis

5.1.1 Erythropoiesis

The erythroid progenitor cells give rise to the erythroid cell line. The *pronormoblast* is the first recognisable cell and is the largest erythroid precursor. Its cytoplasm is deep blue and the nucleus is oval with indistinct nucleus. As the cell matures, there are changes not only in the cell size but also in the cytoplasm and in the nucleus. The pronormoblast gives rise to the *basophilic normoblast* (early) with its basophilic cytoplasm and coarsening of the nucleus and disappearance of the nucleoli. The *polychromatic normoblast* (intermediate) is smaller, and with haemoglobinisation the cytoplasm becomes less basophilic and is of a grey colour and the nucleus dark and condensed. The *orthochromic normoblast* (late) with its eosinophilic cytoplasm and fully condensed nucleus then undergoes karyolysis or karyorrhexis (i.e. it breaks up and is extruded out of the cell) resulting in the formation of the *reticulocyte.* The reticulocyte is characterised by its fine granular or reticular network of ribosomal ribonucleic acid (RNA). The final stage is the release of the mature red cell *(erythrocyte)* into the blood stream. Erythrocyte is a biconcave nonnucleated cell measuring 7–8 um in diameter (Fig. 5.2).

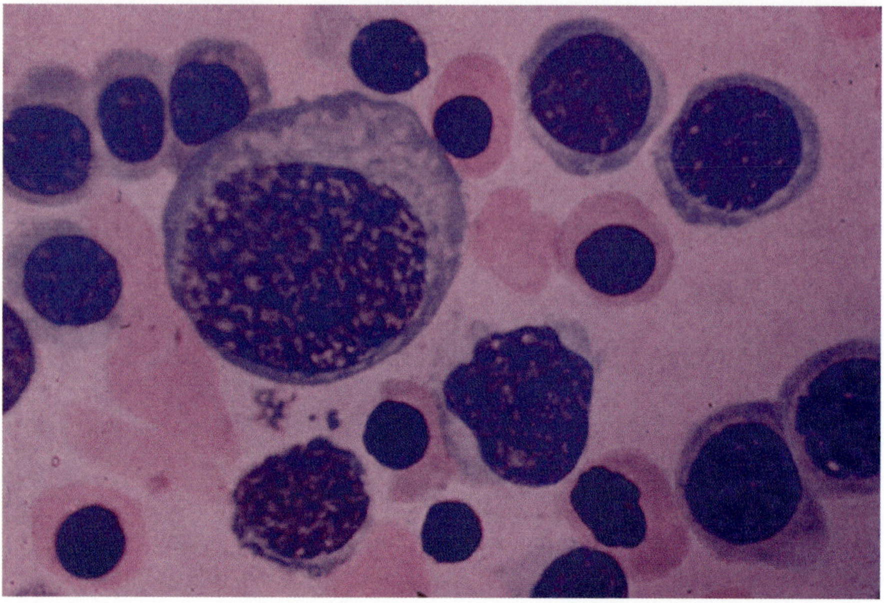

Fig. 5.2 Normoblastic erythropoiesis showing all stages of maturation, pronormoblast, basophilic normoblast, polychromatic normoblast and orthochromic normoblast (Reproduced with permission from Novartis Company Archives, '*Sandoz Atlas of Haematology*' FA Sandoz, 1973)

The erythropoietic process may be abnormal in certain congenital or acquired disorders, for example, in individuals with vitamin B_{12} or folate deficiency states, synthesis of DNA becomes impaired leading to a nuclear/cytoplasm dissociation. The maturation of the nucleus does not keep pace with that of the cytoplasm. The large erythroid precursors with immature nucleus and mature cytoplasm are called megaloblasts. Although called megaloblastic anaemias, there are abnormalities of the white cells and platelets as well (Figs. 5.3 and 5.4).

5.1.2 Myelopoiesis

The neutrophils and monocytes arise from the common committed progenitor cell. Progenitor cells for the eosinophils and basophils have also been identified. The identifiable precursor cell of the myeloid series is the *myeloblast* with a cytoplasm which lacks granules and a nucleus with fine nuclear chromatin and nucleoli. This is followed by the *promyelocyte* which is the most frequent and the largest cell in the series with less prominent nucleoli and coarser chromatin. The cytoplasm is deeply basophilic with non-specific granules. The *myelocyte*, product of the next stage, has a grey-brown cytoplasm with specific granules covering it and the nucleus. The nucleus is round or oval with a slight indentation and indistinct nucleoli. The *metamyelocyte* is characterised by the bean-shaped nucleus and the band formed by the

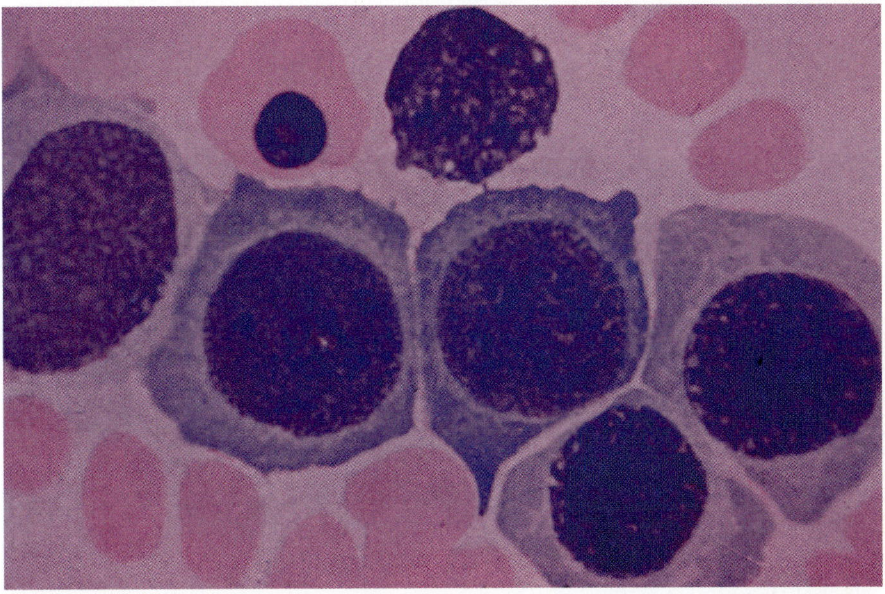

Fig. 5.3 Marrow-megaloblastic erythropoiesis showing promegaloblast, basophilic, polychromatic and orthochromic megaloblasts (Reproduced with permission from Novartis Company Archives, *'Sandoz Atlas of Haematology'* FA Sandoz, 1973)

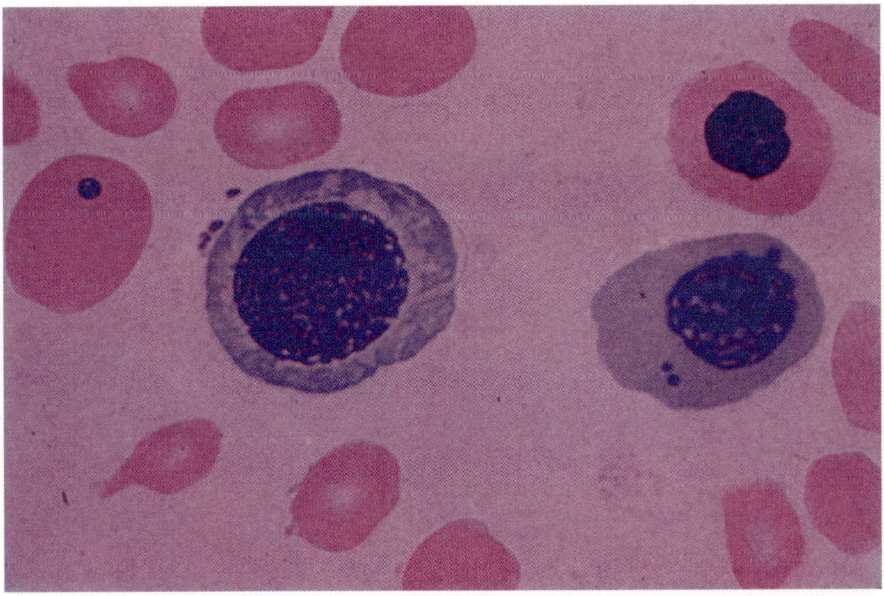

Fig. 5.4 Blood smear. Pernicious anaemia: Showing basophilic, polychromatic, orthochromic megaloblasts. Note nucleocytoplasmic dissociation. Also seen are macrocytes with Howell-Jolly body and poikilocytosis (Reproduced with permission from Novartis Company Archives, *'Sandoz Atlas of Haematology'* FA Sandoz, 1973)

horse-shaped nucleus followed by the segmented neutrophil with its segmented nucleus with 2–5 lobes. The mature *neutrophil* remains in the blood for 12–14 h and then enters the tissues to perform a phagocytic function.

5.1.3 Megakaryocytes and Thrombocytopoiesis

Platelets are anuclear cells arising from the cytoplasm of megakaryocytes. The progenitor cell of the megakaryocyte is the *megakaryoblast* which is a large cell with high nuclear/cytoplasmic ratio. It has a deep blue cytoplasm and contains a nucleus with nucleoli. In the *promegakaryocyte* that follows, the cytoplasm contains some granules and the nucleus is now devoid of nucleoli and is lobulate, and the platelets could be seen on the surface of the cell. Mature *megakaryocyte* is the largest haematopoietic cell in the bone marrow. The cytoplasm is basophilic with azurophilic granules and the platelets can be seen on its surface. The proliferation of the megakaryocytic cell line is unique in that the nuclear division occurs without cytoplasmic division, a process referred to as *polyploidisation.* Platelets are cytoplasmic fragments of their parent cells, the megakaryocytes.

Box 5.1. Key Points. Haematopoiesis and Age-Related Changes

- HSCs reside in the bone marrow in a physical niche, are responsible for the production and replacement of both lymphoid and non-lymphoid blood cells and have the capacity for self-renewal [2].
- The colony-stimulating factors (CSFs) are cytokines that stimulate the production of specific stem cells [8].
- The granulocyte-CSF is specific for cells of granulocyte lineage [10, 11].
- The cytokines secreted by the lymphocytes are lymphokines.

5.2 Age-Related Changes in the Haematopoietic System

Haematopoietic stem cells (HSCs) including the ageing process are controlled by the interplay with the stem cell and niche cells [2]. With increasing age the haematopoietic system undergoes substantial changes. An understanding of the interactions between niche cells and HSCs may provide insights on how the ageing of the HSC compartment contributes to the haematopoietic decline through diverse mechanisms [14]. Age-related changes of the haematopoietic system are very likely the result of age-related alterations in the functions of the HSCs with loss of stem cell activity [15].

The cause of ageing-associated decline in HSC and haematopoietic function is still being debated [16] though a number of mechanisms have been proposed.

Mechanisms put forward for HSC ageing are (i) co-ordinated variation in gene expression of HSC with age – result of epigenetic and genetic changes – and (ii) accumulation of DNA damage with effects of an increase in intracellular reactive oxygen species (ROS) [17, 18]. More recently, the crucial factor considered is changes in the clonal composition of the HSC compartment during ageing [15] and may contribute to or cause the emergence of abnormal clones of haematopoietic cells [19].

There is an age-related decline in haemoglobin from age 70 to 88 among healthy men and less marked in women [20]. Even though the number of stem cells decreases with age, the marrow in older people can repopulate the blood system after serial transplantations [5], and marrow failure in the elderly is rare implying that stem cell exhaustion does not accompany normal ageing [21]. Dysregulation of mechanisms controlling haematopoiesis results in age-associated pathophysiological changes such as diminished adaptive immune competence, greater propensity to anaemia and skewing towards myeloid-biased disorders [15, 22].

An understanding of the interactions between niche cells and HSCs may provide insights on how ageing of the HSC compartment contributes to the haematopoietic decline through diverse mechanisms. The stem cell niche plays an important role in the regulation of cellular ageing in adult stem cells [2]. With age there are striking changes in the functional capacity and quantity of blood cells with decreased competence of the adaptive immune system, elevated incidence of age-associated anaemia and increased haematological malignancies [14].

Box 5.2. Key Points. Age-Related Changes in the Haematopoietic System

- HSCs including ageing process are controlled by the interplay with the stem cell niche [2].
- With ageing there are changes in the clonal composition of the HSC compartment [15].
- Abnormal clones of the haematopoietic cells emerge [19].
- Dysregulation of the mechanisms controlling haematopoiesis results in age-associated changes, diminished adaptive immune competence, greater propensity to anaemia and skewing towards myeloid-biased disorders [15, 22].

5.3 The Anaemias

Introduction

The definition of anaemia in terms of haemoglobin concentration according to the World Health Organization is below 13 g/dl for adult males, below 12 g/dl for women and below 12 g/dl for pregnant women [23]. An Australian study suggested the normal values for haemoglobin to be 12.9–19.4 g/dl and MCV 83.9–100.2 and could be used for assessment of all healthy elderly Australian men [24]. The second National Health and Nutrition Education Survey (NHANES-II) proposed age-specific reference standards for haemoglobin concentrations for elderly persons because of the reduction in haemoglobin levels for males as a consequence of ageing [25]. Some authors have demonstrated that a haemoglobin concentration of <13.7 g/dl in men and <12.6 g/dl in women indicated greater sensitivity than the WHO anaemia criteria [26]. Due to reduced production of testosterone in the elderly, the level of haemoglobin declines, but longitudinal data do not uphold this position that the decline results in anaemia. The diagnosis of anaemia requires measurement of blood haemoglobin level. However, the absolute definition of anaemia in the elderly requires consensus.

Anaemia is common in the elderly and its prevalence increases with age [27, 28]. The third National Health and Nutrition Examination Survey (NHANES-III) [29] revealed deficiencies in iron, folic acid and vitamin B_{12} accounted for approximately 34 % of cases of men in the US elderly, while renal insufficiency and the anaemia of chronic inflammation (ACI) presently known as anaemia of chronic disease (ACD) alone or in combination accounted for an additional 33 % [29]. The remaining 33 % of the anaemias were unexplained (UA). On the basis of the NHANES-III, myelodysplasia which is common in the elderly could account for approximately 20 % of these patients. The most common causes of UA are probably unrecognised renal failure and chronic inflammation. About one-third have anaemia due to deficiencies in iron, folic acid and vitamin B_{12}, another third due to anaemia of chronic disease (renal disease and anaemia of chronic inflammation) and the remaining third is unexplained anaemia which includes myelodysplasia [30].

5.3.1 Microcytic Anaemias

5.3.1.1 Iron Deficiency Anaemia

Total body iron and bone marrow iron stores increase with advancing age because the body cannot excrete the excessive iron. An elderly presenting with iron deficiency is almost exclusively due to blood loss from the gastrointestinal tract. The causes of blood loss in the elderly include neoplasms, drugs such as aspirin and angiodysplasia of the large bowel. Bleeding from the upper gastrointestinal tract due to gastric cancer, peptic ulcers, gastritis and oesophagitis accounts for 20–40 % of cases [31, 32; colon cancer, angiodysplasia or colitis accounts for 10–30 % of cases; and 1–15 % of patients may have bleeding lesions in both upper and lower gastrointestinal tract, and the source of the bleed is not found in 10–40 % of patients [31, 32]. In iron deficiency anaemia, the MCV is usually reduced and the peripheral blood smears show microcytic hypochromic cells. Chronic bleeding also results in elevated platelet count. A transferrin saturation of <16 % may indicate iron deficiency, but this may not always be useful as both serum iron- and total iron-binding capacity decrease in chronic disease.

5.3.2 Macrocytic Anaemias (Vitamin B_{12} and Folic Acid Deficiencies)

5.3.2.1 Vitamin B_{12} Deficiency

Many old people suffer from a deficiency of vitamin B_{12} (cobalamin). About 3–40 % of the general population [33–35] and 15–25 % of the patients in the community, hospital and nursing homes [34, 36] are cobalamin deficient. A Swedish study found 11 % of men and women 75 years or older to be cobalamin deficient [37], and in another study 40.5 % of the elderly people were noted to have a vitamin B_{12} deficiency [38]. In the elderly pure vitamin B_{12} is absorbed but vitamin B_{12} bound to food is inadequately absorbed. In another study the researchers evaluated 548 men and women between the ages of 67 and 96 years. They found that 17.5 % of the elderly had vitamin B_{12} deficiency as opposed to 4.5 % in the younger group, but there were no significant differences with the folate status between the two groups [39].

5.3.2.2 Vitamin B_{12} Absorption

Vitamin B_{12} or cobalamin found in the food is bound to proteins. The absorption process involves an orderly sequence of events [40]. (i) In the stomach the gastric acid and pepsin release cobalamin from their protein complexes. (ii) The released cobalamin binds to the salivary R-protein. (iii) The cobalamin-protein complexes are then degraded by pancreatic proteases [41]. (iv) The released cobalamin combines in the duodenum with the intrinsic factor (IF), another glycoprotein secreted by the stomach parietal cells [41]. (v) The IF-cobalamin complex then attaches itself to the brush border membrane of the terminal ileum and is absorbed. If one of the steps is not functioning properly, anaemia could result [42]:

- Decreased gastric juice – failure to digest protein
- Decreased pancreatic juice – failure to digest R-protein
- In pernicious anaemia, gastrectomy – absence of intrinsic factor
- Ileal resection, Crohn's disease – inadequate absorption
- Bacterial overgrowth – altered intestinal utilisation
- Certain drugs – mucosal or receptor defects [43]

The lack of intrinsic factor due to an autoimmune condition (antibodies targeting either the intrinsic factor or the parietal cells – pernicious anaemia) or surgical gastrectomy is the most frequent cause of vitamin B_{12} malabsorption [41]. Anaemia caused by vitamin B_{12} deficiency is often used synonymously with pernicious anaemia (PA), but typically the term PA characterises vitamin B_{12} deficiency caused by loss of intrinsic factor.

A lack of vitamin B_{12} leads to the development of megaloblastic anaemia and, if untreated, to irreversible neurological damage. There are four stages in the development of vitamin B_{12} deficiency [43]. In stages 1 and 2 biochemical depletion of vitamin B_{12} occurs without any obvious clinical damage and the serum vitamin B_{12} levels may be normal. Stages 3 and 4 represent overt clinical (haematological and neurological), metabolic (raised homocysteine and methylmalonic acid – MMA) or both abnormalities, and serum vitamin B_{12} levels are low.

Box 5.3. Key Points. The Anaemias

- Anaemia is common in the elderly and its prevalence increases with age [28, 29].
- Deficiencies of iron, folic acid and vitamin B_{12} account for one-third of the cases [29].
- One-third is due to anaemia of chronic disease [29].
- In the remaining one-third anaemia is unexplained [29].
- Myelodysplasia could account for 20 % of patients with unexplained anaemia.
- An elderly patient with iron deficiency is almost exclusively due to blood loss from the GI tract.
- About 40 % of the elderly have vitamin B_{12} deficiency [11–13].
- Homocysteine and methylmalonic acid levels are raised in vitamin B_{12} deficiency.

5.4 Haematological Neoplastic Disorders

There has been a change in the nomenclature of myeloproliferative disorders to myeloproliferative neoplasms (MPNs). The MPNs include chronic myeloid leukaemia (CML), polycythaemia vera (PV), essential thrombocythaemia (ET) and primary myelofibrosis (PMF).

5.4.1 Myelodysplastic Syndromes

Myelodysplastic syndromes (MDS) are clonal haematopoietic stem cell disorders in which the haematopoietic process is ineffective [44] resulting in cytopenias, morphologic dysplasia and progression to acute myeloid leukaemia [45]. The incidence of MDS was 3.3 per 100,000 during the years 2001–2004 [46]. On the basis of the NHANES-III data in one-third of elderly patients in the United States with anaemia, the cause was unexplained. Myelodysplasia appeared to be the cause in the unexplained anaemias (UA) in approximately 20 % of these patients [47].

Pathophysiology

MDS is primarily a disease of the elderly with a median age of 74 years [48]. Proliferation of the progenitor and early precursor cells is reduced (hypocellular) or enhanced (hypercellular) in the marrow, but there is a deficit in the circulating mature cells and all three cell lineages, the erythrocyte, granulocyte and megakaryocyte, could be involved. Age is an important risk factor for the development of these disorders [49]. The haematopoietic stem cell injury may be due to radiation exposure, viral infection, chemotherapy or genetic predisposition. In about 40–58 % cytogenetic abnormalities are present [48]. Clonal chromosomal abnormalities are seen in 50 % of the patients with primary MDS patients often involving chromosomes 5, 7 and 8 [50]. MDS is defined further as primary and secondary, the latter related to radiotherapy, chemotherapy or professional exposure to toxic substances [51].

5.4.2 Myeloproliferative Neoplasms

Chronic myeloproliferative disorders include chronic myeloid leukaemia, polycythaemia vera, essential thrombocythaemia and primary myelofibrosis.

5.4.2.1 Chronic Myeloid Leukaemia

Introduction
Chronic myeloid leukaemia (CML) is a clonal disorder with malignant transformation of a pluripotential stem cell resulting in an overproduction of granulocytes (immature and mature). It occurs frequently in young and middle-aged adults with slightly higher incidence in men. In the United States more than 20,000 patients have CML and about 6000 new cases are diagnosed each year [52].

Pathophysiology
In 95 % of the patients with CML, a chromosomal abnormality, the Philadelphia (Ph) chromosome, is present [53, 54] and this abnormality is present in not only in the granulocytes but also in the erythrocytes and megakaryocytes, indicating that CML arises from a pluripotential stem cell. The hallmark for diagnosis is the demonstration of the presence of Philadelphia (Ph) chromosome in the bone marrow cells. In about 5 % of the patients with CML, the Ph chromosome is not detected, and many of these patients with Ph-negative CML are found to have features consistent with myelodysplasia (chronic myelomonocytic leukaemia) [55, 56]. The presence of the Ph chromosome results in the synthesis of the breakpoint cluster region-Abelson murine leukaemia (BCR-ABL) fusion oncoprotein, a constitutionally active tyrosine kinase [57].

The exact cause is not known. A single most important risk factor is radiation exposure. There are three phases of CML, the chronic phase, the accelerated phase and the blast crisis phase. Approximately 80 % of the patients with CML are diagnosed in the chronic phase of the illness which can last from a few months to about 4–5 years. Nearly 80 % of them would progress to the accelerated phase (or transformation) when clinical symptoms and blood abnormalities become more prominent and the survival is less than a year [58]. The third stage is the most advanced stage, the blastic phase, with only a few months survival [58], where more than 30 % of immature cells (the 'blast' cells) are found in the blood and bone marrow.

5.4.2.2 Polycythaemia Vera

Introduction

Polycythaemia vera (PV) is a stem cell clonal disorder in which there is an increased production of red blood cells and increased white blood cells and platelets without significant bone marrow fibrosis [59] together with splenomegaly and hypercellular marrow with hyperplasia of all cell lines. It is rare with a low incidence and high prevalence and occurs more often in males and the peak incidence is between the ages 50 and 70 years [60].

Pathophysiology

PV is a clonal disease in which clonal proliferation of a multipotent haematopoietic stem cells affects all marrow cells resulting in an uncontrolled red cell production and giving rise to an elevated absolute red cell mass, increased white blood cells and platelet production [60]. The cause of the stem cell transformation is still unclear. Physiologic growth factors such as erythropoietin and thrombopoietin [61] stimulate proliferation of the haematopoietic progenitors or differentiation, and many stimulate cellular division in numerous different cell types, while others are specific to a particular cell type. The PV progenitors of the blood cells display abnormal responses to growth factors and are sensitive to multiple cytokines suggesting the deficit may lie in a common pathway downstream from multiple receptors [60]. The clonal cells outgrow the normal precursors of the red blood cell which may still be present in small numbers. The production of red blood cells is not controlled and is independent of erythropoietin, but the stem cells demonstrate hypersensitivity to it and to other growth factors. Genetic mutation has been observed, and a recurrent unique acquired clonal mutation, V617F, in Janus kinase 2 gene (JAK2) had been demonstrated in a vast majority of patients with PV [62, 63] and other myeloproliferative disorders including essential thrombocythaemia and idiopathic myelofibrosis [60].

5.4.2.3 Essential Thrombocythaemia

Introduction

There is an increased production of platelets giving rise to markedly increased in platelet counts. It is rare with a low incidence and high prevalence [64] and occurs more often in males, and the peak incidence is between the ages 50 and 70 years.

Pathophysiology

Essential thrombocythaemia (ET) is a clonal abnormality of a pluripotent haematopoietic stem cell and is one of a group of disorders known as the myeloproliferative disorders.

5.4.2.4 Myelofibrosis and Myeloid Metaplasia

Introduction

Idiopathic myelofibrosis, also known as agnogenic myeloid metaplasia, is a clonal stem cell disorder [65]. The peak of incidence is between 50 and 70 years with a median age of approximately 65 at diagnosis and there is no differences with regard to gender [66].

Pathophysiology

The clonal myeloproliferation is characteristically accompanied by extramedullary haematopoiesis and may occur in any organ but primarily in the spleen and liver [67]. Apart from clonal myeloproliferation, there is an increase in stromal cells, angiogenesis, extracellular matrix proteins and osteosclerosis [60]. The marrow fibroblast arises from the same haematopoietic clone. The cause is unknown.

Box 5.4. Key Points. Myeloproliferative Disorders

- CML is a clonal disorder with malignant proliferation of pluripotent stem cell.
- The hallmark of CML is demonstrating Philadelphia (Ph) chromosome [53, 54].
- Ph-negative CML has features of myelodysplasia [55, 56].
- Polycythaemia vera (PV) is a clonal disease affecting all marrow cells [60].
- Genetic mutation has been observed and a recurrent clonal mutation, V617F, in Janus kinase 2 gene (JAK2) in a vast majority of PV patients [62, 63].
- Myelofibrosis is accompanied by extramedullary haematopoiesis, increase stromal cells, angiogenesis and osteosclerosis [60].

5.4.3 Lymphoproliferative Disorders

5.4.3.1 Chronic Lymphatic Leukaemia

Introduction

Chronic lymphocytic leukaemia (CLL) is derived from mature B lymphocytes [68] and is characterised by a progressive accumulation of lymphocytes in the blood, bone marrow and lymphatic tissues. CLL is a disease of the elderly which increases with advancing age [69] and is twice as common in men.

Pathophysiology

Family history is the greatest risk factor for the development of CLL and a relative risk of CLL among first-degree relatives was 7–8.5-fold [70]. Lymphoid leukaemias are derived from either B lymphocytes or T lymphocytes. The lymphoid leukaemias include chronic lymphatic leukaemia (CLL), prolymphocytic leukaemia, hairy cell leukaemia and less commonly non-Hodgkin's lymphoma [71]. The most common lymphoid leukaemia is chronic lymphatic leukaemia derived from mature B lymphocytes [68].

Observations strongly support the view that antigen plays a crucial role in the pathogenesis of CLL [68]. Furthermore, there is evidence to suggest a genetic component [72] and all CLLs show a common gene expression which suggest derivation from antigen-experienced B cells [73]. CLL lymphocytes coexpress the B-cell antigens CD19 and CD20 along with T-cell antigen CD5 [74]. Most CLL patients carry the mutated immunoglobulin heavy chain variable genes (IGHV) and about 35 % have unmutated IGHV genes [73]. The most common genetic aberration in CLL is deletion of chromosomal region 13q14 [68, 73].

5.4.3.2 Non-Hodgkin's Lymphoma

Introduction

Non-Hodgkin's lymphoma includes a diverse group of haematological disorders which embraces any lymphoma other than Hodgkin's lymphoma and by the absence of Reed-Sternberg cells. Non-Hodgkin's lymphoma (NHL) is the sixth common cancer in Australia. The incidence of non-Hodgkin's lymphoma is increasing by an average of 6.8 % per annum [75] and it increases with age. The average age at the time of diagnosis is around 65 years and is eight times more common than Hodgkin's lymphoma [76] and is more common than leukaemia and multiple myeloma. Epidemiological studies have shown that NHL has been associated with chemicals such as phenoxacetic acid, chlorophenols, and dioxins, among others [77].

Pathophysiology

The most common subtypes are the B-cell follicular lymphoma and the diffuse large B-cell lymphoma (DLBCL) [76]. DLBCL is the largest subgroup and the most common chromosomal translocations affect band 3q27 [78]. In about one-third of the cases of DLBCL, the chromosomal translocations disrupt the normal transcriptional regulation of Bcl-6 [78]. Bcl-6 plays an important role in the repression of genes involved in the control of lymphocyte activation, differentiation and apoptosis within the germinal centre [26]. In NHL chemicals and autoimmune disorders in combination with viruses may impair the immune system and the common mechanism for all these may be immunosuppression [77, 79].

5.4.3.3 Hodgkin's Lymphoma (HL)

Introduction

HL is a malignant tumour of the lymphatic tissues and weakens the immune system. It has a bimodal distribution in people aged 15–25 and a smaller peak after 60 years.

More than 70 % of HL cases in Asia and South America and 20–40 % in the Western world are EBV positive [80].

Pathophysiology
HL is a B-cell lymphoma. The Revised European American Lymphoma (REAL) system classifies HL into two main types: classical and nodular lymphocyte predominant. The classical type includes four subtypes: nodular sclerosing, mixed medullary, lymphocyte depletion and lymphocyte-rich lymphoma [81, 82]. What these lymphomas have in common is the presence of Reed-Sternberg (RS) cells and an extensive immune response [80]. Immunophenotypical studies have demonstrated lymphoid activation markers including CD15, CD25 and CD30, among others [83].

Past infection with Epstein-Barr virus (EBV) is thought to contribute to some cases and has been detected in 40 % of cases of classical HL, and it is clonal and suggests that the virus may play an important role in the pathogenesis of some types of HL [81]. The probable mechanisms whereby the EBV virus may lead to tumorigenesis are by the virus proteins causing genetic instability and by changing the normal processes of apoptosis [84].

Box 5.5. Key Points. Lymphoproliferative Disorders

- All CLLs show gene expression suggesting derivation from antigen-experienced B cells [68].
- The most common genetic aberrant in CLL is the deletion of the chromosome 13q14 [68, 73].
- The most common subtypes of NHL are the B-cell follicular lymphoma and diffuse large B-cell lymphoma (DLBCL) [76].
- In DLBCL the most common chromosome translocations affect band 3q27 [78].

5.4.4 Immunoproliferative Disorders

5.4.4.1 Multiple Myeloma

Introduction
Multiple myeloma is a B-cell neoplastic disease characterised by excessive number of abnormal plasma cells in the bone marrow and overproduction of intact monoclonal immunoglobulins or light chain (Bence Jones) proteins. The cause is not known and the epidemiological pattern remains obscure [85]. Age is the most significant risk factor. Genetic factors, exposure to certain viruses, certain chemicals and radiation and certain occupations have been suggested as possible associations in its causation. It is possible that many factors acting together result in myeloma.

Pathophysiology

The two major lymphocytes which develop from the lymphoid stem cells in the bone marrow are the B cells (B lymphocytes) and T cells (T lymphocytes). When B cells lymphocytes respond to infection they mature and change to plasma cells. The plasma cells produce proteins called immunoglobulins. Each plasma cell line develops in response to a particular foreign substance within the body. There are five classes of immunoglobulins, and each has a heavy chain named by a Greek letter gamma (IgG), alpha (IgA), mu (IgM), epsilon (IgE) and delta (IgD) and the light chains defined as kappa(k) and lambda(l). Each immunoglobulin molecule is made up of two (long) heavy chains and two (shorter) light chains.

Transformation of the normal B cell into a malignant plasma cell (myeloma cell) involves a multistep process and multiple gene abnormalities. The B lymphocytes migrate from the bone marrow to the lymph nodes and plasma cells originate from the postfollicular B cells [86]. In the developing B lymphocyte, genetic damage occurs during the time of isotype switching [87]. The proliferation of B cells and the secretion of antibodies are kept under control by the immune system, and this control is lost when the chromosome and genes are damaged. The genetic instability leads to further translocations and mutations. The mutation results in the dysregulation of the oncogene resulting in proliferation of the plasma cell clone. The myeloma cell expresses the adhesion molecules, insulin-like factor 1 and laminin in order to proceed from the node to the marrow [88]. Multiple myeloma (MM) develops on the B lymphocytes after they leave the lymph node. The myeloma cell is carried in the bloodstream and collects and attaches to the bone marrow stroma. Growth and survival of the MM cells are sustained by the bone marrow stromal cells by way of various cytokines [86]. The cytokines produced by the plasma cells cause bone resorption and increase angiogenesis. The importance of interactions between the MM calls and their bone marrow environment has been emphasised [89]. The myeloma cells grow causing damage to the normal tissue. Recent studies have revealed the osteoclast activity factors, and imbalances between osteoprotegerin, receptor activator of nuclear factor-kappa B (RANK), its ligand RANKL and macrophage inflammatory protein 1 alpha are implicated in osteoclast activation [90] and have important roles in the development of myeloma bone disease [86]. The myeloma cells produce a specific immunoglobulin in large quantities which is monoclonal, i.e. one class of heavy chains and one type of light chains, and is referred to as a monoclonal protein (M protein) or paraprotein. The M protein, unlike the normal immunoglobulin, is of little use to the body.

The frequency of the types of myeloma parallels the normal serum concentrations of the immunoglobulins. The IgG myeloma accounts for about 70 % of all cases of myeloma and IgA for about 20 %. Few cases of IgD and IgE have been reported. About 15–20 % of the patients with myeloma produce incomplete immunoglobulins containing light chain of the immunoglobulin and known as Bence Jones proteins and said to have Bence Jones myeloma or light chain myeloma.

Box 5.6. Key Points. Immunoproliferative Disorders

- Multiple gene abnormalities are involved in the transformation of normal B cell into myeloma cell.
- The immune system controls the proliferation of B cells and secretion of antibodies.
- The B lymphocytes leave the lymph nodes and attach to the bone marrow stroma.
- The cytokines produced by the plasma cells cause bone resorption and increase angiogenesis.
- The myeloma cells produce large amounts of a specific immunoglobulin which is monoclonal.

Multiple Choice Questions

1. The following are true in the formation of blood cells, EXCEPT:
   A. Erythropoietin is also considered a colony-stimulating factor (CSF) as well as a growth factor.
   B. Haematopoietic stem cells (HSCs) reside in the bone marrow in a physical niche with a specific microenvironment which control their destiny.
   C. Cytokines are a unique family of growth factors, secreted primarily from red cells.
   D. Granulocyte-CSF (G-CSF) is a glycoprotein specific for proliferative effects on cells of the granulocyte lineage.
2. The following are true in relation to the relevant anaemias, EXCEPT:
   A. A transferrin saturation of <16 % may indicate iron deficiency, but this may not always be useful as both serum iron and total iron-binding capacity decrease in chronic disease.
   B. A lack of vitamin B_{12} leads to the development of megaloblastic anaemia and, if untreated, leads to irreversible neurological damage.
   C. In the elderly pure vitamin B_{12} is absorbed so does vitamin B_{12} bound to food.
   D. The most common causes of unexplained anaemia are probably unrecognised renal failure and chronic inflammation.
3. The following are true of the following haematological malignancies, EXCEPT:
   A. In 95 % of the patients with CML, a chromosomal abnormality, the Philadelphia (Ph) chromosome, is present.
   B. Polycythaemia vera is a clonal disease in which clonal proliferation of a multipotent haematopoietic stem cells affects all marrow cells.
   C. Lymphoid leukaemias are derived from B lymphocytes only.
   D. Non-Hodgkin's lymphoma includes a diverse group of haematological causes which embraces any lymphoma other than Hodgkin's lymphoma.

4. The following are true in relation to multiple myeloma, EXCEPT:
   A. The lymphocytes migrate to the bone marrow and then to the lymph nodes, and the plasma cells originate from postfollicular B cells.
   B. The cytokines produced by the plasma cells cause bone resorption and increase angiogenesis.
   C. The myeloma cells produce a specific immunoglobulin which is monoclonal.
   D. All patients with myeloma produce incomplete immunoglobulins causing light chains known as Bence Jones proteins.

Answers to MCQs

1 = C; 2 = C; 3 = C; 4 = D.

References

Haematopoiesis-Blood Cell Production

1. Zant GV, Liang Y. Concise review: haematopoietic stem cell aging, life span and transplantation. Stem Cells Transl Med. 2012;1:651–7.
2. Wagner W, Horn P, Bork S, Ho AD. Aging of hematopoietic stem cells is regulated by the stem cell niche. Exp Gerontol. 2008;43(11):974–80 (abstract).
3. Arai F, Hirao A, Suda T. Regulation of hematopoiesis and its interaction with stem cell niches. Int J Hamatol. 2005;82(5):371–6 (abstract).
4. Heissig B, Ohki Y, Sato Y, Rafii S, Werb Z, Hattori K. A role for niches in hematopoetic cell development. Hematology. 2005;10(3):247–53 (abstract).
5. Nagasawa T, Omatsu Y, Sugiyama T. Control of hematopoietic stem cells by the bone marrow stromal niche: the role of reticular cells. Trends Immunol. 2011;32(7):315–20 (abstract).
6. Metcalf D. Hematopoietic cytokines. Blood. 2008;111(2):485–91 (abstract).
7. Robb L. Cytokine receptors and haematopoietic differentiation. Oncogene. 2007;26: 6715–23.
8. Lieschke GJ. Granulocyte colony stimulating factor (G-CSF). Aust Prescriber. http://www.australianprescriber.com.magazine/17/4/96/9.2013. Accessed 22 Apr 2013.
9. Singh VK, Saini A, Chandra K. Role of erythropoietin and other growth factors in viva erythropoiesis. Advances in Regenerative Medicine. 2014(2014):Article ID 426520. 8 pages. http://dx.doi.org/10.11552014/426520.
10. Fleetwood AJ, Cook AD, Hamilton JA. Functions of granulocyte-macrophage colony-stimulating factor. Crit Rev Immunol. 2005;25(5):405–28 (abstract).
11. Hamilton JA, Anderson GP. GM-CSF biology. Growth Factors. 2004;22(4):225–31.
12. Hedley BD, Allan AL, Xenocostas A. The role of erythropoietin and erythropoiesis-stimulating agents in tumor progression. Clin Cancer Res. 2011;17(20):6373–80 (abstract).
13. Zhang CC, Lodish HF. Cytokines regulating hematopoietic stem cell function. Curr Opin Hematol. 2008;15(4):307–11 (abstract).

Age-Related Changes in the Haematopoietic System

14. Beerman I, Maloney WJ, Weissman IL, Rossi DJ. Stem cells and the aging haematopoietic system. Curr Opin Immunol. 2010;22(4):500–6.

15. Woolthuis CM, de Haan G, Huls G. Aging of haematopoietic stem cells: intrinsic changes or micro-environmental effects? Curr Opin Immunol. 2011;23:512–7 (abstract).
16. Henry CJ, Marusyk A, DeGregon J. Aging-associated changers in hematopoiesis and leukemogenesis: what's the connection? Aging (Albany NY). 2011;3(6):643–56 (abstract).
17. Dykstra B, de Haan G. Hematopoietic stem cell aging and self-renewal. Cell Tissue Res. 2008;331(1):91–101.
18. Ergen AV, Goodell MA. Mechanisms of the haematopoietic stem cell aging. Exp Gerontol. 2010;45(4):286–90 (abstract).
19. Rothstein G. Disordered haematopoiesis and myelodysplasia in the elderly. J Am Geriatr Soc. 2003;51:22–6 (abstract).
20. Nilsson-Ehle H, Jagenburg R, Landahl S, Svanborg A. Blood haemoglobin declines in the elderly: implication for reference intervals from age 70 to 88. Eur J Haematol. 2000;65:297–305.
21. Warren LA, Rossi DJ. Stem cells and aging in the haematopoietic system. Mech Ageing Dev. 2006;130:46–53 (abstract).
22. Gazil R, Weissman IL, Rossi DJ. Haematopoietic stem cells and aging haematopoietic system. Semin Hamatol. 2008;45(4):218–24.

Anaemias

23. World Health Organisation. Haemoglobin concentration for the diagnosis of anaemia and assessment of severity. http://www.intvmnis/indicators/haemoglobin.pdf. Retrieved 17 Sept 2014.
24. Magarey M, Tiddy JA, Wilson PC, McCarthy PJ. Normal anthropometric and biochemical values for two groups of healthy males-war veterans and non-veterans. Aust J Nutr Diet. 1992;40:90–5.
25. Yip R, Johnson C, Dallman PR. Age-related changes in laboratory values used in the diagnosis of anemia and iron deficiency. Am J Clin Nutr. 1984;39:427.
26. Zakai NA, Katz R, Hirch C, Shlipak MG, Chaves PHM, Newman AM, et al. A prospective study of anaemia status, haemoglobin concentration and mortality in an elderly cohort: the Cardiovascular Health Study. Arch Intern Med. 2005;165:2214–20.
27. Daly MP. Anaemia in the elderly. Am Fam Physician. 1989;39:129–36.
28. Salive ME, Cornoni-Huntley J, Guralnik JM, Philips CL, Wallace RB, Ostfeld AM, et al. Anaemia and haemoglobin levels in elderly persons: relationship with age, gender and health status. J Am Geriatr Soc. 1992;40:489–96.
29. Guralnik JM, Eisenstaedt RS, Ferrucci L, Klein HG, Woodman RC. Prevalence of anaemia in persons 65 years and older in the United States: evidence for a high rate of unexplained anaemia. Blood. 2004;104:2263–8.
30. Spivak JL. Anaemia in the elderly: a growing health concern. CME. http://www.medscape.com/viewarticle/522647.
31. Gordon SR, Smith RE, Power GC. The role of endoscopy in the evaluation of iron deficiency anemia in patients over the age of 50 years. Gastroenterol. 1994;89:1963–7.
32. Rockey CD, Cello JP. Evaluation of the gastrointestinal tract in patients with iron deficiency anaemia. N Engl J Med. 1993;329:1691–5.
33. Wynn M, Wynn A. The danger of B12 deficiency in the elderly. Nutr Health. 1998;12:215–26.
34. Daharmarajan TS, Norkus EP. Vitamin B12 deficiency in the elderly-population based research. In: Herbert V, editor. Vitamin B12 deficiency. London: Royal Society of Medicine Press Ltd.; 1999:27–33.
35. Stabler SP, Lindenbaum J, Allen RH. Vitamin B12 deficiency in the elderly: current dilemmas. Am J Clin Nutr. 1997;66(4):741–9.
36. Dharmarajan TS, Ugalino JT, Kanagala M, Pitchuoni S, Norkus EP. Vitamin B12 status in hospitalized elderly from nursing homes and the community. J Am Med Dir Assoc. 1999;99(6):725–7.
37. Eggersten R. Prevalence and diagnosis of cobalamin deficiency in older people. J Am Geriatr Soc. 1996;44(10):1273–4.

38. Lindenbaum J, Rosenberg IH, Wilson PW, Stabler SP, Allen RH. Prevalence of cobalamin deficiency in the Framingham elderly population. Am J Clin Nutr. 1994;60:2–11.
39. Allen LH, Casterline J. Vitamin B12 deficiency in the elderly individuals: diagnosis and requirements. Am J Clin Nutr. 1994;60:12–4.
40. Cooper BA, Castle WB. Sequential mechanisms in the enhanced absorption of vitamin B12 by intrinsic factor in rats. J Clin Invest. 1960;39:199–214.
41. Feslen HP. Intrinsic factor secretion and cobalamin absorption. Physiology and pathophysiology in the gastrointestinal tract. Scand J Gastroeneterol Suppl. 1991;188:1–7.
42. Oh R, Brown DL. Vitamin B12 deficiency. Am Fam Physician. 2003;67(5):979–86.
43. Dharmarajan TS, Norkus EP. Approaches to vitamin B12 deficiency. Postgrad Med. 2001;110(1):99–105.

Haematological Malignancies: Myelodysplastic Syndromes

44. Manoharan A, Brighton T, Gemmell R, Lopez K, Moran S, Kyle P. Platelet dysfunction in myelodysplastic syndromes: a clinicopathological study. Int J Hematol. 2002;76:272–8.
45. Zhou J, Orazi A, Czader MB. Myelodysplastic syndromes. Semin Diagn Pathol. 2011;28(4):258–72 (abstract).
46. Rollison DE, Howlader N, Smith MT, Strom SS, Merritt WD, Ries LA, et al. Epidemiology of myelodysplastic syndromes and chronic myeloproliferative disorders in the United States 2001–2004, using data from the NAACCR and SEER programs. Blood. 2008;112:45–52.
47. Guralnik JM, Eisenstaedt RS, Ferrucci L, Eisenstadt RS, Ferrucci L, Klein HG, et al. Prevalence of anaemia in persons 65 years and older in the United States: evidence for a high rate of unexplained anaemia. Blood. 2004;104:2263–8.
48. Saba HI. Myelodysplastic syndromes in the elderly: role of growth factors in management. Leuk Res. 1996;20(3):203–19 (abstract).
49. Ria R, Moschetta A, Reale A, Mangialardi G, Castrovilli A, Vacca A, et al. Managing myelodysplastic symptoms in elderly patients. Clin Interv Aging. 2009;4:413–23.
50. Schmitt-Graeff A, Mattern D, Kohler H, Hezel J, Lubbet M. Myelodysplastic syndromes(MDS): aspects of haematopathologic diagnosis. Pathologie. 2000;21(1):1–15.
51. Flandrin G. Classification of myelodysplastic syndromes. Atlas Genet Cytogenet Oncol Haematol. 2002. URL. http://AtlasGeneticsOncology.org/Anomalies/ClassifMSSID1239.html.

Chronic Myeloid Leukaemia

52. Howlader N, Noone AM, Krapcho M, Garshell J, Neyman N, Altkruse SF, et al., editors. SEER Cancer Statistics Review 1975–2010. National Cancer Institute Bethesda MD http://seer.cancer.gov/csr/1975_2010. Based in November 2012. SEER data submission posted to the SEER website April 2013.
53. Kurzrock R, Kantarjian HM, Druker NJ, Talpaz M. Philadelphia chromosome –positive leukaemias from basic and molecular therapeutics. Ann Intern Med. 2003;138:819–30.
54. Goldman JM, Melo TW. The molecular biology of chronic myeloid leukaemia. Blood. 2000;96(10):3343–56. (abstract).
55. Oscier DG. Atypical chronic myeloid leukaemia: a distinct clinical entity related to the myelodysplastic syndrome. Br J Haematol. 1996;92(3):582–6.
56. Kurzrock R, Bueso-Ramos CE, Kantarijian H, Freirech M, Tucker SL, Siciliano M, et al. BCR rearrangement –negative chronic myelogenous leukaemia. Clin Oncol. 2001;19(11):2915–26.
57. Jabbour E, Cortes J, Kantarjian H. Long term outcomes in the second –line treatment of chronic myeloid leukaemia: a review of tyrosine kinase inhibitors. Cancer. 2011;117(5):897–906.
58. Sawyers CL. Chronic myeloid leukaemia. N Engl J Med. 1999;340(17):1330–40.

Polycythaemia Vera

59. Finazzi G, Barbul T. How I treat patients with polycythaemia vera. Blood. 2007;109(12):5104–11.
60. Besa GC, Woermann V. Polycythaemia vera. http://www.emedicine.com/MED/topic1864.htm.
61. Prchal IF, Axelrad AA. Bone marrow responses in polycythaemia vera. N Engl J Med. 1974;290:1382.
62. Baxter FI, Scott IM, Campbell PI, East C, Fourouclas N, Swanton S, et al. Acquired mutation of the tyrosine kinase JAK2 in human myeloproliferative diseases. Lancet. 2005;352:1054–61.
63. Kralovics R, Passamonti F, Buser AS, Teo S, Tiedt PR, Passweg JR, et al. A gain-of-function mutation of JAK2 in myeloproliferative disorders. N Engl J Med. 2005;352:1779–90.

Essential Thrombocythaemia

64. Penninga EI, Bjerrum OW. Polycythaemia vera and thrombocythaemia: current treatment and strategies. Drugs. 2006;66(17):2173–87.

Myelofibrosis and Myeloid Metaplasia

65. Tefferi A. Myelofibrosis and myeloid metaplasia. N Engl J Med. 2000;342(17):1255–64.
66. Kvasnicka HM, Thiele J, Werden C, Zankovich R, Diehl V, Fischer R. Prognostic factors in idiopathic (primary) osteomyelofibrosis. Cancer. 1997;80:707–19.
67. Ward HP, Block MH. The natural history of agnogenic myeloid metaplasia (AMM) and a critical evaluation of its relationship with the myeloproliferative syndrome. Medicine (Baltimore). 1971;50:357–420.

Lymphoproliferative Disorders: Chronic Lymphatic Leukaemia

68. Klein U, Dalla-Favera R. New insights into the pathogenesis of chronic lymphocytic leukaemias. Semin Cancer Biol. 2010;20(6):377–83.
69. Catovsky D, Fooks J, Richards S. Prognostic factors in chronic lymphatic leukaemia : the importance of age, sex and response to treatment in survival: a report from MRC CLL. Br J Haemat. 1989;72(2):141–9.
70. Goldin LR, Pfeigger RM, Li X, Hemminski K. Familial risk of lymphoproliferative tumours of patients with chronic lymphocytic leukaemia: results from the Swedish Family-Cancer Database. Blood. 2004;104(6):1850–4 (abstract).
71. Foon KA. Chronic lymphoid leukaemias: recent advances in biology and therapy. Stem Cells. 1995;13(1):1–21.
72. Kalil N, Cheson BD. Chronic lymphocytic leukaemia. Oncologist. 1999;4(5):S352–69.
73. Gaidano G, Foa R, Dalla-Favera R. Molecular pathogenesis of chronic lymphocytic leukaemia. J Clin Invest. 2012;122(10):3432–8.
74. DiGiuseppe JA, Borowitz MJ. Clinical utility of flow cytometry in chronic lymphoid leukaemias. Semin Oncol. 1998;25(1):6–10.

Non-Hodgkin's Lymphoma

75. Rolland-Portal I, Tazi MA, Milan C, Couilault C, Carli PM. Non-Hodgkin's lymphoma: time trends for incidence and survival in Cote- D'Or France. Int J Epidemiol. 1997;26(5):945–52.
76. Young GAR, Iland HJ. Clinical perspectives in lymphoma. Int Med J. 2007;37:478–84.
77. Hardell L, Lindstrom G, van Bevel B, Fredikson M, Liljrgren G. Some aspects of the etiology of non-Hodgkin's lymphoma. Environ Health Perspect. 1998;106 Suppl 2:679–81 (abstract).
78. Pasqualucci L, Bereschenko O, Niu H, Klein U, Basso K, Guglielmino R, et al. Molecular pathogenesis of non-Hodgkin's lymphoma: the role of Bcl-6. Leuk Lymphoma. 2003;44 Suppl 3:S5–12.
79. Hardell L, Axelson O. Environmental and occupational aspects on the etiology of non-Hodgkin's lymphoma. Oncol Res. 1998;10(1):1–5 (abstract).

Hodgkin's Lymphoma

80. Poppema S. Immunobiology and pathophysiology of Hodgkin's lymphomas. ASH Education Book. 2005;1231–238. http://asheducationbook.hematologylibrary.org/content/2005/1/231.full. Accessed 23 May 2012.
81. Harris NL. Hodgkin's disease: classification and differential diagnosis. Mod Pathol. 1999;12(2):159–75 (abstract).
82. Foss HD, Msarafioti T, Stein H. Hodgkin lymphoma. Classification and pathogenesis. Pathologe. 2000;21(2):113–23 (abstract).
83. Gruss HJ, Kadin ME. Pathophysiology of Hodgkin's disease: functional and molecular aspects. Baillieres Clin Haematol. 1996;9(3):417–46 (abstract).
84. Meyer RM, Ambinder RF, Stroobants S. Hodgkin's lymphoma: evolving concepts with implications for practice. Hematology Am Soc Hematol Educ Program. 2004;184–202. (abstract).

Immunoproliferative Disorders: Multiple Myeloma

85. Riedel DA, Pottern LM. The epidemiology of multiple myeloma. Hematol Oncol Clin North Am. 1992;6:225–47.
86. Seidl S, Kaulmann H, Drach J. New insights into the physiology of multiple myeloma. Lancet Oncol. 2003;4(9):557–64 (abstract).
87. Jagannath S. Pathophysiological underpinnings of multiple myeloma progression. J Manag Care Pharm. 2008;14(7):S7–11.
88. Menu E, Asosingh K, Van Reit I, Croucher P, Van Camp B, Vanderkerken K. Myeloma cells (5TMM) and their interactions with the marrow microenvironment. Blood Cells Mol Dis. 2004;33(2):111–9.
89. Anderson KC, Carrasco RD. Pathogenesis of myeloma. Ann Rev Pathol. 2011;6:249–74 (abstract).
90. Terpis E, Dimopoulos MA. Myeloma bone disease: pathophysiology and management. Ann Oncol. 2005;16(8):1223–31.

6 Renal and Lower Urinary Tract Disorders in the Elderly

6.1 Anatomical and Physiological Changes with Ageing

The normal function of the kidney includes excretion of waste metabolic products, regulation of water and salt, maintenance of acid balance, regulation of blood pressure and secretion of a variety of hormones. Numerous anatomical and physiological changes occur with ageing [1] resulting in reduced blood flow, reduced GFR and impaired autoregulation [2, 3]. With ageing, there is significant reduction in renal function, yet the kidneys in the elderly function sufficiently to maintain homeostasis of blood composition, volume and pressure. However, the renal reserve is reduced thereby reducing the capacity to adapt in particular during physical stresses. There is a mean decrease in renal mass by about 20 % between the ages of 50 and 80 years [4]. The kidney decreases in size from approximately 250 g in the young adult to 180 g in the eighth decade, and this reduction is primarily due to loss of cortical mass [5]. The cortical loss is due to glomerulosclerosis which increases with age [6], but the severity of the glomerular sclerosis varies from one person to another [4]. The glomerular loops become obliterated [7], and the number of epithelial cells decreases with an increase in the number of mesangial cells thereby reducing the surface area for filtration. There is hyalinization of the basement membrane [7]. There is selective loss of cortical vasculature with age due to decrease in renal blood flow and decrease in function [8, 9]. The medulla is relatively spared. Sclerotic changes occur in the larger renal vessels.

There is a progressive decline in the glomerular filtration rate (GFR) with age [9]: a decrease of about 7 % per decade after the age of 40 years [4] as measured by the creatinine clearance. The creatinine clearance after middle age tends to decline progressively although ageing effect on creatinine clearance varies considerably. After the age of 40 years, there is a yearly decline of about 1 ml/min [10]. The decrease in the GFR with age is less than what was originally thought [11]. The effective renal plasma flow decreases by about 10 % per decade [4] proportionately more than the GFR [12]. In the elderly, there is an increase in the levels of asymmetric dimethylarginine (ADMA); the cause of which is unclear [12].

N. Nagaratnam et al., *Diseases in the Elderly: Age-Related Changes and Pathophysiology*, DOI 10.1007/978-3-319-25787-7_6

Studies in animals have shown that ADMA reduces renal perfusion and increases renal vascular tone and blood pressure [13]. Furthermore, in the elderly, the ability of the postglomerular vasculature to dilate to stimuli such as nitric oxide (NO) is reduced, and it has been shown that the renal microvasculature is particularly sensitive to NO synthase inhibition and NO plays an important role in regulating medullary blood flow [12]. Several changes occur in the tubular structure with age [14] with decrease in the tubular length and size of the proximal tubular epithelial cells [15]. There is tubular dilatation with thickening of the tubular basement membrane and increase in interstitial fibrosis [16, 17]. Resorption and secretion of the solutes are damped by changes in the tubules with ageing. The hormonal regulating mechanisms (renin-angiotensin pathway, aldosterone, antidiuretic hormone) are depressed, and the levels of aldosterone, renin activity and serum renin levels are low in older person [18].

Box 6.1. Key Points. Anatomical and Physiological Changes with Ageing

- With ageing, there is a reduction in blood flow, reduction in GFR and impaired autoregulation [1, 2].
- Renal reserve is reduced thereby reducing the capacity to adapt to physical stress.
- In the elderly, the ability of the postglomerular vasculature to dilate to stimuli such as nitric oxide is reduced, and nitric oxide plays an important role in regulating medullary blood flow [12].
- Resorption and secretion of the solutes are damped by changes in the tubules with ageing.
- The hormonal regulatory mechanisms are depressed [18].

6.2 Glomerular Disease in the Elderly

Introduction

Glomerular disease is characterised by an inability of the kidneys to both filter and retain substances in the blood stream and has many causes. The true incidence of glomerular disease in the elderly may be underestimated as a result of fewer biopsies in those above 65 years and more so in those above the age of 75 years [19]. The incidence of glomerular disease (GD) in the elderly is relatively higher than in young adults [20]. This has been attributed to the increase in malignancies and in the use of a variety of drugs. It is likely that any apparent difference reflects the type of clinical practice rather than any inherent difference in the aged kidney [21].

Pathophysiology

Based on renal biopsy results, there are few histological differences between elderly patients over the age of 60 years and younger patients [20]. As in younger patients, GD can present in a variety of ways, including nephritic syndrome and nephrotic syndrome, and may also present as hypertension, asymptomatic urine changes and chronic kidney disease. In a study of glomerular disease in the elderly (mean age 67.2 ± 6.4), the histopathological changes included extracapillary proliferation, membranoproliferation, membranous nephropathy, focal-segmental glomerulosclerosis, mesangial glomerulonephritis, minimal change disease and diabetic glomerulosclerosis [22]. GD may be primary or secondary to system disease in the ratio of 7:3 in elderly patients [23]. In some patients with GD, extrarenal manifestations suggest a causative disease, and serological markers such as serum anti-neutrophil cytoplasmic autoantibodies (ANCA), anti-nuclear antibodies (ANA), anti-streptococcal antibodies and C3 nephritic factor among others help in the differential diagnosis.

6.3 Renovascular Disease in the Elderly

Introduction
Renovascular disease (RVD) is a progressive condition that causes narrowing or blockage of the renal arteries or veins resulting in reduced renal perfusion [24]. The term renovascular hypertension (RVHT) is applied when blood pressure rises as a result of renal ischaemia. Hypertensive nephrosclerosis (hypertensive nephropathy) refers to damage to the kidneys due to chronic high blood pressure. It should be distinguished from renovascular hypertension which is a form of secondary hypertension. Atheromatous RVD and nephrosclerosis are the most prevalent. In the United States, it is estimated that RVD occurred in 1–5 % of the cases with secondary hypertension in the general population, 30 % in the vascular high-risk group and up to 60 % in those aged 70 years or over [25]. RVD has been the main cause of end-stage renal disease in the elderly with an incidence of 39 % [26]. It has been suggested that 10–40 % of elderly hypertensive patients with newly documented end-stage renal disease (ESRD) with no demonstrable renal disease have significant renal artery stenosis [27]. Several studies have indicated that age is a risk factor for RVD and cause for ERSD [28].

Pathophysiology
RVDs that caused end-stage renal disease (ESRD) are inflammatory vasculitis, nephrosclerosis, RVD atheromatous and embolic disease. Renal artery stenosis is the cause of renovascular hypertension in at least 90 %. Atherosclerotic renal artery stenosis is a disease of older individuals. Other causes include renal atheroembolic and renal thromboembolic disease. Hypertension can cause both vascular and glomerular damage in the kidney and lead to progressive renal insufficiency, a disease called hypertensive nephrosclerosis. It can be benign and associated with mild to moderate hypertension with hyaline thickening of the small arteries and arterioles with slow decline in the GFR over many years. It can be malignant with severe hypertension characterised by fibrinoid necrosis of the small vessels and potentially irreversible renal failure.

Atherosclerosis causes about 70–90 % of RVD. Atherosclerosis involves 80 % of the ostium [29] and the proximal one-third of the renal artery. Renovascular hypertension and ischaemic nephropathy are most commonly seen in patients with atherosclerotic renal artery stenosis [30]. It is commonly associated with other microvascular disease including nephrosclerosis and diabetic nephropathy [31, 32]. It has been proved that high-grade ARVDs have a relationship with extrarenal vascular disease such as carotid and lower extremity arterial disease [31, 33]. One-third of the patients with heart failure exhibit ARVD [34]. In the pathogenesis of renovascular hypertension, the renin-angiotensin system is activated by a decrease in the renal perfusion pressure resulting in the release of renin and the production of angiotensin II. This leads to increased aldosterone secretion resulting in elevation of the blood pressure by expansion of the blood volume. Other mechanisms involved are increased intra-renal prostaglandin concentrations and stimulation of the sympathetic systems (Fig. 6.1).

Box 6.2. Key Points. Renovascular Diseases (RVDs) in the Elderly

- RVDs that cause end-stage renal disease are inflammatory vasculitis, nephrosclerosis, RVD atheromatous and embolic disease.
- Renal artery stenosis is the cause of renovascular hypertension in at least 90% of cases, and atherosclerotic renal artery stenosis is a disease of older individuals [6].
- High-grade ARVDs have a relationship to extrarenal vascular disease such as carotid artery disease and lower extremity arterial disease [3, 33]. One-third of patients with heart failure exhibit ARVD [34].

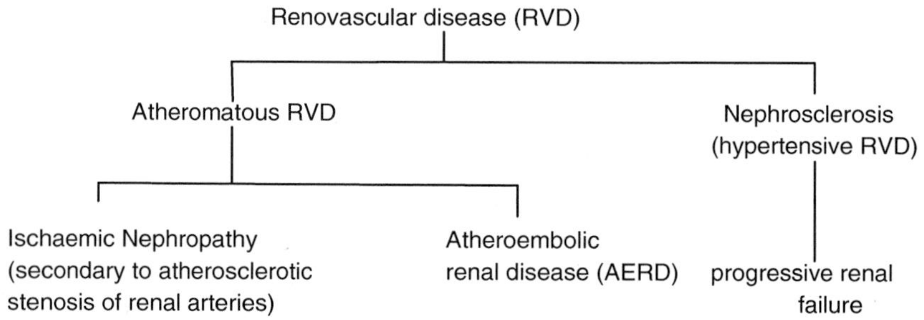

Fig. 6.1 Renovascular disease aetiology

6.4 Acute Kidney Injury (AKI)

Introduction

Acute kidney injury (AKI) also known as acute renal failure (ARF) is the loss of kidney function of abrupt onset resulting in the accumulation of waste products normally excreted by the kidney. The term AKI had been proposed to embrace the entire spectrum of syndrome from minimal changes in renal function to the need for renal replacement therapy (RRT) [35]. The Risk, Injury, Failure, Loss, End-stage Renal Disease (RIFLE) classification provides a graded definition of AKI based on physical measurement of serum creatinine or glomerular function rate (GFR) or urine output [36] and embraces the entire spectrum of acute kidney injury [37]. It has been validated in numerous studies [35]. The Acute Kidney Injury Network (AKIN) is a modification of RIFLE criteria and requires an absolute serum creatinine of 0.3 mg/l in a 48-h period for the diagnosis of AKI [38].

Pathophysiology
ARF comprises three main categories: pre-renal, renal and post-renal. Three important factors in the pathogenesis of pre-renal ARF are volume depletion, decreased effective blood volume and haemodynamic compromise. With ageing, there is an impairment in the ability to concentrate urine and conserve sodium and water. These physiological changes in the elderly make them prone to the risk of volume depletion and the pre-renal type of ARF. In pre-renal type, the kidneys are structurally normal and the impairment of renal function is due to reduced blood flow (RBF). Reduction in RBF results in lowering of the glomerular filtration pressure and decrease in glomerular filtration rate (GFR) regardless of the cause. The GFR and RBF in conditions such as in renal or effective hypovolaemia are particularly sensitive to autoregulatory mechanisms. In the elderly, there is a derangement in autoregulatory defence mechanisms which in combination with volume depletion can lead to ischaemia and AKI [39]. Andreucci et al. [40] used the term 'vasomotor nephropathy' to define ARF due to an ischaemic insult and is associated with retention of nitrogenous waste in the body following haemorrhage, severe salt depletion, burns, shock, sepsis, trauma, rhabdomyolysis, haemolytic reactions or congestive heart failure.

Vasoconstrictive hormones released as a response to systemic hypotension may have a direct effect on glomerular permeability. There is constriction of the renal afferent arterioles due to increased plasma adrenaline and stimulation of the sympathetic nerves. During the period of reduced RBF, the kidneys are vulnerable to other insults. Drugs such as NSAIDs and ACEIs can alter intra-renal haemodynamics in the elderly particularly when associated with salt depletion and hypovolaemia [40] and are can compound the combined effects of nephrotoxic drugs such as aminoglycosides or contrast agents and pre-existing volume depletion [41]. NSAID-induced ARF may be caused by acute interstitial nephritis [42] or haemodynamically mediated and may be related to the reduction of prostaglandin synthesis [43]. By relaxing the preglomerular resistance, the vasodilator prostaglandins preserve renal blood flow and glomerular filtration rate and antagonise the vasoconstrictive action of angiotensin II and norepinephrine [43].

The pathophysiology in renal or intrinsic kidney injury will depend on the specific cause and there are a variety of causes. There are two significant factors in its pathogenesis, namely, ischaemia and nephrotoxins. Acute glomerulonephritis (AGN), rapidly progressive glomerulonephritis (RPGN) and vasculitis give rise to accumulation of inflammatory cells in the glomeruli resulting in reduced glomerular filtration. In interstitial nephritis, the inflammatory reaction is confined to the interstitium. Drugs, infiltrative disease and infectious pyelonephritis are common causes of interstitial nephritis.

Acute tubular necrosis (ATN) is the most important cause of intrinsic AKI [44] and is often initiated by acute injury to the proximal tubular epithelial cells by acute ischaemic or nephrotoxic events [45]. Apart from alteration of autoregulation, the ageing tubular cells are more susceptible to ischaemic damage due to decline in the cellular antioxidant defences [46]. Detachment of the tubular epithelial cells from the basement membrane and the back-leak of the glomerular filtrate cause tubular obstruction resulting in decline in GFR [47]. The pathogenesis of ATN involves interaction of a number of processes that include endothelial injury, microvascular flow disruption, tubular hypoxia, tubular obstruction and apoptosis [44]. In response to the tubular cell injury, there is profound secondary vasoconstriction which is the predominant mechanism [45] and it is the imbalance between vasoconstrictive and vasodilator mediators and vascular obstruction caused by cell aggregation that are involved in the pathophysiology of AKI [47]. Creatinine clearance has both filtration and secretory components [48]. Slight changes in the plasma flow-dependent component of active creatinine secretion by the organic ion transport systems in the proximal tubule may be indicated by moderate changes in the serum creatinine [49] and can be seen as a biomarker for acute tubular injury [50]. Disease of the renal arteries leads to ischaemia of the kidneys resulting in reduced renal function. In the post-renal type, as the back pressure due to renal outflow obstruction increases, the GFR becomes reduced. Furthermore, the increased tubular pressure leads to decreased RBF due to reflex vasoconstriction of the afferent arterioles. Renal hypoperfusion can be reversed with adequate fluid replacement in many but some may progress to ATN and this more frequent in the elderly [51] (Fig. 6.2).

Box 6.3. Key Points. Acute Kidney Injury (AKI)

Pre-renal ARF: volume depletion, decreased effective blood volume and haemodynamic.

With ageing, there is an impairment in the ability to concentrate urine and conserve sodium and water.

These physiological changes in the elderly make them prone to the risk of volume depletion and the pre-renal type of ARF.

In the elderly, there is a derangement in autoregulatory defence mechanisms which in combination with volume depletion can lead to ischaemia and AKI [40].

Vasoconstrictive hormones released as a response to systemic hypotension may have a direct effect on glomerular permeability.

There are two significant factors in its pathogenesis, namely, ischaemia and nephrotoxins [45].

Drugs, infiltrative disease and infectious pyelonephritis are common causes of interstitial nephritis [42].

Acute tubular necrosis (ATN) is the most important cause of intrinsic ARF [44].

The pathogenesis of ATN involves interaction of a number of processes that include endothelial injury, microvascular flow disruption, tubular hypoxia, tubular obstruction and apoptosis [45].

In the post-renal type, as the back pressure increases, the GFR becomes reduced.

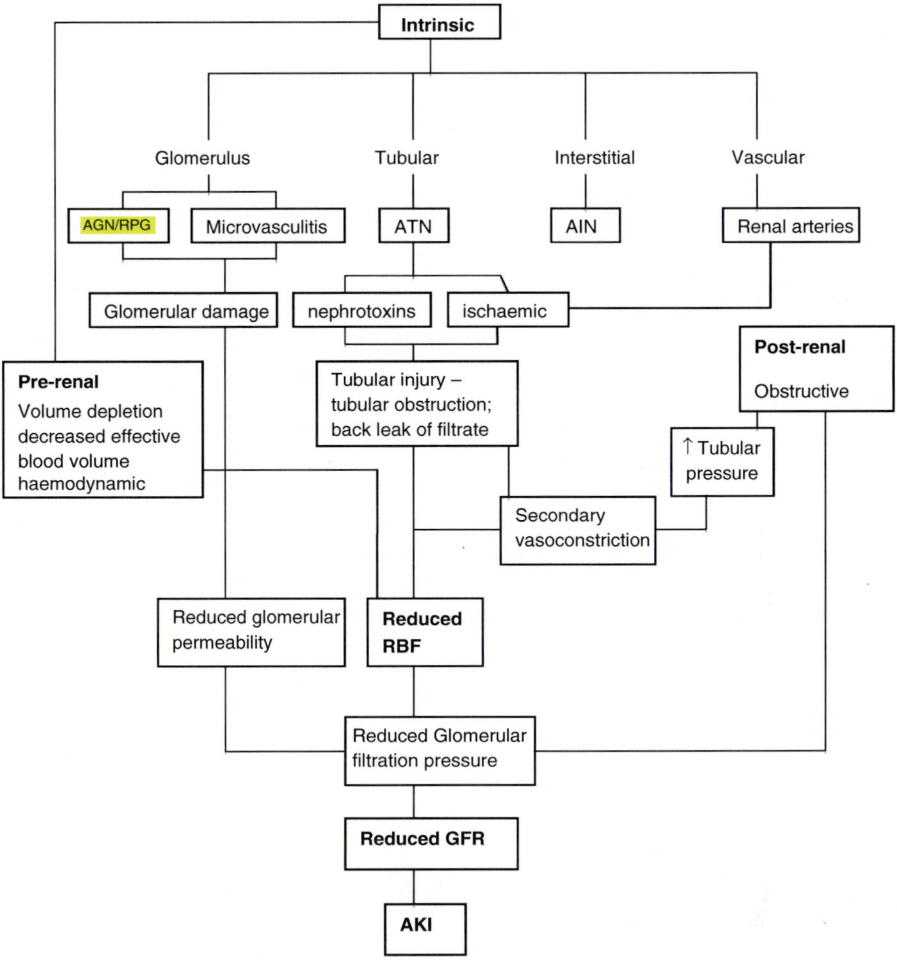

Fig. 6.2 Pathophysiology of AKI (*AGN* acute glomerulonephritis, *RPGN* rapid progressive glomerulonephritis, *ATN* acute tubular necrosis, *AIN* acute interstitial nephritis, *RBF* renal blood flow, *GFR* glomerular filtration rate, *AKI* acute kidney injury)

6.5 Chronic Kidney Disease in the Elderly

Introduction

Chronic kidney disease (CKD) is characterised by a gradual and progressive loss of renal function resulting in permanent renal failure. It is defined as kidney damage or GFR <60 ml/min/1.73 m (2) for 3 months or more irrespective of the cause [52]. According to the United States Data system [53], 48 % of patients starting dialysis were over 65 years and 20 % were over 75 years, and renal vascular disease (RVD) had emerged as the main cause of end-stage kidney disease (ESKD) in the elderly with an incidence of 38 %.

Pathophysiology
In chronic kidney disease (CKD), there is a permanent reduction in the glomerular filtration rate (GFR). Progressive renal failure eventually leads to the uraemic syndrome and end-stage kidney disease (ESKD). The complex of signs and symptoms resulting from the retention of the waste products of nitrogen metabolism is known as the uraemia.

Irrespective of the nature of the initial renal injury, any critical reduction in the functioning renal mass leads to glomerular hyperfiltration and increased single nephron GFR [54]. The single nephron GFR increases to make up for the decline of the GFR by nephron loss. There is an increase in the intraglomerular pressure in the surviving nephrons that causes proteinuria which is considered to be the pathophysiological link between glomerular, interstitial and tubular damage [55]. Furthermore, the increase in intraglomerular pressure contributes to glomerular and tubular hypertrophy [56]. Renal injury also results in the production of angiotensin II, a forceful vasoconstrictor which intensifies the level of intraglomerular pressure [55]. Vascular mechanisms involved in the pathophysiology is the imbalance between vasoconstrictor and vasodilator mediators. Glomerular pressure is controlled by the combined interplay of renal afferent and efferent arterioles. Angiotensin II also increases the glomerular and tubular expression of various factors such as cytokines, growth factors and chemokines which promote tubular interstitial inflammation and fibrosis [57, 58]. Progressive glomerular damage with local inflammation and fibrosis is the result of persistent initial injury and additional factors such as uraemia-associated vasculotoxic and inflammatory insults following endothelial and podocyte cell injury [59, 60]. A reduction in the number of nephrons beyond the critical threshold leads to further failure of the remaining nephrons. In CKD, there is a progressive loss of nephrons irrespective of the primary site of the insult, cortical or medullary. If the damage is severe enough, complete destruction of the nephrons occurs regardless of the primary site whether resulting from glomerular disease or tubular interstitial disease.

CKD is a progressive disease. Hypertension, intraglomerular pressure, proteinuria and renal damage are interrelated in the background of CKD progression. Hypertension is an important risk factor for disease progression [61, 62]. Not only the absolute blood pressure level but also the physiological nocturnal decrease (dipping) may have a role in the progression of the disease [60]. It had been shown that the severity of the proteinuria correlates with the rate of renal failure progression [61], and reduction of the risk of CKD progression seems to be associated with proteinuria reduction [62] (Fig. 6.3).

As the nephrons are lost in CKD and if there is no change in the diet or increase in excretion of solute by the remaining nephrons, sodium, potassium and phosphate would accumulate in the body and will result in symptoms. Humoral and hormonal changes aid these adaptations in the function of the remaining nephrons by decreasing absorption of the solute or increase via its secretion. The total amount of free fluid excreted decreases with the fall of the GFR and decreases in the number of nephrons in the course of the kidney disease. The kidney loses its ability to concentrate with progressive renal disease although dilution ability is well preserved till late.

Serum phosphate level rises with the fall of the GFR especially after eating, resulting in the fall of the serum calcium which promotes increase secretion of parathyroid

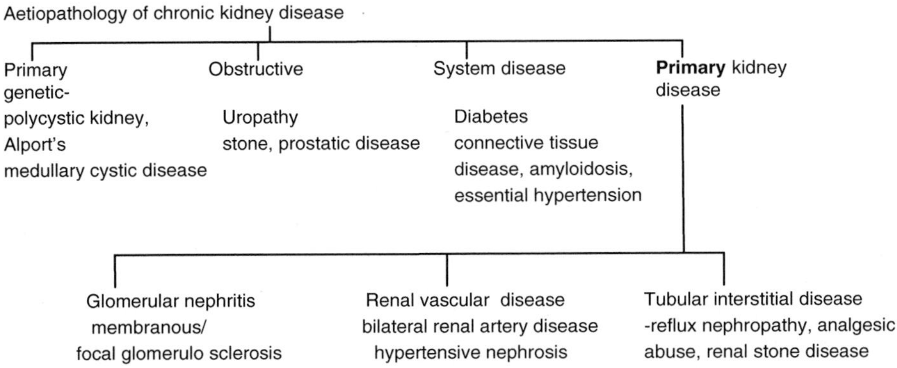

Fig 6.3 Aetiopathology of chronic kidney disease (Information sources: Lopez-Novoa et al. [63])

hormone (PTH) which in turn decreases tubular reabsorption of phosphate and returns calcium to normal. The decrease serum level of 1.25 (OH)2-Vit D3 is due to the loss of nephrons. These changes also lead to decrease in the calcium absorption from the gut. The metabolic acidosis that is present tends to increase the ionised fraction of calcium, and any rapid correction of the acidosis may lead to its fall and precipitate clinical manifestations of hypocalcaemia. Significant acidaemia does not occur until the GFR is very low. Accumulation of phosphate and other titratable acids gives rise to metabolic acidosis with an increase in the anion gap. If the anion gap is greater than about 20 mEq/l, other events such as lactic acidosis or ketosis should be sought. Renal bone disease is caused by abnormalities of calcium, phosphorus and vitamin D metabolism and secondary or tertiary hyperparathyroidism. It is associated with abnormalities in bone turn over, mineralization, linear growth and strength and extravascular complications such as vascular and soft tissue calcification [64].

A five-stage classification of chronic kidney disease by the National Kidney Foundation [65] is as follows:

Stage 1. GFR normal or increased GFR: GFR >90
Stage 2. Mild renal damage decreased GFR: GFR 60–89
Stage 3. Moderately decreased GFR: GFR 30–59
Stage 4. Severely decreased GFR : GFR 15–29
Stage 5. Kidney failure GFR<than 15 (or dialysis)

Box 6.4. Chronic Kidney Disease (CKD)

- Irrespective of the nature of the initial renal injury, any critical reduction in the functioning renal mass leads to glomerular hyperfiltration and increased single nephron GFR [54].
- The single nephron GFR increases to make up for the decline of the GFR by nephron loss.
- In CKD, there is a progressive loss of nephrons irrespective of the primary site of the insult, cortical or medullary.

- Increase in the intraglomerular pressure in the surviving nephrons induces proteinuria which is considered to be the pathophysiological link between glomerular, interstitial and tubular damage.
- Renal injury also results in the production of angiotensin II, a forceful vasoconstrictor [57, 58].
- Vascular mechanism involved in the pathophysiology is the imbalance between vasoconstrictor and vasodilator mediators.
- Hypertension is an important risk factor for disease progression [61, 62].
- Severity of the proteinuria correlates with the rate of renal failure progression [61].
- Serum phosphate level rises with the fall of the GFR.
- Increase secretion of parathyroid hormone (PTH).
- Decrease serum level of 1.25(OH)2-Vit D3.
- Accumulation of phosphate and other titratable acids gives rise to metabolic acidosis with an increase in the anion gap.
- If the anion gap is greater than about 20 mEq/l, other events such as lactic acidosis or ketosis should be sought.

6.6 Ageing and the Reproductive System

Age-related changes

I. Male reproductive system

Structural, hormonal and functional changes occur with ageing in the male reproductive system. There is thinning of the pubic hair, laxity of the scrotal tissues and wasting of the perineal muscles. The testicular mass decreases [66], the tubes undergo sclerosis [67] and the prostate gland increases in size. Benign prostate hypertrophy is an organic manifestation of male ageing and its prevalence closely equals the age [68]. The epididymis and the seminal vesicles may lose some of their surface cells. The amount of seminal fluid may remain the same but the number of living sperms may be reduced [67]. Fertility varies from one individual to another. There may be a decrease in the libido and sexual response may become less intense and slower. The testosterone level declines slowly from the age of 20–30 years [69] and after the age of 50 an approximately 0.4–0.8 % per year [70]. The circadian rhythm in the serum testosterone levels is lost in older men. In the younger men, it is higher in the mornings than in the evenings [71]. It is unclear what proportion of older men experience the low testosterone levels [72]. The LH and FSH levels are increased in older men either due to hypogonadism or to decrease hypothalamic opioid tone [68]. Erectile dysfunction may possibly be due to low testosterone levels. Fertility is not affected in the elderly apart from sperm motility, and other functional semen parameters are not affected by age [68].

II. Female reproductive system
There is atrophy of the labia, thinning of the pubic hair and laxity of the perineal muscles. The vaginal epithelia may thin and the vaginal walls become less elastic and the width and length decrease [67]. The cervix shrinks in size. The ovaries become more fibrotic and less responsive to follicle-stimulating hormone (FSH) [73] and luteinizing hormone (LH). Initially, to compensate for the decreased response, more of the hormones are produced, but they eventually decrease. In the older ovulating females, the oestrogen levels may increase initially probably due to FSH/LH alterations. The hypothalamus-pituitary-gonadal axis eventually will not be able to generate LH surge needed for follicular activity leading to a decline in the level of oestrogen secretion [67]. Menopause is characterised by cessation of menstruation and decline in oestrogen level, and by the mid-1950s, most women would have gone through menopause [67]. It is believed that senescence affects both the ovary (oocyte and granular cell) and uterus [74]. Fertility decreases and there is rapid decrease of fecundity after the age of 35 years, and with menopause the reproductive capacity is lost.

The pelvic muscles may lose tone. Some of the effects of these changes are atrophic vaginitis, dyspareunia, vaginal yeast infections, stress incontinence or frequency and uterine prolapse. Outside the reproductive system, structural targets are skin changes (thinning of the epithelium and atrophy of the sebaceous glands) and the body hair undergoes redistribution. Following menopause, the breasts decrease in size, and the connective tissue supporting the breasts decreases leading to sagging of the breasts [75]. There is cognitive and memory decline [67]. During the first decade after the onset of menopause, there is a normal age-related bone loss due to the diminished oestrogen levels giving rise to osteopenia and osteoporosis [76]. With menopause, cardioprotective effect of oestrogen is removed and these changes correspond to the increase in stroke, coronary artery disease and myocardial infarction [67]. There is loss of sex drive in many women as they go through menopause and this is thought to be related to the reduction in oestrogen and androgens [67]. However, for most women, age-related changes do not interfere with sexual activity or sexual pleasure after menopause [75]. The physiology of coitus has been categorised into four phases: excitement, plateau, orgasm and resolution [77].

6.7 Prostate Gland and Related Disorders

6.7.1 Prostate Gland

Introduction
The prostate gland is a conical structure made up of two lobes and enclosed in an outer tissue, the capsule. It sits between the bladder and the urogenital diaphragm. It is separated from the pubic symphysis by adipose tissue and its posterior surface from the rectum by the Denovilliers' fascia. The normal adult gland weighs about

20–25 g and measures 4.0–4.5 cm across, 2.0–3.0 cm in length and 2.0–2.5 cm in thickness. The adult gland is made up of glandular (70 %) and nonglandular tissue (30 %) [78], and the former is divided into three zones [78, 79]. The central zone comprises about 25 % of the gland, the peripheral zone about 70 % and the transition zone about 5 % [78]. Within the periprostatic fat in the posterolateral part of the peripheral zone are the neurovascular bundles which give off branches into the apex and base of the prostate [80]. Abutting the periurethral glands and the preprostatic sphincter is the anterior one-third of the prostate and the proximal part of the urethra. The urethra then makes an anterior angle of about 30°, and the distal part of the urethra is in contact with the peripheral zone. It secretes an alkaline fluid that comprises a large portion of the seminal fluid [78]. It serves as a conduit for the semen and also prevents retrograde ejaculation into the bladder. Superior and posterior to the prostate gland are the seminal vesicles, and their ducts enter the prostate on its posterior surface below the bladder [81].

Changes with ageing

Changes occur in the structure of the prostate gland and in the different zones in ageing. The central zone is the greatest in the young and atrophies with advancing age. The transition zone enlarges with age by developing benign prostatic hypertrophy, and the proliferative process occurs exclusively in the transition zone and periurethral glands [82, 83]. BPH is a common part of ageing, and by the age of 80 years, about 90 % of men will have histological evidence of BPH [84]. It has been postulated that testosterone plays a role in its development. As man ages, the amount of the testosterone produced decreases with proportionate increase in the oestrogen levels within the gland, and this increases the activity of the substances that promote cell growth [86]. Testosterone is converted to dihydrotestosterone (DHT) by enzyme 5 alpha reductase (5AR), and there are two types of 5 alpha reductase, and type 2 is the primary subtype in the prostate [86]. The androgen 5-alpha dihydrotestosterone (DHT) binds to the androgen receptors and can result in BPH [85]. DHT promotes development and growth of the prostate, but there is no direct correlation between DHT and possible growth [86]. BPH involves both the stromal and epithelial elements of the prostate arising in the periurethral and transition zones and is normally dependent on testosterone and DHT production. Males who are deficient in 5AR will not be able to convert intraprostatic testosterone into DHT [87] and will not develop BPH [88].

Pathophysiology

Static and dynamic factors contribute to the bladder neck obstruction in BPH [89]; the former is due to prostatic enlargement and the latter to the tension in the prostate smooth muscle [82]. In the pathophysiology of clinical BPH, the prostate and/or prostatic urethra plays an important role [82]. In vitro studies have shown that in the capsule of the prostate, the smooth muscle of the stroma and the bladder neck have localised large amounts of alpha-1 adrenergic receptors. Stimulation of these receptors gives rise to increase in the smooth muscle tone which can worsen lower urinary tract symptoms (LUTS) [85]. Some of the LUT symptoms are attributable to the ageing of the bladder and age-matched men and women have similar levels of LUTS [90]. The obstruction of the bladder contributes significantly to the symptoms; the bladder wall becomes thickened, trabeculated and irritable. It hypertrophies to increase its contractile force. Even small volumes of urine in the bladder can cause urinary frequency and LUTS because of the detrusor instability. The bladder gradually weakens and loses its ability to empty completely thus leading to increased residual urine volume.

6.7.2 Acute and Chronic Prostatitis

Introduction
Prostatitis is an inflammatory disorder: bacterial or nonbacterial and can be acute or chronic. The National Institute of Health have classified prostatitis into four categories, namely, acute bacterial, chronic bacterial, chronic nonbacterial, pelvic pain syndrome and asymptomatic inflammatory prostatitis [91, 92].

Pathophysiology
Bacterial prostatitis can be acute or chronic, and in the case of acute prostatitis, the common causal pathogens are *Klebsiella*, *staphylococcus*, *Escherichia coli*, *Pseudomonas aeruginosa* and *Enterobacter* sp [93]. In acute prostatitis, the organisms usually reach the prostate by direct extension from the posterior urethra or the bladder. In otherwise healthy individuals, *E. coli* and *staphylococcus* predominate. Chronic bacterial prostatitis is caused by the same organisms that produce acute prostatitis in addition to *Proteus* [93], and it may be a sequel to acute prostatitis. It is often associated with urinary tract infection (UTI), and relapsing UTI is a hallmark of chronic bacterial prostatitis in men. It is a believed to be due to sequestered bacteria out of reach of antibiotics [94]. There is no infectious component in chronic prostatitis or chronic pelvic pain and is categorised as inflammatory or noninflammatory (CP/CPPS) [93, 94]. Predisposing factors for CP/CPPS include infection, voiding abnormalities, intraprostatic reflux immunological or allergic triggers [95]. Nonbacterial prostatitis is more common than bacterial prostatitis and the cause is unclear. It may be due to dyssynergic voiding and incomplete relaxation of the urinary sphincter [94].

6.7.3 Prostatic Abscess

Introduction
Prostatic abscess is a focal accumulation of pus within the prostate [96]. It is reported most commonly in the age group between 50 and 60 years [97]. There has been a shift in the mortality rate from 6–30 % in the forties to 3–16 % recently [98, 99].

Pathophysiology
It usually results from urinary tract infection (*E. coli* or *Proteus*), acute prostatitis, urethritis and epididymitis. It begins as a localised process usually in the peripheral zone and may involve other areas. It may be caused as a complication of acute prostatitis [100], or a retrograde flow of contaminated urine [101]. Immunosuppressed patients, diabetics [96, 102] and patients with AIDs are vulnerable to develop prostatic abscess. More recently, the causative agents are the gram-negative bacteria such as *Escherichia coli*, whereas in the past *Staphylococcus aureus*, *Neisseria gonorrhoea* and *Mycobacterium tuberculosis* were more common [96].

6.7.4 Carcinoma of the Prostate

Introduction
Carcinoma of the prostate is the commonest known cancer affecting 30 % of men at the age of 50 and 90 % at the age of 90 years [103]. The incidence of prostate cancer increases sharply after the age of 55, peaks at age of 70–74 and slightly declines thereafter [104].

Pathology
The aetiology is not known but it increases with age. It has been suggested that hormonal changes of old age may be associated with its causation. Genetic, environmental and hormonal imbalances have been reported to have a crucial role in the pathophysiology of cancer of the prostate by producing chronic inflammation [105].

It is widely deemed that the prostatic intraepithelial neoplasia (PIN) is the most likely forerunner of invasive prostatic cancer [106]. Cellular proliferation within pre-existing ducts and glands with cytological changes characterises PIN and mimic neoplasm [107]. It is associated with phenotypic and genotypic abnormalities that are in between cancer and normal prostatic epithelium [106, 108]. Not all high-grade PIN develop into invasive disease, but high-grade PIN, age and PSA are decidedly indicative predictors of prostate cancer [108]. Prostate cancer growth and progression are dependent on androgen receptor (AR) signalling [109] and related to a number of genetic abnormalities [106]. The human AR is encoded as a single copy gene located on the X-chromosome [107], and its activity is regulated by its two major ligands, testosterone and dihydrotestosterone [109].

It is usually an adenocarcinoma and begins in the peripheral zone in 70 % of cases but can arise elsewhere and 29 % originate in the transition zone and 19 % in the central zone [110]. Histologically, most lesions are adenocarcinoma with varying degrees of differentiation. It spreads by direct extension and may involve the base of the bladder, rectal wall or the seminal vesicles. It can spread through veins and lymphatics and metastasise to the regional lymph nodes early. The axial skeleton and pelvis ribs are the usual sites of bone metastases from hematogenic spread. The bone metastases are commonly osteoblastic but may be osteolytic.

6.8 Sexuality and Sexual Dysfunction in the Elderly

Introduction
In both men and women, sexuality declines with age. The waning sexuality is more in terms of consistency, frequency and vigour than to desire [111, 112]. For many men and women, the capacity and desire to engage in sex continue throughout life, and sexual relations end only with death. Sexuality is associated with more than procreation and sexual intercourse. It entails an array of facets that includes tenderness, warmth, emotion, passion and touching and sharing feelings.

6.8.1 Sexual Dysfunction with Ageing

The sexual response in both male and female elderly is generally slow and of diminished intensity (Table 6.1).

6.8.1.1 Sexual Dysfunction in the Elderly Male

Anatomy
The penis is made up of the two cylindrical-like structures, the corpus cavernosa enclosed by a tough thick sheath, the tunica albuginea [116]. The corpus spongiosum contains the urethra and lies in the groove created by the corpus cavernosa. As this structure approaches the end, it becomes swollen to become the glans penis [117]. At the other end, it expands to form the bulb. Covering all three structures is a tough membrane, the Buck's fascia [117] and this is covered further by the Colles fascia or superficial layer and is continuous with the abdominal wall. The body of the penis is anchored to the pubic bone. The penile artery branches into the cavernosal arteries which open directly into the cavernous spaces. From here, the post-cavernous venules coalesce to form larger veins which pierce the tunica albuginea to join the deep dorsal vein [116].

In humans, the spinal nuclei for control of erection is situated in the intermediolateral grey matter of S2–S4 and T10–L2 levels [118]. The penis is innervated by the sympathetic, parasympathetic and the somatosensory nerves. The sympathetic originates on the thoracolumbar segments, T_{11}–L_2, and via the white rami of the sympathetic chain ganglia to the superior hypogastric plexus from which arises the hypogastric nerve which in turn joins the pelvic plexus. The parasympathetic arises from the sacral segments S2–S4 and the preganglionic fibres and the pelvic nerves to form the pelvic plexus and together with the hypogastric nerve form the cavernous nerves [118]. The cavernous nerves innervate the cavernous smooth muscles of the penis, the smooth muscles of the arteries and arterioles and the walls of the corpus cavernosa and corpus spongiosum. The parasympathetic input is responsible for tumescence and sympathetic for detumescence [119]. Cerebral impulses travel through sympathetic (inhibiting norepinephrine release), parasympathetic

Table 6.1 Age-related changes in sexual response in the elderly

	Male	Female
Sexual dysfunction	Erectile dysfunction or loss of libido	Dyspareunia, vaginismus
Excitement/arousal	Slow to achieve erection less spontaneous, requiring direct stimulation	Delayed onset of vaginal lubrication, may be induced by stimulation of clitoris
Plateau	Lasts longer and greater ability to stimulate partner	Prolonged
Orgasm	Ejaculation less forceful shorter in duration	Orgasm delayed
Resolution	Erection rapidly lost	Quite rapid
Refractory period	Prolonged 24 h to 1 week	Prolonged
Level of pleasure	No change	No change

Information sources: Applegate [113], Master and Johnson [114], King [115]

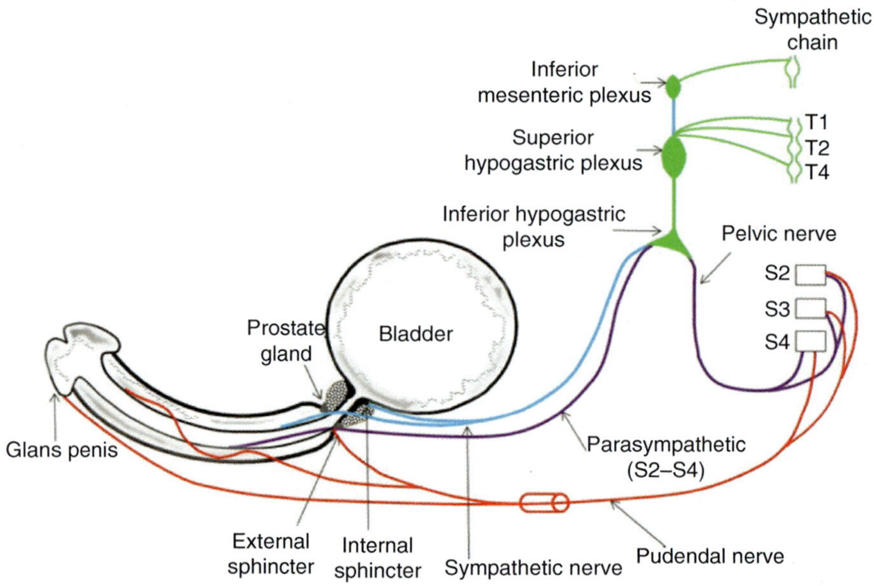

Fig. 6.4 Neuroanatomy and physiology of normal erectile function

(releasing nitric oxide and acetylcholine) and somatic (releasing acetylcholine) pathways to produce normal erection [120] (Fig. 6.4).

The nerve fibres from the sensory receptors situated in the penile skin, glans penis and the corpus cavernosa converge to form the dorsal nerve of the penis which join other nerves to form the pudendal nerve. The pudendal nerve conveys the impulses via the spinal cord, the spinothalamic tract, thalamus and to the sensory cortex for sensory perception [120].

Neurophysiology
The cavernous smooth muscles and the smooth muscles of the arteries and arterioles are in the flaccid state and are tonically contracted by the sympathetic. Relaxation of muscle tone (cavernosa and arterial) will increase the flow of blood into the lacunar spaces of the corpus cavernosa expanding the trabecular walls against the tunica albuginea which compresses the draining venules. The outflow of blood is thereby restricted increasing the intracavernous pressure and raises the penis (full erection phase). Initiation and maintenance of erection is a parasympathetic event [119]. Further increase of pressure with contraction of the ischiocavernosus and bulbospongiosus muscles causes the penis to become rigid (rigid erection phase), and this is achieved with additional pudendal nerve stimulation [119, 121].

Several neurotransmitters are involved in the mediation of supraspinal influences and modulation of the spinal reflex [122]. Nitric oxide is an important neural mediator for penile smooth muscle relaxation and therefore of erection [123, 124] and noradrenaline released by the sympathetic contracts penile smooth muscle fibres [125]. Serotonin and oxytocin are the neurotransmitters involved in the supraspinal control of erection [125]. During detumescence, there is a transient increase in the intracavernous pressure indicating the beginning of smooth muscle contraction. This is followed by reopening of the venous channels and a fast pressure decrease leads to a fully restored venous outflow [120]. The spinal cord is a major site for the neural regulation of penile erection [125]. The thoracolumbar sympathetic and lumbosacral parasympathetic nuclei receive projections from the brain stem, pons and hypothalamus [125]. Genital afferents or descending commands from higher CNS sites may activate the spinal erectile centres [126], but basically erection is a spinal reflex [127].

Sacral centres moderate erections in response to direct genital stimulation and is under sacral parasympathetic control. The trabecular smooth muscle contractions necessary for ejaculation are under sympathetic control. Ejaculation consists of two phases, emission and expulsion under the control of the autonomic and somatocentral nervous system [128]. Emission is made up of secretions and spermatozoa from the seminal vesicles, vas deferens, prostate and epididymis. The neural control is via the sympathetic and parasympathetic, influenced by central mechanisms and activated by stimuli from the genitals mainly the penis [128]. In the second phase, expulsion is considered to be a spinal reflex consisting of afferent and efferent structures made up of sympathetic and parasympathetic fibres. The controlling neural centres are in the lumbosacral and thoracolumbar regions and influenced by supraspinal regions [128]. The striated muscles outside the tunica albuginea are innervated by lumbosacral somatic nerves. The sympathetic impulse via the hypogastric plexus causes contraction of the internal sphincter and prevents retrograde ejaculation. During the sexual arousal phase, the parasympathetic tone increases and sympathetic is inhibited and the penis becomes erect. Nitric oxide (NO) plays an important role in the relaxation of the penile smooth muscle and thereby erection [123, 124], and endothelium NO is essential to maintain erection [127]. The blood flow to the penis increases causing the spongy erectile tissue to swell. The expanding cavernosa compresses the subtunical venous plexus against the tunica albuginea causing obstruction to the outflow of blood and results in penile rigidity. This is the plateau phase, followed by orgasm which is the emotional experience and is accompanied by ejaculation when the semen is expelled through the urethra by the rhythmic contractions of the pelvic muscles. This is followed by resolution when the penis detumescence and the body returns to the non-arousal state. In the refractory period, the penis is unresponsive to sexual stimulation that lasts about 25 min in a male aged 25 years, and this increases as age increases [129], and at the age of 55, the refractory period is between 24 h to about a week [130]. Ejaculation involves a coordinated contraction of many different components including the smooth muscles of the seminal vesicles, vasa deferentia, ejaculatory ducts, and ischiocavernosus and bulbocavernosus muscles.

6.8.2 Erectile Dysfunction (ED)

Introduction

Erectile dysfunction (ED) is characterised by an inability to attain and sustain an erection sufficient for satisfactory sexual intercourse. There is a worldwide increase in erectile dysfunction. The prevalence of ED increases with age. It increases by 10 % per year of age [131]; it increased from 2 % in age group 18–38 years to 48 % in over 70 years and older [132]. In a large population-based study of 108,477 Australian men, the investigators reported that ED increased considerably with age [133]. Approximately one in five Australians over 40 years experience ED [134].

Pathophysiology

Organic causes account for a large proportion of erectile dysfunction in the elderly than in the young. Any reduction to the blood flow (as in atherosclerosis) or injury to nerves or interference of nerve function such as in spinal cord trauma, diabetic neuropathy, pelvic surgery and multiple sclerosis has the potential to cause ED. Ageing, hypertension, smoking, hypercholesterolaemia, diabetes and structural changes in the penile issue conditions that are associated with reduced function of the endothelium can contribute to ED [132]. Organic causes include cardiovascular diseases, diabetes, renal failure, spinal cord trauma, complications of surgery, drug- or alcohol-induced dysfunction, among others. Smoking and heavy consumption of alcohol can cause ED by damaging the nerves and arteries of the penis [135]. Many factors may interfere with erection, and not uncommonly, there may be two or more factors present at the same time (Box. 6.5).

Box 6.5. Risk Factors in Men
Cardiovascular disease
Hormonal disorders
Systemic disease [132]
Neurological disorders
Localised conditions
Psychosocial problems
Drugs/alcohol/smoking

Cardiovascular diseases, hypertension, ischaemic heart disease and peripheral vascular disease are frequently associated with ED. Forty percent of the diabetic men aged 60 years or over had ED all the time [136]. Medications cause erectile problems in about 25 % of clinic patients [137]. Drugs and medications used to treat hypertension, hypercholesterolaemia, depression and psychiatric disorders are often associated with ED. About 10–20 % of patients on thiazide diuretic may be affected by ED [138]. Tricyclic antidepressants and monoamine oxidase inhibitors , benzodiazepines and selective serotonin reuptake inhibitors are known to cause erectile failure, decreased libido and ejaculatory problems [116]. Anabolic steroids either due to a direct effect on the penis or by suppression of normal androgen production can cause ED [139]. Recreational drugs such as cocaine, heroin, amphetamines, marijuana, alcohol and tobacco can cause ED and depress the brain's response to sexual stimulus [135]. Surgery radical prostatectomy and bowel or bladder surgery for cancer can injure arteries and nerves to the penis. Localised disease of the penis such as Peyronie's disease often interferes with erection [116]. Lifestyle changes that contribute to cardiac diseases and vascular disease such as cigarette smoking and overweight can interfere with the functioning of the muscle cells of the penis.

Psychogenic causes though less common are often related to a distinct precipitating event. In older men, often with psychogenic component is usually secondary to an organic cause [140]. Stress, anxiety, feeling of guilt, low esteem, depression, fear of sexual failure, anxiety about sexual prowess and self consciousness are associated with ED. Depression in men is associated with decrease in erectile capacity which may be associated with significant sexual dysfunction [141]. In the elderly, psychogenic cause is often secondary to an organic cause. There may be a physical cause that makes the individual anxious which makes the problem worse. RhoA/Rho kinase place an important role in the regulation of cavernous smooth muscle, and changes in this pathway can contribute to ED in patient subgroups such as diabetes and vascular disease [132].

Box 6.6. Key Points. Erectile Dysfunction

- Erectile dysfunction is a common problem in general medical practice.
- Organic causes account for a large proportion of erectile dysfunction in the elderly than in the young.
- Ageing, hypertension, smoking, hypercholesterolaemia, diabetes and structural changes in the penile tissue conditions that are associated with reduced function of the endothelium can contribute to ED.
- Surgery radical prostatectomy and bowel or bladder surgery for cancer can injure arteries and nerves of the penis.
- Psychogenic causes though less common are often related to a distinct precipitating event.
- The evaluation of nocturnal erections is important which is lost in organic impotence.

Information sources: Weber et al. [133]; Lavelle [135].

6.9 Urinary Incontinence and Voiding Problems in the Elderly

Introduction

The International Continence Society (ICS) had defined urinary incontinence as a condition in which involuntary loss of urine is a social and hygienic problem and is objectively demonstrable [142]. Urinary incontinence is one of the biggest challenges facing the elderly population, and several epidemiological studies have shown a high prevalence of urinary incontinence in the elderly, especially among women. It increases with age and was found to be 17 % in men and 48 % in women 70 years of age, and women had eight times higher odds of having urinary incontinence than men when all ages 70–97 were pooled [143]. At least 15 % of community-dwelling elderly and 50 % of institutionalised elderly have significant incontinence [144]. The prevalence of urinary incontinence among the elderly in rural community in Malaysia is about 9 % [145, 146]. Double incontinence (urinary and faecal) is common in community-residing elderly in Japan [147] and in the Netherlands [148] and increases with age.

Anatomy of the Bladder

The detrusor muscle of the bladder consists of three layers of smooth muscle fibres. A thin layer of areolar tissue separates it from the inner mucosal layer. The mucosal layer is loosely attached to the muscle layer that it falls into folds known as the rugae. Between the two ureteral orifices is an area called the trigone. The internal urethral sphincter is found in the neck of the bladder and is formed by thickening of the detrusor muscle.

Neuroanatomy

The corticoregulatory tract of micturition originates in the frontal cortex (areas 6 and 9) and descends to the pontine micturition centre in the brain stem and then to the neurons of the Onuf's nucleus to finally synapse at the spinal cord centres in the S2, S3 and S4 spinal segments at the lateral horns cells from which emanates the pelvic nerves. The pontine micturition centre also receives input from the periaqueductal grey (PAG) in the hypothalamus. The preganglionic parasympathetic fibres travel with the pelvic nerves through the inferior hypogastric plexus to synapse with the postganglionic neurons in the adventitia of the detrusor and internal sphincter. The prescaral nerves or sympathetic originate from the lower lumbar regions (L1–L2) to travel to the superior hypogastric plexus from which arises the hypogastric nerve. The hypogastric nerve consists of two distinct sympathetic receptors, the alpha-adrenergic receptors to the trigone and proximal urethra (increases tone) and the beta-receptor to the body of the urinary bladder (reduces tone causing relaxation). The somatic innervation is from the pudendal nerve which is from the primary rami of S2–S4 and supplies the external sphincter. Three important components that play a major role in the maintenance of continence are the detrusor muscle, internal sphincter and the external sphincter.

Neurophysiology

Normal micturition occurs in two phases. In the first phase of bladder filling, the bladder detrusor muscle relaxes and the urethral sphincter contracts. The parasympathetic system through its cholinergic fibres from the pelvic nerve and stimulation of the beta-adrenergic fibres of the sympathetic system relaxes the detrusor muscle. The sympathetic system through its alpha-adrenergic fibres contracts the smooth muscle sphincter. The somatic nerve system contracts the striated muscle sphincter through the cholinergic fibres of the pudendal nerve. When the bladder fills, the stretch receptors of the detrusor muscle are stimulated and afferent impulses are conveyed to the brain via the pelvic nerves. The brain inhibits voiding until an appropriate time and place and then promotes input from the bladder to initiate and complete voiding. The first phase actually involves relaxation of the pelvic floor muscles, which precedes contracture of the detrusor muscle. The second phase is the voiding when the detrusor muscle contracts through the parasympathetic cholinergic fibres and the sphincters relax through the inhibition of the alpha fibres (Fig. 6.5). Modulation of the micturition reflex in the central nervous system is through various transmitters such as dopamine, serotonin, norepinephrine, GABA acetylcholine, neuropeptides, among others [149]. The parasympathetic pelvic nerve stimulates the detrusor muscle of the bladder to contract and is mediated by M3 muscarinic receptors being activated by acetylcholine and the purinergic receptors activated by adenosine triphosphate and the urethral smooth muscle is mediated by nitric oxide (NO) to relax (Fig. 6.5) [150].

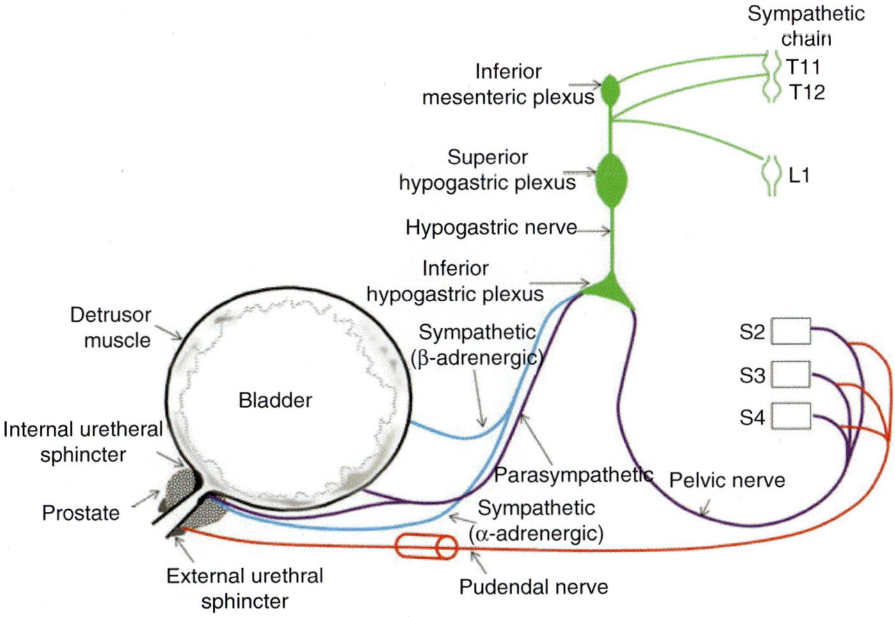

Fig. 6.5 Neuroanatomy and physiology of normal micturition

Age-related changes
The urinary bladder and pelvic structures undergo specific alterations which are related to the ageing process even without disease. In both men and women, the ability to postpone voiding, bladder capacity and urinary flow rate decline with age. The number of sporadic contractions of the bladder that are not blocked rises with age resulting sometimes with episodes of incontinence [151]. The postvoid residual urine increases to no more than 50–100 ml. In women, the urethral closure pressure and urethral length and the ability of the urinary sphincter to close tightly probably decline [149], and in men, there is enlargement of the prostate. These result in increased risk of urinary urgency, incontinence, urinary tract infection and nocturnal polyuria [152]. However, urinary incontinence should not be considered as a part of the ageing process.

In the elderly, the risk factors for urinary incontinence are multifactorial, among them being age-related changes, comorbidity, polypharmacy and functional impairments [153]. Urinary incontinence is often attributable to medical problems or disease and general impairment of health [154, 155], many of which are more common among older adults and could disrupt the mechanisms of continence. Medications, impaired mobility, falls, and comorbidity such as depression, stroke, transient ischaemic attacks, dementia and heart failure are risk factors for urinary incontinence in older people [156]. Damage to the bladder efferent nerves in the pelvis, as in infiltrative cancer, produces a flaccid bladder and sphincter, with constant dribbling. In men, stress incontinence is uncommon and may be associated with neurological disease, tumour or prior surgery to the prostate. Radical prostatectomy is complicated by urinary incontinence in a range of 5–34 % [157] and following transurethral resection in less than 1 % of patients [158]. In a study of a large cohort [159] of 64,396 women, Mathews et al. found that incontinence was primarily associated with advanced age, decompensating medical conditions, depression and multiparity. Men mostly tend to have urge incontinence, but women suffer from both urge and stress incontinence. Men do not have stress incontinence for the anatomical reason in that their urethra is long and tortuous with the sphincter and prostate helping to prevent urine loss [160]. In women, the short and straight urethra and the less effective sphincter together with pregnancies are reason for the stress incontinence [161]. In frail elderly, detrusor hyperactivity with impaired contractility (DHIC) leads to increased postvoidal residual urine [162].

Types of Incontinence
It is useful to categorise the problem into urge, stress, mixed and overflow incontinence. With urge incontinence, there is a strong desire to void and an inability to inhibit leakage of urine at unexpected times. The detrusor may also contribute to urgency due to increased afferent signalling, and urge incontinence is the most common form in older men and increases with age [163]. In stress incontinence, the loss of urine is caused by activities such as exercise, coughing, laughing and sneezing and associated with increased intra-abdominal pressure and decreases with age [163]. In older women, parity hardly contributes to stress incontinence compared to the younger and middle aged [163]. Combination of both stress and urge is mixed incontinence and common in the younger-old women, and with increasing age, it remains stable [163]. The third type of incontinence is overflow incontinence. Overflow incontinence

is the involuntary loss of small amounts of urine, or a constant leak from a full bladder. This results from inability of the bladder to empty completely or when the flow of urine is blocked. The causes include benign hypertrophy of the prostate, medications such as sedatives, antidepressants, antipsychotics and anticholinergics, neurological causes such as spinal cord injuries and medical conditions such as diabetes and multiple sclerosis. They have frequent or constant dribbling of urine. Another type of incontinence is functional incontinence. Persons with physical disability or a medical condition may have difficulty in reaching the toilet (Table 6.2).

Box 6.7. Key Points. Urinary Incontinence

- Urinary incontinence should not be considered as a part of the ageing process.
- Urinary incontinence is often attributable to medical problems or disease and general impairment of health, many of which are more common among older adults and could disrupt the mechanisms of continence [154–156].
- It is useful to categorise the problem into urge, stress, mixed and overflow incontinence.
- In frail elderly, detrusor hyperactivity with impaired contractility (DHIC) leads to increased postvoidal residual urine [162].
- Men mostly tend to have urge incontinence, but women suffer from both urge and stress incontinence [163].

Table 6.2 Types of urinary incontinence, cause and effect

Type	Pathophysiology	Cause	Effect
STRESS	Malfunction of the urethral sphincter	Pelvic prolapse, urethral hypermobility, intrinsic sphincter deficiency due to alpha-adrenergic-blocking drugs, surgical trauma	Urine leak with increase of intra-abdominal pressure, e.g. coughing, laughing, sneezing, lifting
URGE	Uncontrolled bladder contractions (detrusor overactivity)	Infection, calculi, malignancy, atrophic vaginitis/urethritis	Involuntary leakage of large amounts of urine, with a strong desire to void
	Impaired central system	Drugs, hypoxaemia, encephalopathy, neurological conditions like stroke, Parkinson's, dementia	
OVERFLOW	Urine retention, bladder distension	Obstruction to outflow – prostate, faecal impaction, bladder denervation (tumours, radiation, surgery, diabetic neuropathy medications) – anticholinergics, Ca channel blockers	Loss of small amounts of urine, frequent or constant dribbling

Information sources: Kuchel and Du Be [163]

Multiple Choice Questions

1. In the elderly, the following age- related changes in renal function are true, EXCEPT:
   A. There is a decrease in the glomerular filtration rate (GFR) with ageing.
   B. The ability of the postglomerular vasculature to dilate to stimuli such as nitric oxide is reduced.
   C. The effective renal plasma flow increases with ageing.
   D. After the age of 40, there is a decline in the creatinine clearance of about 1 ml/min per year.
2. The following causes of acute kidney injury (AKI) are true, EXCEPT:
   A. Volume depletion from vomiting and diarrhoea.
   B. Acute tubular necrosis (ATN) is not a common cause in the elderly.
   C. The use of ACE inhibitors in patients with small- and large-vessel renal arterial disease.
   D. Postrenal obstructive causes with increase in age and is important.
3. The distinction between acute and chronic kidney disease may not be clear. Which of the following suggest chronic rather than acute?
   A. History of chronic kidney disease.
   B. Presence of normocytic normochromic anaemia.
   C. Low serum phosphatase.
   D. Ultrasound may reveal bilaterally small kidneys.
4. The following in relation to acute kidney injury (AKI) are true, EXCEPT:
   A. 50–60 % of patients with AKI treated with some form of RRT die.
   B. Acute tubular necrosis (ATN) is the result of acute injury to the distal renal tubular epithelial cells.
   C. NSAID-induced AKI is often haemodynamically mediated but may be caused by acute interstitial nephritis.
   D. The diagnosis today of AKI rests on the serum creatinine which is a perfect marker of GFR.
5. The following are true in relation to the benign hypertrophy of the prostate (BHP), EXCEPT:
   A. BPH is a common part of ageing, and by the age of 80 years, about 90 % of the men will have histological evidence of BPH.
   B. Testosterone is converted to dihydrotestosterone (DHT) by enzyme, 5 alpha reductase (5AR).
   C. Males who are deficient in 5AR will not be able to convert intraprostatic testosterone into DHT and will develop BPH.
   D. BPH involves both the stromal and epithelial elements of the prostate arising in the periurethral and transition zones.
6. The following are true in relation to cancer of the prostate, EXCEPT:
   A. The incidence of prostate cancer increases sharply after the age of 55 and peaks at the age of 70–74 and increasing thereafter.
   B. Genetic, environmental and hormonal imbalances have been reported to have a crucial role in the pathophysiology of cancer of the prostate.

C. It is widely deemed the prostatic intraepithelial neoplasia (PIN) is the most likely forerunner of invasive prostatic cancer.
D. It is usually an adenocarcinoma and begins in the peripheral zone in 70 % of cases but can arise elsewhere and 29 % originate in the transition zone and 19 % in the central zone.

7. In the elderly, erectile dysfunction may be associated with the following, EXCEPT:
   A. In the elderly, psychogenic cause is often secondary to an organic cause.
   B. Ageing, hypertension, smoking, hypercholesterolaemia, diabetes and structural changes in the penile tissue.
   C. Surgery radical prostatectomy and bowel or bladder surgery.
   D. Drinking alcohol occasionally.
8. A 68-year-old woman complains of 'bladder problems'. She revealed that the urinary loss occurred when coughing or laughing. She was obese and had hypertension which was well controlled on amlodipine . On examination, she was alert and her blood pressure was 130/ 84 mmHg. The MMSE was 29/30. Which additional finding would suggest a diagnosis of stress incontinence rather than urge incontinence?
   A. In stress incontinence, the urine incontinent volume will be smaller than urge incontinence.
   B. In stress incontinence, there is a strong desire to void.
   C. In stress incontinence, there is obstruction to outflow.
   D. Stress incontinence is due to uncontrolled bladder contractions.
9. A 78-year-old woman was accompanied by her daughter with inability to hold her urine. She had suffered a stroke 6 months ago which had left her with restricted mobility. She has had three incidents of urinary incontinence and in all three occasions she had been out in the garden watering the plants. She has in all probably:
   A. Stress incontinence
   B. Mixed incontinence
   C. Overflow incontinence
   D. Functional incontinence

Answers to MCQs

1 = C; 2 = B; 3 = C; 4 = D; 5 = C; 6 = A; 7 = D; 8 = C; 9 = D

References

Anatomical and Physiological Changes with Ageing

1. Epstein M. Aging and the kidney. J Am Soc Nephrol. 1996;7(8):1106–22 (abstract).
2. Lameire N, Hoste E, Van Lo A, Dhondt A, Bernaert P, Vanholder R, et al. Pathophysiology, causes and prognosis of acute renal failure in the elderly. Ren Fail. 1996;8:333–46.

3. Abdel-Kader K, Palevsky P. Acute kidney injury in the elderly. Clin Geriatr Med 2009;25(3): 331–5.
4. Godin M, Moulin B, Etienne I, Fillastre JP. Renal aging in man. Presse Med. 1992;21(26):1246–8 (abstract).
5. Dunnill MS, Halley W. Some observations on the quantitative anatomy of the kidney. J Pathol. 1973;11:121.
6. Porush JG, Faubert PF. Renal disease in elderly patients. Rev Clin Gerontol. 1997;7(4):299–307 (abstract).
7. Bolton WK, Sturgill BC. Spontaneous glomerular sclerosis in aging Sprague–Dawley rats. Am J Pathol. 1980;98:339–50.
8. Hollenberg NK, Adams DF, Solomons HS, Rashid A, Abrams HL, Merrill JP. Senescence in renal vasculature in normal man. Circ Res. 1974;34:309–76.
9. Martin JE, Sheaff MT. Renal ageing. J Pathol. 2007;211(2):198–205 (abstract).
10. Lubran MM. Renal function in the elderly. Ann Clin Lab Sci. 1995;25(2):122–33.
11. Lindeman BD, Tobin I, Shock NW. Longitudinal study in the rate of decline in renal function with age. J Am Geriatr Soc. 1985;33:278–85.
12. Kleiston JT, Bode-Boger SM, Haller H, Fliser D. Functional changes in the ageing kidney: is there a role for asymmetric dimethylarginine? Nephrol Dial Transplant. 2003;18(7):1245–8.
13. Gardiner SM, Kemp PA, Bennett T, Palmer RM, Macada S. Regional and cardiac haemodynamic effects of NG, NG,dimethyl-L-arginine and their reversibility by vasodilators in conscious rats. Br J Pharmacol. 1993;110:1457–62.
14. Darnmady EM, Offer J, Woodhouse MA. The parameters of the aging kidney. J Pathol. 1973;109:195–207.
15. Spitzer A, Brandis M. Functional and morphological maturation of the superficial nephrons. J Clin Invest. 1974;53:279–87.
16. Mudler WJ, Hillen HF. Renal function and renal disease in the elderly: part 1. Eur J Intern Med. 2001;12:86–97.
17. Inserra F, Romano LA, de Cavanagh EM EM, Ercole L, Ferder LF, Gomez RA. Renal interstitial sclerosis in aging: effects of enalapril and nifedipine. J Am Soc Nephrol. 1996;7:676–80.
18. Luckey AE, Parsa CJ. Fluid and electrolytes in the aged. Arch Surg. 2003;138:1055–60.

Glomerular Disease in the Elderly

19. Abrass CK. Renal biopsy in the elderly. Am J Kidney Dis. 2000;35:544–6.
20. Sabins SG, Antonoiych TT. A study of 500 cases of kidney diseases in the elderly. Geriatr Nephrol Urol. 1993;3(1):15–22.
21. Davison AM. Renal disease in the elderly. Nephron. 1998;50:6–16 (abstract).
22. Sanchez-Fructuoso A, Macia M, Blanco J, Barrientos A. Glomerular disease in the elderly: incidence and clinicopathologic findings: a 20 year retrospective study. Geriatr Nephrol Urol. 1993;3(2):65–70.
23. Prakesh J, Singh AK, Saxena RK, Usha. Glomerular diseases in the elderly in India. Int J Urol Nephrol. 2000;353:283–8.

Renovascular Disease in the Elderly

24. American College of Cardiology/American Heart Association. ACC/AHA. Pocket Guidelines-Management of patients with peripheral arterial disease. American College of Cardiology Foundation and American Heart Association, Inc. March 2006.
25. Schmidt RT, Siman SS. Renovascular hypertension. eMedicine. 2008.
26. United States Renal Data System 1997. Annual data report. Am J Kidney Dis. 1997; 30(Suppl 1):S1–213.

27. Textor SC, Wilcox CS. Renal artery stenosis: a common treatable cause for renal failure? Annu Rev Med. 2001;52:421–42 (abstract).
28. Woolfson RG. Renal failure in atherosclerotic renovascular disease: pathogenesis, diagnosis and intervention. Postgrad Med J. 2001;77:68–74.
29. Eardley KS, Lipkin GW. Atherosclerotic renal artery stenosis: is it worth diagnosing? J Hum Hypertens. 1999;13(4):217–20 (abstract).
30. Bośmans JL, De Broe ME. Renovascular hypertension: diagnostic and therapeutic challenges. JBR-BTR. 2004;87(1):32–5 (abstract).
31. Olin JW, Melia M, Young JR, Graor RA, Risius B. Prevalence of atherosclerotic renal artery stenosis in patients with atherosclerosis elsewhere. Am J Med. 1990;88:46N–51.
32. Sawicki PT, Kaiser S, Heinemann L, Frenzel H, Berger M. Prevalence of renal artery stenosis in diabetes mellitus-an autopsy study. J Intern Med. 1991;229:489–92.
33. Zierler RE, Bergelin RO, Polissar NL, Beach KW, Caps MT, Cantwell-Gab K, et al. Carotid and lower extremity arterial disease in patients with renal artery atherosclerosis. Arch Intern Med. 1998;158:761–7.
34. Zoccali C, Mallamaci F, Finocchiaro P. Atherosclerotic renal artery stenosis: epidemiology, cardiovascular outcomes and clinical prediction rules. JASN. 2002;1:S179–83.

Acute Kidney Injury (AKI)

35. Kellum JA. Acute kidney injury. Crit Care Med. 2008;36:S141–5.
36. Peacock Jr PR, Sinert R. Renal failure, acute. http://emedicine.mediscape.com/article/777845-overview.
37. Kellum JA, Heste EA. Acute kidney injury: epidemiology and assessment. Scand J Clin Lab Invest. 2008;241(Suppl):6–11 (abstract).
38. Chung KK, Stewart IJ, Gisler C, Simmons JW, Aden JK, Tolley MA, et al. The Acute Kidney Injury Network (AKIN) criteria applied in burns. J Burns Care Res. 2012;33(4):483–94.
39. Lameire N, Van Hoste E, Loo A, Dondt A, Bernaert P, Vanholder R. Pathophysiology, causes and prognosis of acute renal failure in the elderly. Ren Fail. 1996;18:333–46.
40. Andreucci VE, Fuiano G, Russo D, Andrecucci M. Vasomotor nephropathy. Nephrol Dial Transplant. 1998;13 Suppl 7:17–24.
41. Anderson S. Fluid and electrolyte disorders in the elderly. In: Kokko JP, Tannen RL, editors. Fluid and electrolytes. Philadelphia: Saunders; 1996. p. 831–9.
42. Mandal AK, Baig M, Koutoubi Z. Management of acute renal failure in the elderly. Treatment options. Drugs Aging. 1998;9(4):219–50 (abstract).
43. Rose BD, Post TW. NSAIDS: acute kidney injury (acure renal failure). And nephrotic syndrome. http://wwwupdate.com/patients/content/topic.do?topicKey=gjS/LK_CKVuPo. Retrieved 18 May 2009.
44. Cheung CM, Ponnusamy A, Anderton JG. Management of acute renal failure in the elderly patient: a clinicians guide. Drug Aging. 2008;25(6):455–76 (abstract).
45. Bidani A, Churchill PC. Acute renal failure. Dis Mon. 1989;35:57–132.
46. Miura K, Goldstein RS, Morgan DG, Pasino DA, Hewitt WR, Hook JB, et al. Age-related differences in susceptibility to renal ischaemia in rats. Toxicol Appl Pharmacol. 1987;87:284–96.
47. Halfer M, Schelling G. Acute kidney failure. Physiopathology-clinical diagnosis-therapy. Anaesthetist. 2000;49(4):349–52 (abstract).
48. Serdar MA, Kurt I, Ozcelik E, Urhan M, Ilgan S, Yenicesu M. A practical approach to glomerular filtration rate measurements: creatinine clearance estimation using cimetidine. Ann Clin Lab Sci. 2001;31:265–73.
49. Urakami Y, Kimura N, Okuda M, Inui K. Creatinine transport by basolateral organic cation transporter hOCT2 in the human kidney. Pharm Res. 2004;21:976–81.

50. Warnock DG. Towards a definition and classification of acute kidney injury. J Am Soc Nephrol. 2005;16:3149–50.
51. Macias-Nunez JF, Lopez-Novoa JM, Mariinez-Maldonado M. Acute renal failure in the aged. Semin Nephrol. 1996;16(4):330–4.

Chronic Kidney Disease in the Elderly

52. Levey AS, Eckardt KU, Tsukamoto Y, Levin A, Coresh J, Rossert J, et al. Definition classification of chronic kidney disease: a positive statement from Kidney Disease: Improving Global Outcomes (KDIGO). Kidney Int. 2005;67(6):2089–100.
53. United States Renal Data System 1997. Annual Data Report. Am J Kidney Dis. 1997;30(Suppl. 1):S1–213.
54. Hostetter TH, Olson TL, Renuke HG, Venkatachalam MA, Brenner BH. Hyperfiltration in emanant nephrons: a potential adverse response to renal ablation. Am J Physiol. 1981;241:F85–93.
55. Remazzi G, Bratam T. Pathophysiology of progressive nephropathies. NEJM. 1998;339: 1448–56.
56. Wuhl E, Schaefer F. Managing kidney disease with blood pressure control: pathophysiology of CKD progression. Medscape. http://www.medscap.org/viewarticle/744528_3. Retreived 2/07/2013.
57. Wang SN, Hirschberg R. Growth factors ultrafiltration in experimental diabetic nephropathy contributes to interstitial fibrosis. Am J Physiol Renal Physiol. 2000;218:F554–60.
58. Zoja C, Donadelli S, Colleoni M, Figiuzzis S, Bonazzola M, Morigi M, et al. Proximal tubular cell synthesis and secretion of endothelin-I on challenge with albumin and other proteins. Am J Kidney Dis. 1995;26:934–41.
59. Lee LK, Meyer TW, Pollock AS, Lovett DH. Endothelial injury initiates glomerulosclerosis in the rat permanent kidney. J Clin Invest. 1995;96:959–60.
60. Takano T, Brady HR. The endothelium in glomerular inflammation. Curr Opin Nephrol Hypertens. 1995;4:277–86.
61. Peterson JC, Adler S, Burkart JM, Greene T, Herbert LA, Hunsicker LG, et al. Blood pressure control, proteinuria and the progression of renal disease. The modification of diet in renal disease study. Ann Inter Med. 1995;123:754–62.
62. Ruggenenti P, Echieppati A, Remuzzi G. Progression, remission, regression in chronic renal diseases. Lancet. 2001;357:1601–8.
63. Lopez-Novoa JM, Rodriguez-Pena AB, Oritz A, Marinez-Salgado C, Hernandez FJ. Etiopathology of chronic tubular, glomerular and renovascular nephropathies: clinical implications. J Trans Med. 2011;9:13. doi:10.1186/1479-5876-9-13.
64. Moe S, Drueke T, Cunningham J, Goodman W, Martin K, Olgaard K, et al. Definition, evaluation and classification of renal osteodystrophy. A position statement from Kidney Disease: Improving Global Outcomes (KDIGO). Kidney Int. 2006;69:1945–53.
65. National Kidney Foundation. K/DOQI clinical practice guidelines for chronic kidney disease: evaluation and stratification. Am J Kidney Dis. 2002;39(2):S1–266 [Medline].

Ageing and the Reproductive System

66. Chahal HS, Drake WM. The endocrine system and ageing. J Pathol. 2007;211:173–80.
67. Knight J, Nigam Y. The physiology of ageing 8-the reproductive system. Nurs Times. 2008;104(46):24–5.
68. Hermann M, Untergasser G, Rumpold H, Berger P. Aging of the male reproductive system. Exp Gerontol. 2000;35:1267–79 (abstract).

69. Tsitoura P, Bulat T. The aging male reproductive system. Endocrinol Metab Clin N Am. 1995;24:295–315.
70. Gray A, Berton JA, McKinley J, Longcope C. An examination of research design effects on the association of testosterone and male ageing. Results of a meta analysis. J Clin Epidemiol. 1991;7:671–84.
71. Bremner WJ, Vitiello MV, Prinz PN. Loss of circadian rhythmicity in blood testosterone levels in aging normal me. J Clin Endocrinol Metab. 1983;56:1278–81.
72. Bagatell CJ, Bremner WJ. II. Changes in reproductive hormones during the aging process. J Clin Endocrinol Metab. 1998;83:34–6 (abstract).
73. Montague SE, Watson R, Herbert R. Physiology for nursing practice. 3rd ed. Oxford: Bailli Tindall; 2005.
74. Pellicer A, Simon C, Remohi J. Effects of aging on the female reproductive system. Hum Reprod. 1995;10 Suppl 2:77–83 (abstract).
75. Brzyski RG, Knudtson J. Effects of aging on the female reproductive system. The Merck Manual Home edition. 2013. http://www.merckmsanuals.com/home/womens_health_issues/biology_of_the_female.retrieved. 13 Sep 2014.
76. Riggs BL, Melton LJI. Involutional osteoporosis. NEJM. 1986;314:1676–86.
77. Masters WH, Johnson VE. Sex and aging process. J Am Geriatr Soc. 1981;29:385.

Prostate Gland an Related Disorders

78. Weerakkody Y, Maingard J. Prostate. http://radiopaedia.org/artcles/prostate. Accessed 26 Jan 2015.
79. Canadian Cancer Society. Anatomy and physiology of the prostate. http://www.cancerca/en/cancer-information/cancer-type/prostate/anatomy and physiology.?region+on. Retrieved on 26 Jan 2015.
80. Villiers GM, Verstraete K, De Neve WJ, Meerleer GO. Magnetic resonance imaging anatomy of the prostate and the periprostatic area: a guide for radiotherapists. Radiother Oncol. 2005;76(1):99–106.
81. Sinnathamby C. Last's anatomy 10. Churchill Livingstone. Elsevier; 2005.
82. Lepor H. Pathophysiology of benign prostatic hyperplasia in the aging male population. Rev Urol. 2005;7 Suppl 4:S3–12.
83. McNeal JE. The prostate gland. Morphology, pathobiology. Monogr Urol. 1983;4:5–13.
84. Berry SJ, Coffey DS, Walsh PC, Ewing LL. The development of human prostatic hyperplasia with age. J Urol. 1984;132:474–9.
85. Levelliee RJ, Patel VR, Bird VG. Prostate hypertrophy, benign. eMedicine Update. 2006.
86. Lepor H. Pathogenesis, epidemiology and natural history of benign prostate hypertrophy. Rev Urol. 2004;6 Suppl 9:S3–10.
87. Walsh PC, Madder JD, Harrod M. Familial incomplete male pseudohermaphroditism type 2: decreased dihydrotestosterone formation in pseudovaginal perineoscrotal hypospadias. NEJM. 1974;291:944–9.
88. Diamond DA. Sexual differentiation normal and abnormal. In: Walsk PC, Retik AB, Vaughan Jr ED, Wein AJ, editors. Campells urology. 8th ed. Philadelphia: WB Saunders Co; 2002. p. 2395–527.
89. Caine M. The present role of alpha-adrenergic blockers in the treatment of benign prostate hypertrophy. J Urol. 1986;136:1–6.
90. Editor' summary of meeting presentation in Lepor H. Pathophysiology of benign prostatic hyperplasia in the aging male population. Rev Urol. 2005;7(Suppl. 4):S3–S12.
91. Krieger JN. Classification, epidemiology and implications of chronic prostatitis in North America, Europe and Asia. Minerva Urol Nefrol. 2004;56:99–107.
92. Ramakrishnan K, Salinas RC. Prostatitis acute and chronic. Prim Care Clin Office Pract. 2010;37(3):547–63.

93. Maitre S. Prostatitis: prevalence classification and treatment. Virtual Mentor. 2006;8(11):748–51.
94. Andriole GL. Prostatitis. The Merck Manual Professional Edition. http://www.merckmanuals.com/ptofessional/geitourinary_disorders/benign-prostate. Accessed 27 Jan 2015.
95. Anothaisintawee T, Attin J, Nickel JC, Thammaraisom S, Numthavaj P, McEvoy M, et al. Management of chronic prostatitis/chronic pelvic pain. JAMA. 2011;305(1):78–86.
96. Faris G, Metz Y, Friedman B, Stein A. Prostatic abscess –diagnosis and treatment. Harefuah. 2008;147(7):594–6, 663 (abstract).
97. Venyo A. Prostatic abscess: case report and review of literature. WebmedCentral Urol. 2011;2(11):WMC002433.
98. Oliveira P, Andrade JA, Porto JE, Filho LE, Vinhaes AF. Diagnosis and treatment of prostatic abscess. Int Braz J Urol. 2003;29:30–4.
99. Grndios EA, Caffaralti J, Farina L, Hoesman H. Prostatic abscess drainage clinical-sonography correlation. Urol Int. 1992;48:358–61.
100. Jameson RM. Prostatic abscess, carcinoma of the prostate. Br J Urol. 1968;40:288–92.
101. Trauzzi SJ, Kay CJ, Kaufman DG, Lowe JC. Management of prostatic abscess in patients with immunodeficiency syndrome. Urology. 1994;93:629–33.
102. Bansal P, Gupta A, Mongha R, Bera M, Ranjit K, Kunda AK. Minimally –invasive management of prostatic abscess. The role of transrectal ultrasound. Urol Ann. 2009;1:56–60.

Prostatic Cancer

103. McNeal JE. The prostate gland. Morphology, pathobiology. Monogr Urol. 1983;4:5–13.
104. Gann PH. Risk factors for possible prostate cancer. Rev Urol. 2002;14 Suppl 5:S3–70.
105. Balistreri CR, Candore G, Lio D, Carruba G. Prostate cancer: from the pathophysiologic implications of some genetic risk factors to translation in personalized cancer treatments. Cancer Gene Ther. 2014;21:2–11. doi:10.1038/cgt.2013.77.
106. Dreicer R, Garcia J. Prostate cancer. http://www.clevelandclinicmeded.com/medicalpubs/diseasemanagement/hematology. Accessed 16 Mar 2015.
107. Bostwick DG. High grade prostatic intraepithelial neoplasia: the most likely precursor of prostate cancer. Cancer. 1995;75:1823–36.
108. BMJ Best Practice. Prostate cancer. http://bestpractice.bmj.com/best-practice/monograph/254/basics/path0physiology.html. Retrieved 16 Mar 2015.
109. Velcheti V, Karnik S, Bardot SF, Prakash O. Pathogenesis of prostate cancer: lessons from basic research. Ochsner J. 2008;8(4):213–8.
110. Stamey TA, Donaldson AN, Yemoto CE, McNeal JE, Soezen S, Gill H. Histological and clinical findings in 896 consecutive patients treated with radical retropubic prostatectomy: epidemiologic significance of annual changes. J Urol. 1998;160:2412–7.

Sexuality and Sexual Dysfunction in with Aging

111. Kinsey A, Pomeroy W, Martin C. Sexual behaviour in human male. Philadelphia: WB Saunders; 1948.
112. Kinsey A, Pomeroy W, Martin C. Sexual behaviour in the human female. Philadelphia: WB Saunders; 1948.
113. Applegate WB. Sexuality in the elderly. In: Calkins E, Davis PJ, Ford AB, editors. The practice of geriatrics. Philadelphia: Pub WB Saunders Company; 1986.
114. Masters WH, Johnson VE. Sex and aging process. J Am Geriatr Soc. 1981;29:385–8.
115. King R. Handbook of erectile dysfunction. Middle Cove: Intimate Solutions Pty; 2007.
116. Wagner G, de Tejafda IS. Update on male erectile dysfunction. BMJ. 1998;316:678–82.

117. Andersson K, Wagner G. Physiology of penile erection. Physiol Rev. 1995;75:191–236 (abstract).
118. Lue TF, Zeineh SJ, Schmidt RA, Tanagho EA. Neuroanatomy of penile erection: its relevance to iatrogenic impotence. J Urol. 1984;131(2):273–80 (abstract).
119. Junemann KP, Persson-Junemann C, Lue TF, Tanagho EA, Aiken P. Neurophysiological aspects of penile erection: the role of the sympathetic nervous system. Br J Urol. 1989;64(1):84–92 (abstract).
120. El-Sakka AI, Lue TF. Physiology of penile erection. Digital Urology Journal Articles website: http://www.duj.com/Article/Lue.html. Accessed 25 Aug 2008.
121. Junemann KP, Lue TF, Melchor H. The physiology of penile erection. Neurophysiology of penile erection. Urologe A. 1987;26:289–93 (abstract).
122. Ramopin O, Bernabe J, Giuliano F. Spinal control of penile erection. World J Urol. 1997;15(1):2–13 (abstract).
123. Burnett AL. Role of nitric oxide in the physiology of erection. Biol Reprod. 1995;52:485–9 (abstract).
124. Priviero FB, Leite R, Webb RC, Teixeira CE. Neurophysiological basis of penile erection. Acta Pharmacol Sin. 2007;28(6):751–5 (abstract).
125. Giuliano F, Rampin O, Jardin A. Physiology of erection. La Rev de Med interne/fondee. 1997;18 Suppl 1:3s–9 (abstract).
126. McKenna KE. Central control of penile extraction. Int J Impot Res. 1996;10 Suppl 1:S25–34 (abstract).
127. Andresson KE. Erectile physiological and pathophysiological pathways involved in erectile dysfunction. J Urol. 2003;170(2 Pt 2):S6–13 (abstract).
128. Giuliano F, Clement P. Physiology of ejaculation: emphasis on serotonergic control. Eur Urol. 2013;48:408–17 (abstract).
129. Haake P, Exton M, Haverkamp J, Kramer M, Loygraf N, Hartmann U, et al. Absence of orgasm-induced prolactin secretion in healthy multi-orgasmic male subject. Int J Impot Res. 2002;14:133–5.
130. Gentili A, Mulligan T. Sexual dysfunction in older adults. Clin Geriatr Med. 1998;14:383–93.

Erectile Dysfunction in the Male Elderly

131. Nicholson A, Moreira Jr ED, Shirai M, Bin Mohd Thambi MI, Glasser DB. Epidemiology of erectile dysfunction in four countries: cross international study of the prevalence and correlates of erectile dysfunction. Urology. 2003;61:201–6.
132. Parazzini F, Munchini FF, Bortolotti A, Calabro A, Chatenond L, Colli E, et al. Frequency and determinants of erectile dysfunction in Italy. Eur Urol. 2000;37:43–9.
133. Weber MF, Smith DP, O'Connell DL, Patel M, de Souza PL, Sitas F, et al. Risk factors for erectile dysfunction in a cohort of 108477 Australian men. MJA. 2013;199(2):107–11.
134. Holden C, McLachlan RI, Pitts SM, CummingR Wittert G, Agius PA, et al. Men in Australia: Telephone Survey (MATEeS): a national survey of the reproductive health and concerns of middle- aged and older Australian men. Lancet. 2005;366:218–20.
135. Lavelle P. Erectile dysfunction. ABC Health & Wellbeing. http://www.abc.net.au/health/library/stories/2008/02/14/2160484.htm. Retrieved 29 Aug 2008.
136. Chew KK, Earle CM. Stuckey BGA erectile dysfunction in general medical practice: prevalence and clinical correlations. Int Impot Res. 2000;12:41–5.
137. O'Keefe M, Hunt DK. Assessment and treatment of impotence. N Med Clin N Am. 1995;79:415–34.
138. Buffum J. Pharmacosexology update: prescription drugs and sexual function. J Psychoactive Drugs. 1986;18:97–106.
139. Guay AT. Erectile dysfunction-are you prepared to discuss? Postgrad Med. 1995;97: 127–43.

140. Krane RJ, Goldstrin I, Saenz de Tejada I. Impotence. N Engl J Med. 1989;321:1648–9.
141. Thase MG, Reynolds CF, Jennings JR. Nocturnal penile tumescence ids diminished in depression in men. Biol Psychiatry. 1988;24:33–46.

Urinary Incontinence

142. Abrams P, Blaivas JG, Stanton SI, Andersen JT. The standardization of terminology of lower urinary tract function. The International Society Committee in Standardization Terminology. Scand J Urol. 1988;114(Suppl):5–19.
143. Mollander U, Sundh V, Stein G. Urinary incontinence and related symptoms in older men and women studied longitudinally between 70 and 97 years of age. A population study. Arch Gerontol Geriatr. 2002;35:237–44.
144. Mayo Foundation for Medical Education and Research Geriatric Medicine. Urinary Incontinence (Internet) USA Mayo Clinic. 2010. http://www.mayo.edu. Accessed 4 Aug 2013.
145. Sidik SM. The prevalence of urinary incontinence among elderly in rural community in Selangor. Malays J Med Sci. 2010;17(2):18–23.
146. Poi P. Giants of geriatrics II-incontinence. In: Srinivasas P, editor. Proceedings of First National Symposium on Gerontology 1995. Kuala Lumpur: University of Malaysia; 1995. p. 92–7.
147. Nakanishi N, Tatara K, Naramura H, Fujiwara H, Takashima Y, Fulkuda H. Urinary and faecal incontinence in a community residing older people in Japan. J Am Geriatr Soc. 1997;45(2):215–9 (abstract).
148. Teunissen TA, van den Bosch WJ, van den Hoogen HJ, Largo-Jansson AL. Prevalence of urinary and faecal incontinence among community dwelling elderly patients in Nijmegen, The Netherlands. Ned Tidschr Geneeskd. 2006;150(44):2430–4 (abstract).
149. Yoshimura N. New insights into the neural mechanisms controlling the micturition reflex. Nihon Yakuurigaku Zasshi. 2003;121(5):290–8 (abstract).
150. Yoshimura N, Kaiho Y, Miyazato M, Yunoki T, Tori C, Chancellor MB, et al. Therapeutic receptor targets for lower urinary tract dysfunction. Naunyn Schmiedebergs Arch Pharmcol. 2008;377(4–6):437–48 (abstract).
151. Jaipaul N. Effects of aging on the urinary tract. The Merck Manual Home Edition. 2012. http://www.merckmanuals.com/home/kidney_and_utinary_tract_disorders/biology_of. Accessed 12 Sep 2014.
152. Smith CM, Cotter VT. Age related changes in health. Hartford Institute for Geriatric Nursing. http://consultgerirn.org/topics/normal_aging_changes/want_to_know_more. Accessed 12 Sep 2014.
153. Inouye SK, Studenski S, Tinetti ME, Kuchel GA. Geriatric syndromes: clinical research and policy implications of a core geriatric concept. J Am Geriatr Soc. 2007;55:780–91.
154. Yu LC, Rohner TJ, Kaltreider L, Hu TW, Igou JF, Dennis PJ, et al. Profile of urinary incontinent elderly in long term care institutions. J Am Geriatr Soc. 1990;38:433–9.
155. Vehkalalahti I, Kivela S-L. Urinary incontinence: and its correlates in very old age. Gerontology. 1985;31:391–5.
156. DuBeau CE. Beyond the bladder " management of urinary incontinence in older women. Clin Obstet Gynecol. 2007;50:720–34.
157. Bocon-Gitod L. Urinary incontinence after radical prostactectomy. Eur Urol. 1997;6:112–6.
158. McConnell JD, Barry MS, Bruskewitz RC. Proatatic hyperplasia, diagnosis, treatment. Clinical Practice Guide-Line No. 8. Rockville: US Dept Health and Human Services Public Health Service Aging for Health Care Policy and Research.
159. Mathews CA, Whitehind WE, Townsend HK, Grodstein F. Risk factors for urinary and faecal incontinence on Nurses' Health Study. Obstet Gynecol. 2013;122(3):539–48.

160. Schulman C, Claesin H, Matthijs J. Urinary incontinence in Belgium: a population based survey. Eur Urol. 1997;32:315–20.
161. Milson I, Ekelund P, Molander U, Arvidsson L, Areskong B. The influence of age, parity, oral contraception, hysterectomy and the menopause in the prevalence of urinary infection in women. J Urol. 1997;149:1459–62.
162. Resnick NM, Yalla SV, Laurino E. The pathophysiology of urinary incontinence among institutionalized elderly persons. NEJM. 1989;320:1–7.
163. Kuchel GA, DuBeau CE. Chapter 30. Urinary incontinence in the elderly. Geriaric Nephrology Curriculum. Am Soc Nephrol. 2009. p. 1–4.

Neurological Disorders and Related Problems in the Elderly

7

7.1 Anatomical and Physiological Changes in the Nervous System with Ageing

Normal ageing appears to be associated with both structural and functional changes in the brain with cerebral atrophy, neuronal loss, decrease in neurotransmitters and blood flow reductions. With ageing, there is an overall decline in brain weight and volume [1], the decline increases with age [2] more so over the age of 70 years [3] together with enlargement of the ventricles [4]. Ageing affects different brain regions differently [5, 6]; similarly the effect of ageing on the type of cell (neurons or glial cells, their numbers and branching) and the site of action (synapse) varies. There are considerable individual variations in the loss of neurons which are limited to certain areas in old people with no apparent functional or pathological deficits. With the advent of neuroimaging, the major age-related changes have been shown to include a decrease in the grey and white matter density, atrophy of specific brain regions and focal abnormalities in the white matter and basal ganglia. The hippocampus shows the most significant age-related atrophy with advancing age. White matter may decline with age, the myelin sheath deteriorates after the age of 40 years, even in normal ageing [2]. Age-related changes in the white matter (leukoaraiosis) occurs as zones of low density, and these changes are better appreciated on T2-weighted MRI as increased signal MRI white matter hyperintensities [5] and shows a predilection for the frontal regions [7] and may progress with increasing age to the posterior areas [8]. With ageing leukoaraiosis increases and may denote subclinical ischaemia [2].

After the age of 60, there is a reduction in muscle volume and muscle strength, and this is largely due to continuous denervation and reinnervation due to a reduction of functioning motor units mediated through the motor units and the spinal cord [9]. As age advances, there is an increasing diminution in the number of motor neurons [10, 11] in the spinal cord. There is gradual age-related loss of neural tissue from the spinal cord, and up to 46 % may be lost over the age of 50 years [12]. Sensory stimuli reaching the central nervous system can be reduced by increased

N. Nagaratnam et al., *Diseases in the Elderly: Age-Related Changes and Pathophysiology*, DOI 10.1007/978-3-319-25787-7_7

pressure on the spinal cord and its branch nerve roots by changes in the intervertebral discs [13].

Changes in the peripheral nerves are less well known. The morphological and functional features of the peripheral nervous system are deeply affected by ageing [14]. The myelin sheaths undergo slow progressive degeneration, with loss of myelinated and nonmyelinated fibres and axonal atrophy [14]. This degeneration with ageing results from decreased blood flow, pressure on the nerves or both resulting in decreased co-ordination, strength, balance and agility. There is a reduction in reaction time and decline in conduction velocity [14]. There is marked reduction in vibratory sense resulting in decreased co-ordination and balance. There is age-related decline in nerve regeneration [14] and regrowth of peripheral axons take longer in elderly subjects [15].

Evidence of age-related changes in elements of several neurotransmitter systems is important for effective functioning in health and disease. There are several neurotransmitters but the well known ones include the amino acids (glutamic acid, GABA, aspartate), glycine, monoamines (norepinephrine, dopamine, serotonin), acetylcholine, peptides (vasopressin, somastatin, substance P) and gases (carbon monoxide and nitric oxide). The peripheral nervous system has two neurotransmitters: acetylcholine and norepinephrine. The monoamines and acetylcholine perform specialised modulating function and often confined to specific structures. The acetylcholine synapse is said to decline by 4 % per decade of adult life span [16]. There is loss of striatal dopamine with ageing. In general dopamine appears to decline with age in parts of the brain associated with thinking. Reduction at D1 receptor occurs at the rate of 7 % per decade with ageing [17] and 1 % annual decrement at D2 receptor. The serotonin synapse also declines with age, for instance, the 5HT transporter declines approximately by 4 % per decade [18]. The peptides have special function in the hypothalamus and act as neuromodulators, and with age, both increases and decreases occur. In the spinal cord, the loss of neurons and reduction in the neurotransmitters slow nerve conduction; thereby, some tasks may take longer with advanced age. GABA and certain amino acids such as glutamate and aspartate have important roles, of these GABA transmits inhibitory impulses and aspartate and glutamate usually moderate excitatory synaptic transmissions. Changes in the spinal cord lead to reduction in reaction times as a result of reduction in impulse velocity [19]. Decline in sensory and motor conduction increases the chance of injury due to poor co-ordination and balance [13].

Cerebral blood flow has been shown to decrease with age. The cerebral vessels undergo the same atherosclerotic lesions seen in other arterial vasculature. This progresses with age and compromises the neural tissues which are dependent on oxygen and glucose for their metabolism and function. The structural changes have functional implications. Normal physiological changes occur in sleep with advancing age, and probably the most common is a decline in slow wave or delta sleep and increases in stage 1 and 2 non-rapid eye movement sleep [20]. As age advances, it is the quality of sleep rather than the quantity that changes. The clinical manifestations include morning wakening, increased night-time wakefulness and increased fragmentation of sleep periods with decrease in sleep time that impedes daytime performance and optimal functioning. Due to a phase advance in their normal circadian sleep cycle, the elderly tend to go to sleep earlier in the evening and wake earlier [20]. Memory is the most widely seen cognitive changes with ageing [2]. With normal ageing, there is a linear decline in memory and reasoning. There is loss of short-term memory and is probably the earliest indication of age-related changes within the brain [13].

Box 7.1. Key Points. Anatomical and Physiological Changes in the Nervous System with Ageing

- Structural and functional changes include cerebral atrophy, decrease in neurotransmitters and blood flow reductions.
- Ageing affects different brain regions differently [6, 7].
- Hippocampus shows significant age-related changes.
- Age-related changes occur in the white matter.
- Denervation and reinnervations of the motor units in the spinal cord result in reduction of muscle volume and strength [9].
- Peripheral nervous system is deeply affected by ageing [14].
- Age-related elements of several neurotransmitter systems, for example, reduction of D1 receptor occurs at the rate of 7 % per decade of ageing [17].
- Cerebral blood flow decreases with age.
- Ageing influences electrical activity and cognitive (especially memory), sensory and affective processes [13].
- There is reduction in reaction time as a result of reduction in impulse velocity due to changes in the spinal cord [19].

7.2 Parkinson's Disease, Secondary Parkinsonism and Parkinson Plus Syndromes

Introduction

Parkinson's disease is a progressive disorder caused by degeneration of the dopaminergic neurons of the substantia nigra and is the second most frequent neurodegenerative disorder in the elderly. In idiopathic Parkinson's disease, there is accumulation of alpha-synuclein in neuronal perikarya (Lewy bodies) and neuronal processes (Lewy neuritis) [21]. Secondary parkinsonism describes the syndrome of parkinsonism when it occurs as the result of a known cause, for example, certain medications, strokes and tumours among others. Parkinson plus syndromes embrace a number of disorders characterised by degeneration of neurons in different parts of the brain. They include progressive supranuclear palsy (PSP), striatonigral degeneration, multisystem atrophy (MSA) and normal pressure hydrocephalus (NPH). The most common of the parkinsonian tauopathies is PSP, and the other major alpha-synucleinopathy is MSA [21]. Based on epidemiological studies, the prevalence of Parkinson's disease ranges from 146 to 780 per 100,000 [22, 23]. In a study

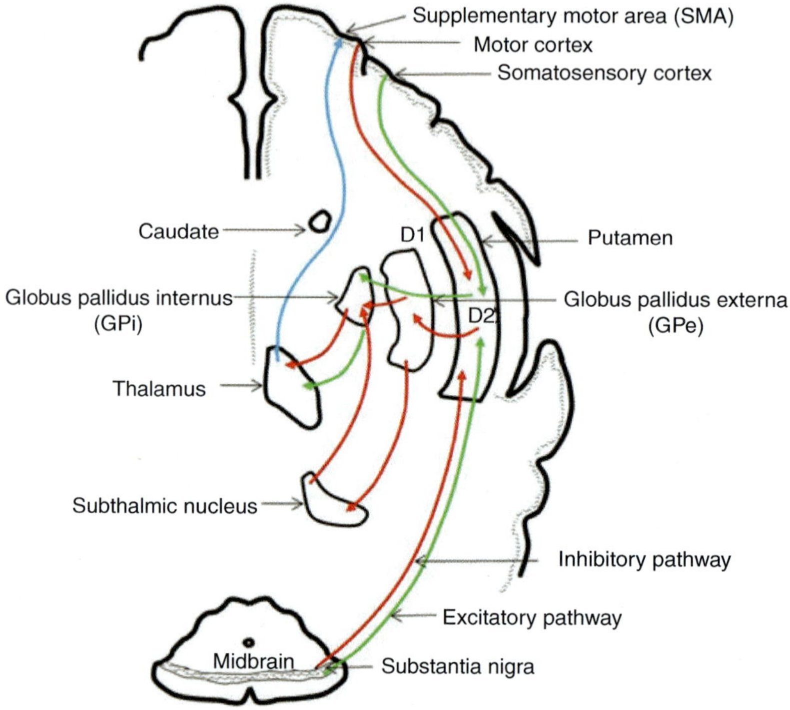

Fig. 7.1 Dopaminergic pathways. Direct pathway (*green*) (D1). Projections from the caudate/putamen GPi thalamus premotor cortex. Excitatory inputs from the substantia nigra and cortex to the putamen/caudate are also shown. Indirect pathway (*red*) D2. Projections from the caudate/putamen GPe subthalamic nucleus, GPi thalamus motor cortex. GPe also receives excitatory input from the cortex and inhibitory from the substantia nigra. There is an excitatory input from the subthalamic nucleus to the GPi

of 588 newly diagnosed cases of PD, an overall annualised age- and gender-adjusted rate was 13.4 per 100,000 with only 4 % below the age of 50 years [24]. PD affects about 1 % of the people beyond the age of 65 years [25].

Pathophysiology
The striatum consisting of the caudate and the putamen together with the subthalamic nucleus, intralaminar nuclei of the thalamus and the globus pallidus form the basal ganglia. The dopamine receptors are situated in the striatum. The pars compacta of the substantia nigra (SNpc) contains the pigmented dopamine-secreting (dopaminergic) cells. The putaminal neurons of the direct pathway have dopamine D1 receptors that facilitate movement, while the putaminal neurons of the indirect pathway have D2 receptors that inhibit movement. Projections from the dopamine neurons in the substantia nigra (SN) modulate the motor production of the basal ganglia circuits. The striatonigral pathway plays a regulatory role in the system of positive and negative pathways that serve to modulate feedback from the thalamus to the motor cortex (Fig. 7.1).

The projection of the neurons to the striatum is just a component of a complex network of neural pathways. The putamen receives excitatory input from the cerebral cortex via the direct pathway to the internal division of the globus pallidus (GPi) and the indirect pathway to the external division of the globus pallidus (GPe) to the subthalamic nucleus (STN) and then to the GPi. The GPi projects to the thalamus (ventrolateralis), and the thalamus in turn transmits the increased activity to the motor cortex perhaps via the supplementary motor area (SMA). From the cortex, it descends via the corticospinal tract. The GPi also projects to the substantia nigra (SN). According to Braak et al. [26], years before the substantia nigra compacta (SNc) and cortex are involved, there is pathological evidence of PD as defined by the presence of Lewy bodies in the medulla oblongata, pontine tegmentum and olfactory bulb. Once the SNc is affected by the initial pathological process, it hastens acceleration of the cell loss in the SNc causing symptoms in advance of the earlier affected areas [27].

Increased knowledge and better understanding of the organisation of the basal ganglia in both health and disease have led to the hypothesis of direct and indirect pathways of the flow through the basal ganglia of cortical information [28]. Genetic and environmental toxins have been linked with PD [29], and other factors responsible are neurodegeneration, oxidative stress and mitochondrial dysfunction [30], but what leads to the cell death remains unclear [29]. Lotharius and Brunden [29] proposed that defective sequestration of dopamine into the vesicles is the foremost event in the death of dopaminergic neurons in PD. Recent studies have disclosed that several genes may be involved [31] which can result in the misfolding of proteins and dysfunction of the ubiquitin-proteasome pathway. This in turn plays an important role in PD pathogenesis [30].

In PD dopaminergic cells in the SN degenerate, and severe involvement of these cells interferes with the normal function of the striatum and probably responsible for the motor dysfunctions in PD [32]. SN degeneration results from accumulation of the protein alpha-synuclein which forms proteinaceous cytoplasmic inclusions called Lewy bodies and other additional processes such as reduced levels of glutathione, accumulation of iron and altered calcium homeostasis [27]. Alpha-synuclein is a presynaptic neuronal protein linked genetically and neuropathologically with PD [33] and other neurodegenerative disorders [34]. Two other neurodegenerative diseases, dementia with Lewy bodies and multisystem atrophy, have also been found to be associated with alpha-synuclein dysfunction [35]. Alpha-synuclein dysfunction is brought about by a chain of events, triggered by either environment or genetic resulting in dopaminergic neuronal death. In the surviving dopaminergic neurons and in other affected regions of the central nervous system, alpha-synuclein misfolds resulting in the formation of cytoplasmic inclusions called Lewy bodies [34]. The mechanism of dopaminergic neuronal death is not clearly understood. More recent data indicate these events lead to disruption of the neuronal membrane traffic and selectively blocking endoplasmic reticulum (ER)-to-Golgi transport, thus causing ER stress [36].

Age influences both the development and progression of PD [37, 38]. Several studies have shown an association between advancing years and faster rate of progression of PD, more severe gait and postural abnormalities and reduced levodopa responsiveness [38]. Degeneration of the dopaminergic cells within the substantia nigra and subsequent dopamine depletion result in the striatonigral-thalamic outflow dysfunction which leads to alterations in the activity of the neural circuits in the basal ganglia. The lack of dopamine leads to inhibition of the direct pathway and excitation of the indirect pathway and increased inhibition of the ventrolateral nucleus of the thalamus (the relevant neurotransmitter probably is gamma-aminobutyric acid (GABA)) which sends projections to the motor cortex. From the cortex, it descends via the corticospinal tract to cause increased tone (rigidity) and slowed movement (bradykinesia).

There is evidence that neural oscillations and synchronisation within the basal ganglia play a vital role in the generation of the disease [39]. Weakly coupled neural networks of the basal ganglia-thalamocortical loops are the likely movers for the oscillations [40]. Changes in the firing patterns and oscillatory activity are crucial in PD pathophysiology [41]. The loss of dopaminergic inputs to the basal ganglia increases the oscillatory firing and synchronisation also in basal ganglia nuclei, namely, the globus pallidus and subthalamic nuclei [42].

Oscillating neuronal activity within the CNS is believed to be the cause of parkinsonian tremor, but the underlying mechanism remains unclear [43]. Results of studies suggest that the altered balance between beta and gamma oscillations in the motor circuits in the subthalamic nucleus (STN) is associated with the tremor in PD [41]. PD tremor has been shown not to be strictly correlated with the abnormal synchronous oscillations of the basal ganglia but leads to rigidity and akinesia [44]. The indirect pathway via the STN is important in understanding (i) the mechanism of the hemiballismus and (ii) the benefit of deep brain stimulation of the STN to relieve the dyskinesias in late stage PD treated with L-dopa.

The three major dopaminergic tracts in the brain comprise the (i) nigrostriatal, substantia nigra to the stratum; (ii) mesocortical, ventral tegmental area to the neocortex especially the prefrontal cortex; and (iii) mesolimbic, ventral tegmental area to many components of the limbic system. The neuropsychiatric symptomatology is likely due to disruption of the non-striatal pathways.

The intraneuronal enzymes required for dopamine synthesis are markedly diminished in PD. The dopaminergic neurons synthesise dopamine from the amino acid tyrosine through an intermediate compound to form dopamine which is stored in the neuron's storage vesicles. It is then released into the synaptic cleft where it may bind to the postsynaptic receptors (D1 is stimulatory and D2 is inhibitory) in the striatum or is inactivated by binding to the autoreceptor in the same neuron, sequestered and stored to be released again (Fig. 7.2). Furthermore, it is also inactivated by the enzymes monoamine oxidase type B (MAO-B) and by catechol-O-methyltransferase (COMT). The enzyme glutamic acid decarboxylase (GAD) responsible for the synthesis of GABA is also reduced in the substantia nigra and the cortex. In PD apart from the selective degeneration of the pigmented dopaminergic neurons of the substantia nigra, there are scattered neurons containing eosinophilic inclusion bodies known as Lewy bodies. This is the pathologic hallmark of the disease.

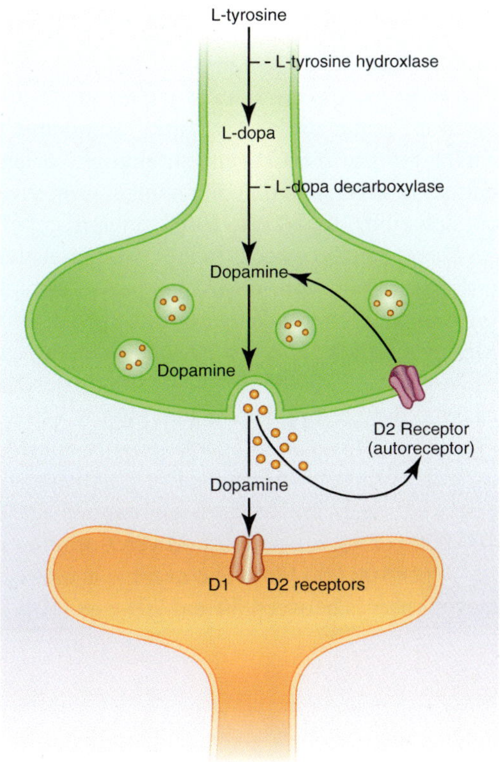

Fig. 7.2 Dopamine synthesis

Box 7.2. Key Points. Parkinson's Disease (PD)

- Lewy bodies are present in the medulla oblongata, pontine tegmentum and olfactory bulb long before pathological evidence of PD [26].
- Defective sequestration of dopamine into vesicles is the foremost event in the death of dopaminergic neurons in PD [29].
- Several genes are involved in the misfolding of proteins and dysfunction of the ubiquitin-proteasome pathway [30].
- Substantia nigra degeneration results from accumulation of alpha-synuclein and forms proteinaceous cytoplasmic inclusions called Lewy bodies [34].
- Age influences both development and progression of PD [37, 38].
- The intraneuronal enzymes required for dopamine synthesis are markedly reduced.
- Lack of dopamine leads to inhibition of the direct pathway and excitation of the indirect pathway [39, 41].
- Evidence that normal oscillations and synchronisation within the basal ganglia plays a vital role in the generation of the disease.
- In PD besides degeneration of dopaminergic neurons, there are scattered neurons called Lewy bodies, and this is the hallmark of the disease.

7.3 Multisystem Atrophy (MSA)

Introduction

The term multisystem atrophy was coined to embrace most cases of Shy-Drager syndrome, pure autonomic failure, autonomic failure associated with olivopontocerebellar atrophy (OPCA) and striatonigral degeneration [45]. It is now a well-defined entity; however, it is one of a number of multisystem degenerations. MSA can cause combinations of parkinsonism, autonomic, pyramidal and cerebellar symptoms. All four characteristics occur in the vast majority of patients with MSA but with considerable variation with regard to specific symptoms, and any one of the four could predominate. Presently if parkinsonian features predominate, it is referred to as MSA-P and accounts for two-thirds of the cases in the Western hemisphere [46]. MSA-C cerebellar symptoms predominate and accounts for about two-thirds of the cases in the Eastern hemisphere [46]. MSA-A is now the term used for Shy-Drager syndrome. Most patients were initially considered to have Parkinson's disease, and even at death, one-third still carry that diagnosis [47]. In the population aged 50 years and over, the incidence has been reported as 0.6 per 100,000 per year, rising to 3 per 100,000 per year in patients 50 years or more [48, 49]. The age-adjusted prevalence is 4.4 per 100,000 [46]. The average age of onset is around 50 years, and the mean age of onset is between 50 and 70 years [50].

Pathophysiology

MSA is a neurodegenerative disorder and the histopathological hallmark is the formation glial cytoplasmic inclusions (GCIs) in the oligodendroglia [51–53] and staining positive for alpha-synuclein [52]. Apart from this, in MSA there is an aggregation of filamentous alpha-synuclein in the neurons in the olivopontocerebellar and striatonigral systems but also in the fibres connecting their affecting lesions [54].

Box 7.3. Key Points. Multisystem Atrophy (MSA)

- MSA is a neurodegenerative disease [51–53].
- Formation of glial cytoplasmic inclusions in the oligodendroglia and staining positive for alpha-synuclein [51–53].
- Aggregates of filamentous alpha-synuclein are found in the neurons in the olivopontocerebellar and striatonigral systems but also in the fibres connecting their affected lesions [54].

7.4 Motor Neuron Disease

Introduction

The term motor neuron disease (MND) encompasses a group of disorders that result from degeneration of the motor neurons in the brain and/or spinal cord. Amyotrophic lateral sclerosis (ALS) commonly occurs between the ages of 40 and 60 years, and males are affected more than females, but several studies suggest the incidence peaks around the age 75–79 and thereafter decreases [55].

Pathophysiology
ALS affects both upper and lower motor neurons and is characterised by a progressive degeneration and death of the anterior horn cells, corticospinal tracts and/or bulbar motor nuclei. The other disorders in the group include progressive bulbar palsy, progressive pseudobulbar palsy, progressive muscular atrophy (primarily involving the lower motor neurons), primary lateral sclerosis (pure UMN), spino-bulbar muscular atrophy (Kennedy disease) and post-polio syndrome. After the onset of the disease, the cellular processes involved include protein aggregation, generation of free radices, mitochondrial dysfunction excitotoxicity and apoptosis [56, 57]. There is an association between frontotemporal dementia (FTD) and ALS. Most cases with both are characterised by neuronal inclusions immunoreactive for ubiquitin but not tau, and the ubiquitinated protein has been identified as TDP-43 and linked to chromosome 9p [58]. About 10 % of the familial cases of ALS result from a specific genetic defect which gives rise to mutation of the gene Cu/Zn, superoxide dismutase 1 (SOD1) [59–61]. Primary lateral sclerosis (PLS) is characterised with pure UMN signs 4 years after the onset of symptoms and is slowly progressive [62].

Box 7.4. Key Points. Motor Neuron Disease (ALS)
- Progressive degeneration and death of anterior horn cells, corticospinal tract and/or bulbar motor nuclei.
- The cellular processes include protein aggregation, generation of free radicals, mitochondrial dysfunction, excitotoxicity and apoptosis [56, 57].
- FTD and ALS are characterised by neuronal inclusions immunoreactive for ubiquitin but not tau [58].

7.5 Peripheral Neuropathy

Introduction
Peripheral neuropathy can be defined as a syndrome characterised by muscle weakness and wasting, altered or loss of sensation and vasomotor symptoms occurring singly or in various combinations. It may be acquired or hereditary, restricted to the peripheral nerve or be part of a systemic illness. In the elderly, diabetes is the most common cause of neuropathy. It is less common in the old-old (>80 years) compared to the young-old (65–79 years), 25 % vs. 46 % [63]. Idiopathic neuropathies are common in the old-old as compared to young-old (39 vs. 9 %) [63].

Pathophysiology
There are four basic degenerative processes. (I) Axonal degeneration follows a diffuse neural injury resulting in axonal damage starting in the distal portion of the

axon and proceeding proximally towards the cell body, with breakdown of the myelin sheath, a process called 'dying back' [64]. It is believed that the pathology begins in the neuronal body which is unable to meet the metabolic needs of the axon [65]. Recovery is slow and incomplete. (II) Wallerian degeneration involves the axon at a specific point distal to the injury resulting in degeneration of the axon and myelin sheath, and changes also occur in the neuronal body [65]. Recovery is incomplete similar to that in axonopathy. Both diffuse demyelination and axonal degeneration [64] tend to affect the longest axons first and produce a syndrome of neuropathy [65]. All the motor fibres are large myelinated axons; the sensory nerves however contain all sizes of myelinated and nonmyelinated axons. (III) Neuronal degeneration is caused by damage to the motor or sensory cell bodies followed by degeneration of their peripheral and central processes. Recovery is often poor because of the involvement of the cell body. (IV) Segmental demyelination results from multifocal injury to the myelin sheath with preservation of the underlying axon [64, 65]. Recovery is usually rapid and complete because the axons are spared [66].

Pathologically neuropathy can be classified on the basis of specific cell type involved, namely, neurons or Schwann cells or mixed. Those that involve the neurons are the neuronopathies or its axon, the axonopathies. Those that involve the Schwann cells or its myelin sheath are the demyelinating neuropathies. This classification is useful for it correlates well with the electrophysiological findings. In demyelinating neuropathies, there is decreased nerve conduction velocity for the conduction velocity depends on the integrity of the myelin sheaths, thickness of the nerve and the distance between the nodes of Ranvier. In axonopathies there is little or no loss of nerve conduction velocity.

Most of the elderly diabetic patients have axonal type of neuropathy. *Neurological abnormalities of B_{12} deficiency* include a myelopathy with or without neuropathy [67]. The neurological symptoms include subacute combined degeneration, ataxia and mononeuropathies (optic neuropathy or olfactory atrophy and central visual scotomas) [68]. *Nutritional neuropathy* other than due to vitamin B_{12} deficiency can be due, more importantly, to vitamin B_1 (thiamine) and pyridoxine deficiencies. About 50 % of the elderly have been found to be thiamine deficient. Thiamine deficiency in the elderly is associated with low intake and decreased activation of thiamine. Chronic disease, hospitalisation, institutionalisation and dialysis contribute to the risk of deficiency. Low-thiamine intake or chronic alcoholism can lead to beriberi and Wernicke-Korsakoff syndrome and is characterised by confusion, ataxia, confabulation and coma. Thiamine pyrophosphate is an essential coenzyme in the glycolytic and pentose phosphate pathways of glucose metabolism. Deficiency of thiamine leads to degeneration of the axonal sheaths with subsequent impairment of the axon giving rise to a polyneuropathy in about 3 months [69].

The principal manifestation of pyridoxine deficiency is peripheral neuropathy which is potentially severe in alcoholics. Pyridoxine deficiencies are usually associated with increased excretion due to isoniazid ingestion and cause a sensorimotor neuropathy and seizures. It may rarely be associated with a vasculitic mononeuropathy multiplex [69]. A pure sensory neuropathy could result following long-term excessive pyridoxine consumption due to its toxic effect on the dorsal root ganglions [67]. The pathogenic role of alcohol in the development of neuropathy remains controversial. It usually presents as a sensorimotor polyneuropathy with numbness, weakness and sensory ataxia [70]. It has been attributed to three processes, direct toxicity from the metabolites, nutritional deficiency and indirect toxicity, for example, from hepatic dysfunction resulting in damage to the axon itself [68]. It is very likely that direct toxicity of alcohol and its metabolites is involved in the pathogenesis of pure alcoholic neuropathy, and nutritional deficiency largely due to associated B group of vitamins [71] may be superimposed and additive. The main pathological feature is distally accentuated axonal degeneration of both myelinated and unmyelinated fibres [70]. *Paraneoplastic neuropathies.* Many anti-neuronal antibodies have been described to date. Patients with anti-Hu antibodies usually present with paraneoplastic subacute sensory neuropathy [72]. Anti-Hu antibodies are often seen with small cell lung cancer and are most pertinent to autoimmune dysfunction. Paraneoplastic sensorimotor polyneuropathies may cause confusion with chronic inflammatory demyelinating polyneuropathy (CIDP) and with lymphomas with direct infiltration of the nerves [73].

An acute attack in *acute intermittent porphyria* could involve any part of the nervous system. The pathophysiology of porphyric neuropathy is unclear and develops when reduced activity of the Na^+/K^+ pump results in membrane depolarisation [74]. *Sepsis and multiple organ failure* now called the systemic inflammatory response syndrome (SIRS) [75] is often accompanied by a form of sensorimotor axonal polyneuropathy referred to as critical illness neuropathy (CIN). CIN occurs in 70 % of patients with the septic syndrome [76].

Toxic neuropathies occur following exposure to various drugs, heavy metals and industrial toxins. They are usually axonopathies and often resemble neuropathies due to metabolic abnormalities, nutritional deficiencies and systemic illness both clinically and electrophysiologically [77]. Pathological features in some agents damage the nerve cell, others induce demyelination, and the vast majority produce distal axonal degeneration [78]. Anticancer drugs especially vinca alkaloids, cis plastin and isoniazid, amiodarone, dapsone, nitrofurantoin, metronidazole and phenytoin have been commonly implicated. Isoniazid causes a sensorimotor neuropathy due to pyridoxine deficiency associated with increased excretion. Chronic lead exposure predominantly gives rise to motor neuropathy characterised by symmetrical radioneuropathy and wrist drop. A delayed-onset progressive polyneuropathy may follow exposure to arsenic either intentional or from insecticide.

Box 7.5. Key Points. Peripheral Neuropathy

- Classified on the basis as to the specific cell type involved, namely, neurons, Schwann cells or mixed.
- In axonopathies there is little or no loss of nerve conduction velocity.
  In demyelinating neuropathy, there is decreased nerve conduction velocity.

- Most elderly patients have axonal neuropathy.
- Deficiency of thiamine leads to degeneration of axon sheath with subsequent involvement of the axon [67].
- Direct toxicity of alcohol and its metabolites is involved in the pathogenesis of pure alcoholic neuropathy with distally accentuated axonal degeneration of both myelinated and unmyelinated fibres [68].
- Patients with anti-Hu antibodies usually present with paraneoplastic subacute sensory neuropathy [72].
- In toxic neuropathies there is damage of nerve cells, others induce demyelination, and the vast majority produce distal axonal degeneration [78].

7.5.1 Guillain-Barre Syndrome (GBS) or Acute Inflammatory Demyelinating Polyradiculopathy (AIDP)

Introduction
GBS is an immune-mediated peripheral neuropathy causing limb weakness that progresses over a time period of days or at the most up to 4 weeks [79]. GBS consists of different subtypes [80, 81] and can be divided into demyelinating and axonal forms based on pathological and electrodiagnostic findings [82]. They are the acute inflammatory demyelinating polyradiculopathy (AIDP), acute motor axonal neuropathy (AMAN), acute motor sensory axonal neuropathy (AMSAN), Miller-Fisher syndrome and panautonomic neuropathy [83]. The Miller-Fisher syndrome, Guillain-Barre syndrome with ophthalmoplegia, Bickerstaff's brain stem encephalitis and acute ophthalmoparesis without ataxia are closely related forming a continuous range and have been confirmed clinically [84]. It has been suggested that there is a bimodal incidence in adult life [85, 86] with peaks seen in late adolescence and in the elderly. The age-incidence rise approximating fourfold between the under 20 age group and the over 60 year age group [87, 88] and the reason for the peaking in the elderly are not clear (Table 7.1).

Pathophysiology
It has been suggested that it may be due to the defective immune suppressor mechanisms [82]. It is considered an autoimmune disease triggered by preceding viral or bacterial infection. The autoimmune response is directed against the Schwann cells or myelin and in some cases the axon [89]. The association of clinical characteristics of GBS with specific infections have been reported [90, 91]. The commonly identified pathogens are the *Campylobacter jejuni* [80, 81, 92–94], cytomegalovirus (5–15 %) [91], Epstein-Barr virus (2–10 %) [91] and *Mycoplasma pneumoniae* (1–5 %) [91]. Axonal forms are caused by antibodies to gangliosides, and quarter of them are associated with *Campylobacter jejuni* infection [80]. The pathophysiology

Table 7.1 Common acquired neuropathies in the elderly

	Physiological abnormality	
Clinical presentation	Axonal	Demyelinating
Acute/subacute	AMAN, AMSAN Alcoholic Critical illness Vitamin deficiency Porphyria Carcinoma (late)	AIDP Diphtheria Carcinoma Hodgkin's/lymphoma
Chronic	Diabetes Uraemia B12 deficiency HIV Hodgkin's/lymphoma Vitamin deficiencies Lyme disease Toxic	Paraprotein demyelinating Chronic liver disease Hypothyroidism Chronic inflammatory demyelinating

Information sources: Ludolph and Spencer [78], Uncini and Kuwabara [98]
AIDP acute inflammatory demyelinating polyneuropathy, *AMAN* acute motor axonal neuropathy, *AMSAN* acute motor and sensory axonal neuropathy

of the syndrome was recently determined with the presence of anti-GQ1b antibodies [95]. The Miller-Fisher subtype is particularly associated with antibodies to GQ1b [87, 96]. GBS is now considered to embrace a number of subtypes with evidence of different immunological mechanisms [97]. Besides the antibodies against the peripheral nerve gangliosides, new antibodies against other nerve antigens such as neurofascin have been described [97]. T cells are also involved, and experimental autoimmune neuritis has been induced by T-cell responses to one or more of the three myelin proteins, P2, PO and PMP22 [91]. GBS is reclassified based on different electrodiagnostic criteria [98] into acute inflammatory demyelinating polyradiculoneuropathy (AIDP), acute motor and sensory axonal neuropathy (AMSAN) and acute motor axonal neuropathy (AMAN) [94, 98].

Box 7.6. Key Points. Guillain-Barre Syndrome (GBS)

- May be due to defective immune suppressor mechanisms [82].
- Autoimmune response is directed against the Schwann cells or myelin and in some cases the axon.
- Axonal forms are caused by antibodies to gangliosides [1].
- Miller-Fisher subtype is associated with antibodies to GQ16 [87, 96].
- GBS is reclassified based on different electrodiagnostic criteria into acute inflammatory demyelinating polyradiculopathy (AIDP), acute motor and sensory axonal neuropathy (AMSAN) and acute motor axonal neuropathy (AMAN) [94, 98].

7.6 Disorders of Neuromuscular Transmission

Introduction

Myasthenia gravis (MG) is an autoimmune disorder characterised by fluctuating muscle weakness and fatigue caused by antibodies directed against the nicotine acetylcholine (ACh) receptor (AChR) or against the muscle-specific tyrosine kinase (MuSK) receptor [99]. In the general population, the incidence is about 1 in 100,000, whereas the prevalence varies from 5 to 15 in 100,000 [100, 101]. In the United States, the prevalence rates have increased to about 20 per 100,000 [102], and the prevalence has increased over the past four to five decades [103]. MG is probably underdiagnosed in the elderly population [104–106]. The incidence is age and sex related [106, 107]. About one-third of all cases occur in the older population [108], and over the past 40 years, the occurrence after the age of 50 years is not uncommon [109]. In the early onset cases, most are between the ages of 15 and 40, with a predilection for females. In the late onset cases, between ages 60–70 years, the males predominate [105–107]. In general women are affected twice as often as men, and men formed two groups one group with peak of onset between 25 and 30 years and the other between 60 and 70 years [110].

Physiology of normal neuromuscular transmission

The neuromuscular junction comprises the nerve terminal, the muscle fibre, the presynaptic membrane, the postsynaptic membrane and the synaptic cleft. In normal neuromuscular transmission, acetylcholine (ACh) is the neurotransmitter and is contained in vesicles in the presynaptic terminal [111]. In the axonal terminal, there are voltage-gated calcium channels which open to release calcium ions with the arrival of the nerve action potential. Vesicles containing ACh then fuse with the cell membrane releasing ACh into the synaptic cleft. The ACh then crosses the synaptic cleft to bind to the nicotine acetylcholine receptor (AChR) in the postsynaptic muscle fibre. This results in generating an action potential brought about by the opening of the voltage-gated sodium channels. Rapsyn, an intracellular adaptor, binds AChRs and attaches them to a contractile protein, F-actin, allowing AChR to cluster densely at the top of the postsynaptic membrane folds [112]. A high concentration of AChR is necessary for effective neurotransmission. There is an inflow of sodium ions into the muscle cell from the sodium channels. The entry of sodium ions into the muscle cell depolarises the cell membrane and triggers a regenerative muscle action potential spreading throughout the cell releasing calcium from the sarcoplasmic reticulum and initiating the process of muscle contraction. The unbound ACh is then broken down by acetylcholinesterase into choline and acetyl group. The choline passes into the sarcoplasmic reticulum and is repackaged into vesicles [113]. The muscle-specific kinase (MuSK), a tyrosine kinase receptor, is necessary for the postsynaptic differentiation and clustering of acetylcholine receptors. Agrin [114] released from the motor nerve interacts with LRP4 [115] which then associates with MuSK and stimulates a signalling pathway that promotes the clustering of AChR [116] and preparing the way to anterograde signalling by subsequent phosphorylation of DOK7, an intracellular adapter [112]. The agrin/LRP4/MuSK/DOK7

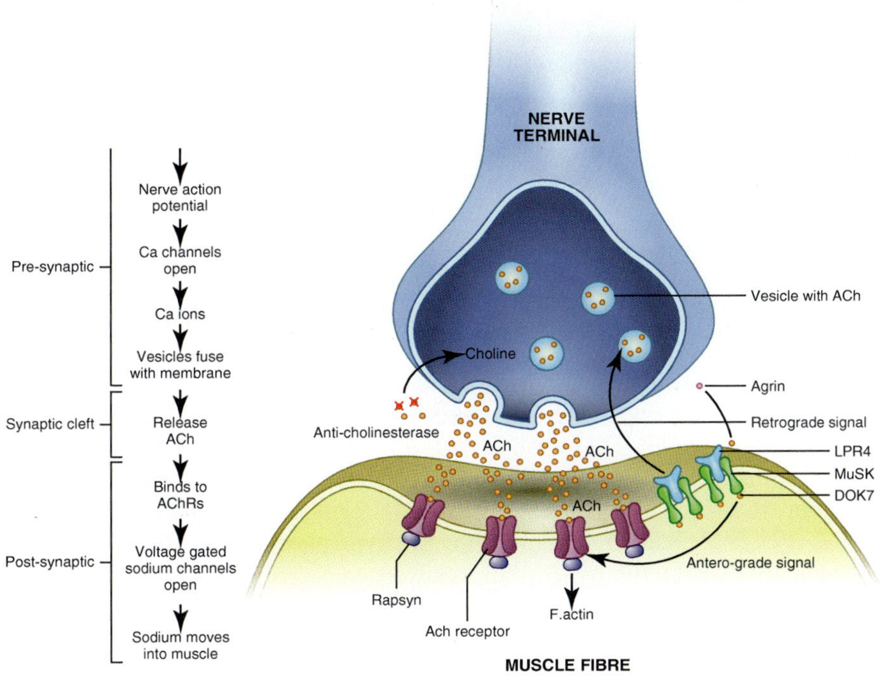

Fig. 7.3 Neuromuscular transmission (Information sources: Koneczy et al. [112], Reddel [118])

pathway is crucial for the clustering process [112]. It is believed that LRP4 sends a retrograde signal to the presynaptic site which includes clustering of voltage-gated calcium channels [112] (Fig. 7.3).

Pathophysiology

In MG antibodies to the AChR cause a functional blockade of the binding site for ACh [117]. The autoantibodies in MG are either directed to the muscle nicotine acetylcholine receptor (AChR) or to the muscle-specific tyrosine kinase (MuSK) [99, 117]. In MG there is a reduction in the number of functional AChRs, and several mechanisms have been proposed as to the mechanism for AChR impairment [117]. There is a reduction in its surface expression and initiation of complement and inflammatory cascades [118] leading to reduction in the postsynaptic folding [99]. AChRs and Na(+) channels are concentrated in the neuromuscular junction postsynaptic folds. There appears to be a causal relationship between the binding of antibody to AChR, the reduction in muscle AChR and impairment of neuromuscular transmission [119]. It has also been shown that autoantibodies against MuSK decrease the patency of the neuromuscular junction, resulting in the symptoms of MG. The agrin-induced AChR clustering in the muscle myotubes is inhibited by the MuSK antibodies directed against the extracellular domain of MuSK [120].

Some MG patients do not have detectable AChR antibodies and are termed seronegative MG [120]. In 2–3 % of AChR seronegative patients, there was seropositivity of anti-MuSK antibody [121]. It had been reported that anti-AChR antibodies were seen in 65 % with early-onset MG compared to 85 % in the late-onset MG, and elevated titres of anti-MuSK antibodies were similar [121]. In vitro studies have shown that some seronegative patients' plasma often contains a factor, most likely an immunoglobulin antibody that alters AChR function [120]. Some MG patients without antibodies against AChR have instead antibodies to MuSK [122]. In patients with non-AChR antibodies, there are two major antigens, the Ca(2+) release channel of the sarcoplasmic reticulum and the ryanodine receptor (RyR) and titin which is essential for muscle function and structure [123]. Titin and ryanodine receptor antibodies are seen in 95 % of thymic MG and in 50 % of late-onset MG and are associated with severe disease [123, 124]. Antibodies against LRP4 were found in some patients who had no antibodies directed against AChR or MuSK [125, 126].

The role of the thymus in MG is not known. Its content of AChR, skeletal muscle elements and the presence of germinal centres in MG suggest that the thymus could be the site of autosensitisation [117, 119]. In nearly 75–85 % of AChR-positive MG, the thymus shows pathological abnormalities [127]; thymoma is found in 10–20 % of MG cases [117] and 65 % showed thymic hyperplasia [128]. HLA-haplotypes predominate with thymic hyperplasia (and different from that of thymoma). A familial disposition is found in 5 % of the cases with an increased frequency of HLA-B8 and DR3 [129]. It is an autoimmune disorder, and individuals with family members who suffer from disorders such as rheumatoid arthritis, scleroderma or lupus erythematosus have an increased risk of myasthenia gravis. Ocular MG and generalised MG are sometimes associated with thyroid ophthalmopathy or thyroid autoimmunity [130] and thyroid function abnormality ratio is higher in the early-onset group [131].

7.6.1 Eaton-Lambert Syndrome

Introduction

Eaton-Lambert syndrome (E-LS) is a disorder of neuromuscular transmission characterised by a reduction in the release of acetylcholine from the motor nerve terminals. Its prevalence has been reported as 2.3 per million with an annual incidence rate of 0.5 per million [132]. It is a rare condition and is a disease of middle age and the elderly and the average of diagnosis is about 60 years of age.

Pathophysiology

More than half the patients with E-LS are associated with malignancies such as small cell lung cancer (SCLC), non-small cell lung cancer [133], lymphoma, T-cell leukaemia and transitional cell carcinoma of the bladder and possibly thymic malignancies. It was first described as a paraneoplastic syndrome in patients with lung cancer. There are two main subgroups E-LS combined with SCLC and E-LS with non-SCLC [133].

The antibodies are directed against the presynaptic voltage-gated calcium channels (VGCC) in the presynaptic cholinergic nerve terminals at the neuromuscular junction which are responsible for the release of ACh [134–137]. The antibodies in E-LS prevent the opening of the calcium channels and hence the release of ACh. The ACh release is mediated by a synaptic fusion complex which consists of three soluble fusion attachment protein receptors (SNARE proteins) [138]. SCLC is found in 60 % of the E-LS, and the calcium channels also present a cell line derived from the tumour [135]. In some patients with E-LS, there are no antibodies, and the exact mechanism underlying the disorder remains unclear.

Box 7.7: Key Points. Disorders of Neuromuscular Transmission: Myasthenia Gravis (MG)

In MG antibodies to AChR cause a functional blockade of the binding site for ACh [117].

- The autoantibodies are directed either against the muscle nicotine AChR or the muscle-specific tyrosine kinase (MuSK) [99, 117].
- Autoantibodies against MuSK decreases the potency of neuromuscular junction.
- Some MG without antibodies against ACHR have instead antibodies to MuSK [122].
- Titin and ryanodine receptor antibodies are seen in 95 % of thymic MG and in 50 % of late-onset MG [123, 124].
- Antibodies against LRP4 were found in some patients who had no antibodies directed against AChR or MuSK [125, 126].
- *In nearly 75–85 % of AChR-positive MG, the thymus shows pathological abnormalities* [127].

Box 7.8. Key Points. Eaton-Lambert Syndrome

- Characterised by reduction in the release of Ach from the motor nerve terminal.
- Associated with malignancies in more than half the patients [133].
- Antibodies are directed against the presynaptic voltage-gated Ca channels (VGCC) in the presynaptic cholinergic nerve terminals at the neuromuscular junction responsible for the release of ACh [134–137].

7.7 Stroke in the Elderly

Introduction

The incidence of stroke rises exponentially with increasing age. About half of all strokes occur in the group aged >70 years and nearly a quarter occur in those who are >85 years of age [139, 140]. The incidence rates of first-ever stroke rose markedly with age and will keep increasing even at 90 years and over [141]. The incidence of all stroke doubles with each decade after the age of 55 years.

Pathophysiology and pathogenesis
Approximately 15 % of strokes are due to primary intracerebral haemorrhage and the remaining 80–85 % to cerebral infarction. About 25 % of the ischaemic strokes are due to atherosclerosis and may follow hypoperfusion or atherogenic embolism. Small vessel disease giving rise to lacunar infarcts amounts to 25 %. A further 25 % are due to cardiac embolism and the remaining to a number of causes, namely, cryptogenic, arteritis and dissection, among others.

7.7.1 Large Vessel Atherosclerosis

Atherosclerosis is by far the commonest pathological feature resulting in stroke. Atherosclerosis is primarily typified by the formation of intimal plaques called atheroma. A chain of events leads up to the formation of the plaque. Many of the events are linked at least initially to chronic injury to the endothelium [142]. According to the insudation theory, the focal accumulation of fat in the vessel wall is derived from the plasma lipoproteins. This begins with endothelial dysfunction which may be triggered by factors such as shear stress and turbulent flow, oxidative stress, hyperlipidaemia, hypertension, smoking and impaired glucose metabolism, among others [142, 143]. The endothelium has two important roles: one is that it prevents the passage of substances in the blood into the vessel wall and the other prevents intravascular clotting. Insudation of lipoproteins especially the low-density lipoproteins (LDL) into the intima undergoes modification and initiates monocyte migration. The lipoproteins are taken up by the monocytes to become lipid-filled foam cells, the hallmark of atherosclerosis.

As the plaque evolves, denudation of the endothelium occurs followed by platelet deposition giving rise to the release of platelet-derived growth factor (PDGF) which further enhances the proliferation of smooth muscle cells. Thrombi are formed over the plaque as a result of (i) loss of endothelium, where the thrombus forms on the plaque surface (superficial), and (ii) by plaque rupture where the thrombus forms within the plaque (deep). The fibrous cap of the plaque tears to expose the lipid core containing large amounts of cholesterol crystals, fragments of collagen and tissue factor and thrombus forms rapidly within the plaque itself [144].

The thrombogenic cascade is triggered as the result of endothelial injury. Injury (erosion/denudation) to the endothelium exposes the collagen allowing platelets to adhere to it as a result of the Ia/Ib receptor [144]. At the same time, the coagulation is initiated by the formation of thrombin and fibrin which triggered by the tissue factor is independent of vWF and glycoprotein. Under these conditions, von Willebrand factor (vWF) appears to play an important role in both platelet adhesion and aggregation.

7.7.2 Small Vessel Disease

It is widely surmised that disease of the small intracranial vessels is responsible for the small deep-seated (lacunar) infarctions and primary cerebral haemorrhage [145]. About 25 % of ischaemic strokes are due to small vessel disease following occlusion of the small penetrating arteries. Fisher [146] distinguished two types of underlying vascular pathology, lipohyalinosis and microatheromatosis.

I. Ischaemic stroke

Cerebral infarction can be classified as lacunar, territorial and watershed infarctions. The lacunar infarctions lie in the deeper non-cortical parts of the cerebrum, brain stem and cerebellum and result from occlusion of the penetrating branches of the large cerebral arteries. The territorial infarction is in turn subdivided into cortical and subcortical. The watershed infarction is subdivided into cortical and internal. In cerebral infarction, the mechanisms are (i) embolism, the embolic material originating from the heart (cardio-embolic) or from non-cardiac source, for instance, the carotid arteries (artery to artery embolus). Embolism due to fat, tumour cells or air is a rare occurrence. (ii) Thrombotic formation of a thrombus or clot within a cerebral vessel. (iii) Thromboembolic-embolic material originating from a thrombus. (iv) Haemodynamic, hypoperfusion giving rise to border zone/watershed infarction. Cellular mechanisms of neuronal death: occlusion emboli, atherosclerotic or other vascular diseases of the cerebral artery lead to focal cerebral infarction (Fig. 7.4).

Ischaemia is rapidly followed by neuronal cell death. Thus, cerebral ischaemia may result in a central core of infarcted tissue surrounded by a region which is potentially salvageable, the penumbra. There has been a new understanding of the mechanisms by which ischaemic neurons die. In cerebral ischaemia, there are three cellular mechanisms for cell death: necrosis, apoptosis and necroptosis. The last is a mechanism which embraces both necrotic and apoptotic components.

Within an hour of the ischaemic insult, there is an area of severe ischaemia known as the 'core zone' where the CBF is 10–25 % of the normal. There is necrosis of the neurons as well as the supporting glial cells. Surrounding this area is an ischaemic zone of oligaemia called the 'penumbra'. Changes that may occur following cellular injury during the ischaemia are brain oedema. There are two types of oedema, cytotoxic and vasogenic. Cytotoxic oedema occurs within minutes to hours and may be reversible. Hypoxia resulting from acute cerebral ischaemia causes the neurons, glia and endothelial cells to swell due to failure of the ATP-dependant (Na and Ca) transport. The rapid accumulation of sodium within the cells results in flow of water to maintain osmotic equilibrium causing swelling of all the cellular elements of the brain. The vasogenic oedema occurs over hours to days and is considered to be irreversible. It is characterised by increase in the extracellular fluid volume due to increased permeability of the capillary endothelial cells to macromolecular serum proteins like albumin giving rise to plasma protein containing fluid leaking into the extracellular space. It can give rise to midline shift and to cerebral herniation. The larger the infarct, the greater the potential to develop cerebral oedema.

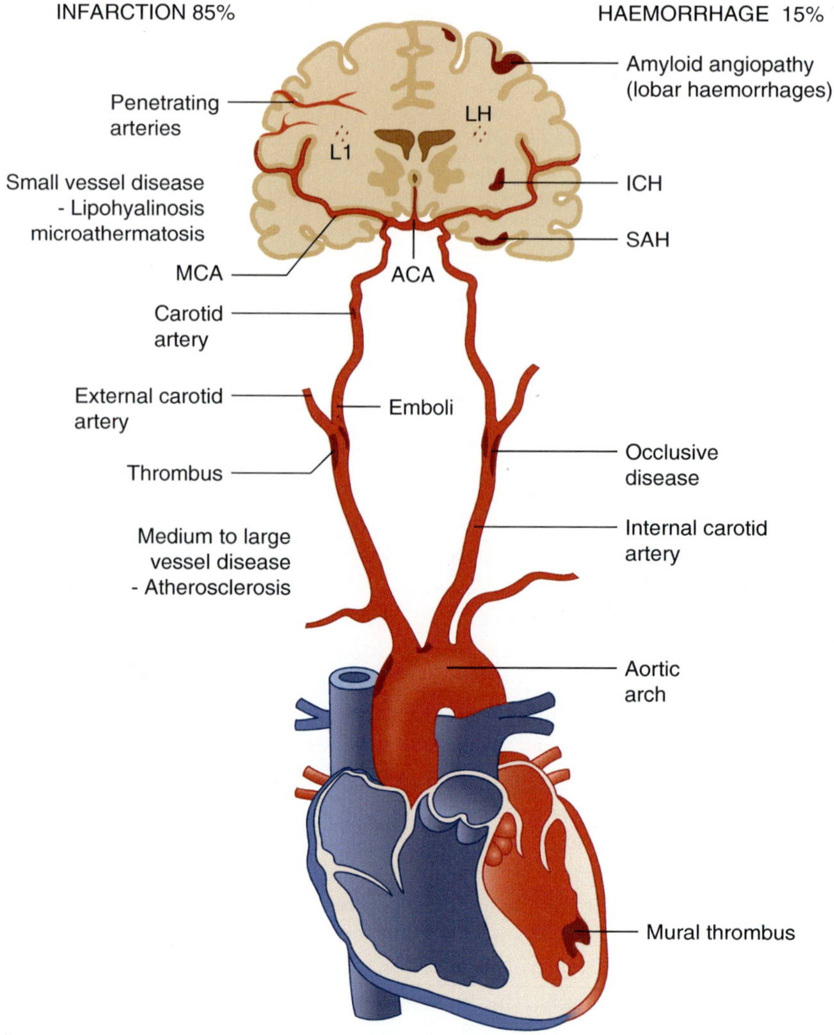

Fig. 7.4 Pathophysiology of stroke. Diagram shows atherosclerosis in the medium and large vessels and lipohyalinosis in the penetrating arteries. Mechanisms involved are thrombosis, embolism and haemodynamic giving rise to territorial (cortical and subcortical), lacunar and water-shed infarcts

An ischaemic infarct can undergo haemorrhagic conversion or transformation. Haemorrhagic conversion can take two forms, haemorrhagic infarction (HI) or less commonly parenchymatous haematoma (PH). Some haemorrhagic transformation may be of indeterminate form with features of both HI and PH. HI is confined within the vascular territory, is asymptomatic and on CT scan appears as hyperdense areas ranging from a few petechiae and patchy to confluent areas of bleeding. PH differs from HI in that it extends beyond the vascular territory, is symptomatic, often exerts mass effect and on CT appears as hyperdense homogenous collection of blood. In most instances PH is due to rupture of an ischaemic vessel which has been subject to reperfusion pressures.

II. Cerebral Haemorrhage

Pathophysiology
Approximately 80 % of primary intracerebral haemorrhage (PICH) is due to spontaneous rupture of small vessels damaged by hypertension. The second most common cause is cerebral amyloid angiopathy. Secondary intracerebral haemorrhages are due to either congenital causes or acquired conditions such as vascular anomalies, coagulopathies and various drugs, among others.

7.7.3 Cellular Mechanisms of Neuronal Death

Cerebral haemorrhage is a dynamic process and continues for several hours. Many of the haemorrhages continue to expand over several hours after the onset of symptoms. In a third of the patients, it occurs within the first 24 h, and in two-thirds of them, it is evident within the first 4 h [147]. The expansion is likely to be due to continued bleeding from the primary source and to mechanical disruption of the surrounding vessels. A local coagulation deficit and acute hypertension may be associated [148]. Inflammation caused by thrombin and end products of coagulation causes most of the brain injury and swelling [149]. Haematoma initiates neuronal damage and oedema which accumulates in the extravascular space [150]. The latter results from the osmotically active proteins in the haematoma which develops over the first 24–96 h and slowly resolves over several weeks. The late-onset oedema which persists for several weeks after the initial haemorrhage is the result of disruption of the blood-brain barrier, lysis of red cells and formation of free radicals and direct cytotoxicity [149]. Neuronal death occurs in the regions surrounding the haematoma and is predominantly necrotic, and there is evidence to suggest the presence of programmed cell death (apoptosis) [149] (Fig. 7.5).

(i) Small vessel disease
In microvascular disease, the small penetrating arterioles of the subependymal and pial microvasculature tend to become stenosed and undergo lipohyalinosis, or they may dilate to form microaneurysms. Patients with microvascular brain disease can have recurrent events which can be either ischaemic or haemorrhagic. It is not clear why some vessels affected by fibrinoid necrosis rupture, some occlude and some heal without any obvious sequelae. It is surmised that sudden alterations in cerebral blood flow or pressure cause fibrinoid necrosis and cause vessel wall to rupture [145].

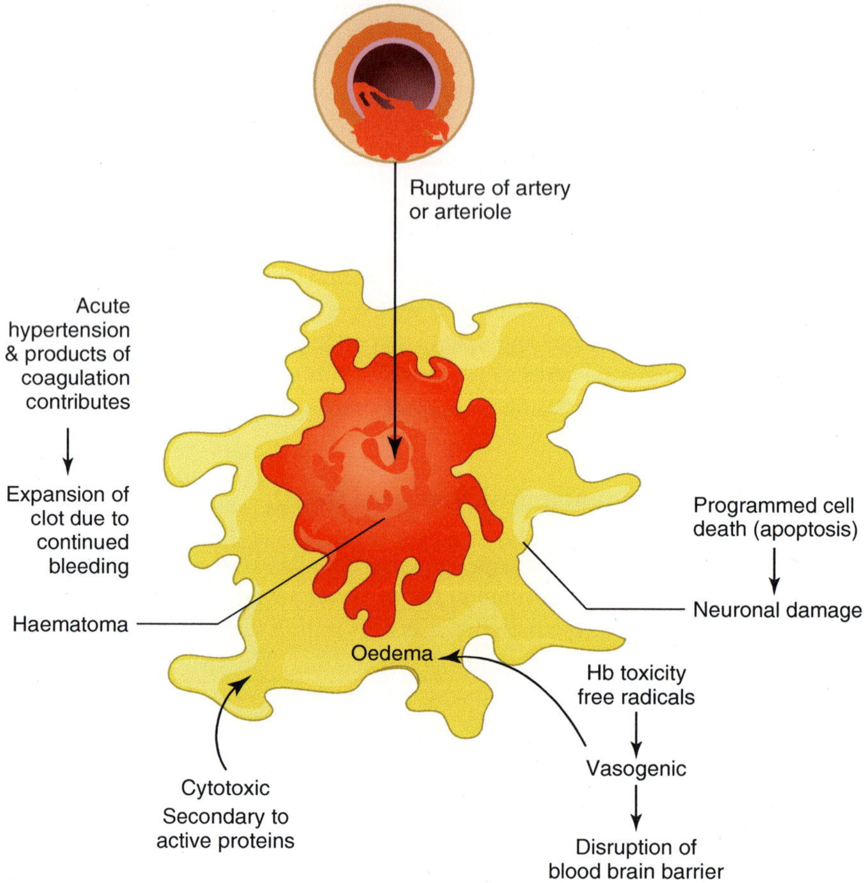

Fig. 7.5 Modified schematic illustration of neuronal death at molecular level in cerebral haemorrhage (Information sources: Brott et al. [147], Qureshi et al. [148], Chakravathy and Sivane [149], Butcher [150])

(ii) Cerebral amyloid angiopathy (CAA)
CAA results from extracellular deposition of fibrillar proteins (b-amyloid or Ab) on the walls (tunica media and adventitia) of small- and mid-sized blood vessels of the brain and meninges. It damages the cortical and leptomeningeal vessels causing stenosis of the vessel lumen, fragmentation of the arterial elastic lamina and thickening of the basement membrane. These processes result in fibrinoid necrosis and formation of microaneurysms. Age is the strongest risk factor for CAA and is a major cause of ICH. The haemorrhages are superficial, lobar cerebral and cerebellar and often breach the cortical surface resulting in secondary subarachnoid haemorrhage. They can be multiple and recurrent. The most frequent sites of CAA-related haemorrhages are the occipital and frontal lobes with subcortical haemorrhages. Other features are leucoencephalopathy and small cortical ischaemic infarcts. Sporadic CAA is common in the elderly and is often found in association with Alzheimer's disease. The Boston Criteria aided and differentiated lobar intracerebral haemorrhage into possible, probable or definite based on the likelihood of underlying CAA [151].

Box 7.9. Key Points. Stroke in the Elderly

- 25 % of ischaemic strokes are due to atherosclerosis and may follow hypoperfusion or atherogenic occlusion.
- 25 % are due to small vessel disease.
- 25 % are due to cardio-embolism.
- Remaining due to a number of causes.
- The mechanisms in ischaemic stroke are embolism (cardio-embolic/artery to artery), thrombotic, thrombo-embolic and haemodynamic.
- Many of the cerebral haemorrhages continue to expand for several hours after the onset of symptoms [147–149].
- Cerebral amyloid angiopathy results from extracellular deposition of fibrillary protein in the walls of small- and mid-sized blood vessels.

7.8 Related Disorders

7.8.1 Insomnia and Related Sleep Disorders in the Elderly

Introduction

Insomnia is characterised by the perception that sleep has not been restorative as the result of imperfect sleep due to difficulty in falling asleep [152–154], maintaining sleep or awakening too early in the morning. Insomnia is common in elderly people [155, 156], and chronic insomnia is more common in this group [157]. Population studies have revealed that insomnia has a high prevalence in the old age groups and ranges from 30 to 50 % [158, 159], depending on definitions, methods used and populations studied [160, 161]. Two epidemiological studies found a high prevalence of insomnia in those over 60 years, especially among women [162]. However true sleep disorders are less prevalent in older people [159]. Another study found that 49.9 % of men and 69.2 % of elderly women complained of insomnia [163], and women complained more about sleep difficulties than elderly men [164].

Physiology of sleep

There are five phases of sleep: REM (rapid eye movements) and stages 1, 2, 3 and 4 of non-REM (NREM). More recently these stages have been identified as N1, N2 and N3 [165]. A complete sleep cycle takes 90–110 min; the second and later cycles take longer in normal adults [166]. About half the sleep time is spent in stage 2 and about one-fifth in REM and the remaining in the other stages. REM period length increases [167] and predominates in the last one-third of the night [168]. As the sleep progresses, stage 2 accounts for most the NREM sleep, and stages 3 and 4 may sometimes disappear. During REM, muscle tone decreases with rapid eye movements, and breathing becomes more rapid, irregular and shallow. During stages 1 and 2, muscle tone is moderately reduced, and on the encephalogram, there is gradual slowing of the background activity. In stages 3 and 4, extremely slow waves appear interspersed with smaller faster waves. Stages 3 and 4 together are called

Table 7.2 Pathophysiology of sleep in the elderly

Age-related changes	Primary sleep disorders	Secondary sleep problems
1. Total sleep time little change; 'deep' stage (4) markedly reduced Nocturnal awakenings – fragmentation and disruption of sleep increase 2. Changes in circadian rhythm	Sleep apnoea syndrome PLMS PLS, RBD, central apnoea, sleep bruxism	Associated with (i) psychiatric alterations – Anxiety, depression Psychosis, fear of dying (ii) Organic diseases-and Symptoms – nocturia Pruritus, pain, respiratory disorders (iii) Neurological diseases dementia, Parkinson's (iv) Drug and alcohol (v) Inadequate sleep Hygiene (vi) Environmental factors

Information source: Avidan [154], Bombos et al. [159], Culebras [173], Dement et al. [174]

deep sleep and provides the subjective feeling of restful sleep. The circadian rhythm is the major determinant of sleep and is regulated by an internal biological clock over a 24-h period [169]. The important factors which determine the amount and timing of sleep and sleep architecture (sleep stages) are the circadian rhythms, environment and time awake [170].

Pathophysiology

The changes in the sleep-wake patterns in insomnia have been attributed to the (i) physiological changes that are part of normal ageing. The sleep patterns that follow advancing age suggest age-related disturbances of the circadian sleep-wake rhythm as well as (ii) primary sleep disorders such as obstructive sleep apnoea, periodic limb movement (PLM), restless leg syndrome (RLS) and circadian rhythm disorders [154]. These together with REM and sleep apnoea syndrome (SAS) are the most common sleep disorders in relatively healthy elderly people [171] and (iii) secondary sleep problem resulting from one of a variety of causes, such as psychiatric, medical conditions and psychosocial factors [154] or a combination of all three [172] (Table 7.2):

(i) Physiological changes with ageing

Sleep requirements and patterns change throughout life. As age advances, it is the quality of sleep rather than the quantity that changes. Stage 4 sleep is markedly reduced or even lacking, and whereas an adult experiences about two awakenings, the elderly show increase in duration as well as the number [168] of these as many as five to ten [152]. In the first half of the night, stages 3–4 predominate, and in the second half, REM and later stages 1 and 2 prevail. The elderly manifest early morning awakening, increased night-time wakefulness and increased fragmentation of sleep periods with corresponding decrease in total sleep time [175] that impedes daytime performance and optimal functioning. The increase in overnight arousal due to sleep fragmentation may be exacerbated by medical conditions of the elderly including sleep apnoea, cardiopulmonary disease and musculoskeletal disorders

[168]. The increased night-time wakefulness is followed by daytime tiredness, daytime napping and falling asleep during the day [176–178] which can have consequences in function the following day [157, 178]. These age-related changes in sleep are independent of any medical or psychiatric disorders, and elderly who have no symptoms and no known disease do have these changes in the sleep-wake patterns as compared with younger persons [179].

(ii) Sleep disorders
There are two distinct forms of sleep apnoea, obstructive (OSA) and central, and the former is more common. In the former breathing is interrupted, and airflow is absent because of occlusion of the upper airways. Obesity, nasal congestion, large neck, upper airway muscular weakness and sedating drugs are some of the risk factors for OSA [180]. In central apnoea breathing is interrupted due lack of effort, and there is no evidence of respiratory activity. Symptoms could be present for years without recognition during which time the individual may have become conditioned to the daytime sleepiness and fatigue.

Due to changes in the blood gas tensions during sleep, normal subjects experience brief periods of apnoea during sleep, and they are less than 10 s and ten times a night and occur during sleep stages 1 and 2 and in REM. In individuals where airflow is reduced to a degree where the O_2 level falls, neurological mechanism triggers a sudden interruption of sleep called neurological arousal. These may or may not have a significant negative effect on the restorative quality of sleep. In obstructive sleep apnoea repetitive disruption of sleep results in sleep deprivation.

(iii) Sleep-related disorders
Disorders of partial arousal and those that interfere with sleep stage transitions are known as parasomnias. They occur during transition from wakefulness and NREM sleep or wakefulness and REM sleep. The former includes sleep walking (somnambulism), bruxism, restless leg syndrome and periodic limb movement. NREM parasomnias such as sleep walking typically occur in the initial third of the night with the presence of stage 3 sleep [168]. The latter includes REM sleep behaviour (RBD) and catathrenia. Two sleep-related disorders, the restless leg syndrome (RLS) and the periodic limb movement disorder (PLMD), affect the elderly [172] with increasing severity. RBDs, RLS and PLMD increase with age [159]. The prevalence of RLS varies from 5 to 20 % in the general population in North America [181]. The cause is not known. RLS is characterised by unpleasant sensations in the legs, 'creepy and crawly' [182] and an uncontrollable urge to move when at rest and the symptoms are activated by lying down or when relaxing resulting in an inability to fall asleep [172]. Older patients experience these more frequently and for longer periods of time. People with RLS have difficulty in falling asleep.

The prevalence of periodic leg movements (PLMS) is estimated to be 4–11 % in adults, and it occurs with sleep disturbances in the elderly [183]. PLMS is most frequently seen in RLS and often occur in narcolepsy [183]. Periodic leg movement disorder (PLMD) is characterised by involuntary leg twitching or jerky movements during sleep, with rhythmic extension of the toes and with bending of the ankle, knee and hip [182] and typically anywhere from 10 to 50 times an hour and sometimes throughout the night. These symptoms cause repeated awakenings [172] and cause excessive daytime sleepiness. PLMD has been seen in patients with healthy sleep patterns, and some studies have shown there is no greater incidence in patients with insomnia than in those with sleep-wake conditions like excessive day-time sleepiness.

REM sleep behaviour disorder (RBD) is a parasomnia characterised by loss of normal muscle tone together with simple and complex behaviours while dreaming and occurring during REM-associated sleep which occurs in the last half of the night [168]. It occurs most frequently in the elderly over the age of 60 years [180]. The patients have striking and often frightening dreams and appear to 'act out their dreams' often causing self-injury or injury to the partner [184]. The behaviours are usually nondirected and include punching, kicking and running from bed during REM sleep [184]. At least one of the criteria laid down by the American Sleep Disorder Association [185] must be satisfied to make the diagnosis which includes potential harmful sleep behaviour, dreams that appear acted out and sleep behaviour that disrupts sleep continuity.

RBD maybe idiopathic or may be associated with various neurological conditions [184] (see Box 7.11). It may coexist or precede Parkinson's disease (PD) or dementia of the Lewy body type (LBD) and can be an early marker of these diseases [186]. Neuroimaging and pharmacological studies suggest that the dopaminergic systems are involved in RBD and RLS [184]. In RLS besides abnormality of dopaminergic metabolism, abnormality of iron metabolism is implicated in its pathophysiology [180].

(iv) Environmental factors notably influence sleep

Good sleeping habits should be encouraged. The elderly are easily roused from night-time sleep by auditory stimuli. Physical illnesses could disrupt sleep and produce symptoms mistaken for insomnia. Psychiatric problems, depression, anxiety, psychosis and stress could be the cause and/or effect of insomnia. Medical illnesses, for instance, prostatic problems in elderly men, arthritic pain, nocturnal angina and paroxysmal nocturnal dyspnoea, are common causes of awakening in the night. Lifestyle influences that include the use of stimulants, alcohol, caffeine and nicotine could trigger awakenings, as do erratic work practices and sleep schedules.

7.8.1.1 Narcolepsy

Narcolepsy is a sleep disorder characterised by uncontrollable episodes of falling asleep during the daytime. It is associated with other symptoms, namely, cataplexy, sleep paralysis and hypnagogic and hypnopompic hallucinations, and together they form the classical tetrad. It results from irregular sleep cycling; individuals with narcolepsy enter sleep directly into REM sleep instead of entering sleep through NREM [187]. It occurs in the elderly, and in one review of 41 consecutive patients, 38 % were in their 60s and 70s [188]. Those that occur later in life are usually associated with Parkinson's disease or multiple sclerosis and are referred to as secondary narcolepsy [189]. All four symptoms are usually present in less than 50 % of the cases.

Box 7.10. Key Points. Insomnia and Related Disorders

- The elderly manifest early morning awakening, increased night-time wakefulness and increased fragmentation of sleep periods with corresponding decrease in total sleep time that impedes daytime performance and optimal functioning [155].
- Parasomnias are disorders of partial arousal or those that interfere with sleep stage transition.
- Those that occur during transition from wakefulness and NREM sleep are sleep walking, sleep terrors, bruxism, RLS and PLMD. Those that occur during transition from wakefulness and REM sleep are RBD and catathrenia [168, 172].

Box 7.11. Causes of REM Sleep Behaviour Disorder

(i) Idiopathic
(ii) Neurodegenerative and neurological
Disorders
DLB disease
Parkinson's disease
Progressive supranuclear palsy
Alzheimer's disease
Shy-Drager syndrome
Multiple sclerosis affecting the brain stem
Multisystem atrophy
Brain stem neoplasm

Information sources: Matheson [180]; Uddin and Jarmil [184]; Tachebana [186]

7.8.2 Headache in the Elderly

Introduction

Headache is pain or discomfort in the head caused by pressure or stimulation of the structures of the head. The prevalence varies with age. In one study 92 % of women and 74 % of men between the ages of 21 and 34 years had headaches as compared with the over 75 age group when the prevalence decline to 55 % and 22 %, respectively [190, 191]. Among the 65 years and over attending the outpatients, 8 % had headaches of which 13.4 % were women and 6.5 % men [192, 193]. Severe recurrent or constant headaches are experienced by approximately 10 % of women and 5 % of men at the age of 70 [194, 195]. In a study to assess

Table 7.3 Showing classification of chronic and recurrent headaches

Chronic (recurrent and persistent) headaches[a]	
Migraine	Giant cell arteritis[a]
Cluster headaches	Chronic open-angle glaucoma[a]
Tension headaches	Chronic sinusitis[a]
Trigeminal neuralgia	Ice-pack paroxysmal hemicrania
Intracranial tumours[a]	Substance abuse
Post-traumatic headaches	Cervical radiculopathy
Subdural haematoma	Chronic obstructive lung disease
Hypnic headache	Rebound headache
AVM, giant aneurysms	Hydrocephalus

Sources of information: Hershey and Bednarczyk [202], Edmeads [209], Evans [215]
[a]Many of these could begin acutely

the 1 year prevalence of headache in an elderly population, the prevalence rates were 44.5 % for tension type of headache, 11 % for migraine headaches 2.2 % for symptomatic headaches and 0.7 % for the remaining [196]. The incidence of primary headache declines with ageing with increase in organic causes especially in the 55–60 years of age [197].

The Headache Classification Committee of the International Headache Society (HIS) listed 13 major headache categories and more than a 100 subdivisions [198] which makes it cumbersome for clinical use. The second edition of The International Classification of Headache Disorders 2004 classifies headache into primary and secondary disorders [199]. Headaches classified as primary headaches due generally to benign neurochemical factors within the nervous system include migraine, tension-type headache, cluster headache may persist in the elderly [200], hypnic headache [191] and other primary headaches. Secondary headaches are symptomatic to some underlying condition [201] which include trigeminal neuralgia, temporal arteritis, post-herpetic neuralgia, cervical spondylosis, sleep apnoea and glaucoma [194, 202]. Headaches can also be classified as headaches of acute onset and those that are persistent and recurrent. Chronic headache is characterised by the occurrence of headache lasting 15 days or more per month [203] and for more than 3 months [204]. It is important to distinguish those that are life-threatening from those that are benign.

In the elderly, the prevalence of acute headaches, include accelerated hypertension, subarachnoid haemorrhage, intracranial disorders (meningitis, encephalitis strokes, ischaemia, haemorrhage), infections (acute viral illness, acute sinusitis) and acute of primary headache such as migraine, tension type and cluster decline. On the other head, prevalence of secondary headaches such as intracranial mass lesions, system disease and temporal arteritis increase. Furthermore headache symptomatology may also change; for example, migraine may evolve into a pattern of chronic daily headache, and aura may occur without headache [205] (Table 7.3).

7.8.2.1 Primary Headaches

Benign dysfunctional headaches
In the elderly only 2 % of migraines begin after the age of 50 years [206]. More often than not, the symptomatology changes as age advances, for instance, the auras may disappear [207] or the aura can occur in isolation [195] and create difficulties in diagnosis. Scintillating visual disturbances, marching paraethesias, dysphagia or hemiplegia characterise the late-life migraine accompaniments [208]. Change in symptomatology and other auras such as hemiparesis, sensory disturbance and monocular or hemianopic visual loss produce more difficulty in diagnosis, and imaging study is then mandatory [209] to rule out an infarct or bleed. In acephalic migraine, neurological symptoms such as hemiparesis, visual impairment or sensory disturbances occur in the absence of headache, rendering differentiation from cerebral infarction or TIA difficult. If the patient has not had typical migraine headaches in the past, this diagnosis should not be made until all other possibilities are excluded [210].

Tension headache is common and occurs at any age and is more common in women. The headache is of a pressing character, band-like and of mild to moderate severity. Nausea is rare and is not aggravated by physical activity nor is there any aura but like migraine is associated with photophobia and phonophobia.
Cluster type is rare and occurs, less than 0.5 % of the population and affects mainly men.

Hypnic headache first described by Raskin in 1988 [211] is a rare primary headache also known as 'clockwise' or 'alarm clock' headache [212, 213]. It is exclusively sleep related and usually starts after the age of 50 years [211, 213]. The pathophysiological mechanism is unclear and continues to be debated but is thought to be associated with hypothalamic dysfunction [214].

7.8.2.2 Secondary Headaches

(i) Temporal arteritis
Temporal arteritis (giant cell arteritis, cranial arteritis) (TA) is a chronic inflammatory disease of the large vessels. It presents more often than not after the age of 50 years, abruptly or insidiously. Headaches have been reported in 60–90 % of patients with TA and are felt over the temple [215]. Typically the symptoms are severe headache localised in the arteries of the scalp (temporal and occipital), claudication in the jaw and muscles of the tongue in two-thirds to half the patients and visual disturbances. The last are due to involvement of either the ophthalmic or posterior ciliary arteries. Visual loss has an abrupt onset and is often preceded by transient visual symptoms such as amaurosis fugax, diplopia, field defects and blurred vision. In more than half the patients, it is accompanied by polymyalgia rheumatica. Systemic symptoms include fever, joint pains, fatigue and loss of weight occur in the majority of the patients. A low-grade anaemia and subtle changes on the liver function tests may be present. It is another cause of pyrexia of unknown origin or unexplained weight loss. Physical examination reveals the affected scalp vessels to be swollen, tender, thickened, nodular and pulseless.

(ii) Intracranial headaches

Brain tumours. The incidence of brain tumours in the over 70s has increased sevenfold [216], and the average annual percentage increases with age [217, 218]. In the elderly the incidence of primary brain tumours is higher [219]. Headaches and seizures are the most common symptoms at presentation [220]. Posterior fossa tumours are more likely to produce headache than supratentorial tumours [221]. Headaches which are indeterminate are not particularly aggravated by coughing, exertion or the head-low position and is seldom accompanied by nausea or other symptoms [222, 223]. Patients may wake up with headache which soon settles. They are localised and become intense in severity as the tumour progresses and the seizures, focal or generalised may develop [220]. Neurological signs include localised limb weakness, sensory changes, speech, behavioural difficulties and visual and gait difficulties, depending on the location of the tumour. Focal neurological deficits may be helpful to localise the tumour [220]. In the elderly patients, clinical signs that may suggest the presence of a brain tumour are gait disorders, short-term memory deficits and intellectual decline over a short period of time [224]. In the elderly primary tumours (meningiomas, malignant gliomas, astrocytoma, primary central nervous system lymphomas) and secondaries from the lung and breast are common.

CT scans showing a meningioma and secondaries

Chronic subdural haematoma. The chronic syndrome is common in the elderly [225]. A study in North Wales showed the incidence of chronic subdural haematoma (cSDH) in the over 65 years to be 8.2 per 100,000 in that population [226]. The common presentations are altered mental state (42–52 %) and focal neurological deficits (46–50 %) [225–228]. It often resembles vascular dementia with focal neurological signs and cognitive impairment. There is an increased tendency for fall (57 %) [225] and together with cerebral atrophy (which stretches the dural veins) and impaired haemostasis (33 %) [226].

CT scan showing subdural haematoma

(iii) Cerebrovascular disease

Cerebral haemorrhage (subarachnoid and intracerebral) can produce sudden and excruciating headaches and are potentially life-threatening and may be accompanied by reduced level of consciousness, neurological signs, papilloedema and convulsion. In the case of subarachnoid haemorrhage, meningism, retinal haemorrhage and fever may also be present. A very good clinical axiom is that any person presenting with acute onset of severe headache, the worst in his/her life, is presumed to have an acute subarachnoid haemorrhage, until proven otherwise.

Cerebral ischaemia. The headaches are non-specific, dull and usually not severe and may precede to the more flagrant signs of brain ischaemia such as hemiparesis, aphasia and sensory changes. About half the patients with vertebrobasilar insufficiency and quarter of those with middle cerebral artery ischaemia have a recurrent but unremarkable headache [222]. A more prominent headache with impairment of consciousness occurs 1–4 days after the onset of cerebral infarction due to surrounding oedema. Headache at the onset of infarction occurs often in cerebral embolism for reasons that are not clear.

Acute meningitis. The elderly are at high risk of having acute bacterial meningitis (ABM) than the younger adults [229]. Due to co-morbid conditions and the clinical symptoms at presentation, the diagnosis is often delayed [229]. In the elderly there is a greater variety of organisms for the meningitis, and viral causes are less common [230, 231]. The organisms responsible are *Streptococcus pneumoniae* being the most common followed by *Listeria monocytogenes* [232, 233], and case fatality for the former is 24 % and for latter 40 % [234].

Rebound headache occurs as a result of overusing medications for headache. It is increasingly common and preventable. Drug-induced headaches tend to be dull, diffuse and sometimes throbbing [197]. Medications containing caffeine as an ingredient are especially hazardous.

Box 7.12. Key Points. Headaches in the Elderly

- Useful to classify headaches into those with acute onset and those that are persistent and recurrent.
- It is important to distinguish those that are life-threatening from those that are benign.
- With advancing years, the prevalence of primary headaches decline while that of the secondary headaches such as intracranial mass lesions and temporal arteritis increase.
- Most alarming complication of temporal arteritis is blindness.
- Urgent ophthalmological evaluation is mandatory if visual impairment is reported.
- Chronic subdural haematoma is common in the elderly and may resemble vascular dementia [225].
- In the elderly primary tumours and secondaries are common [216, 219].

7.8.3 Memory and Memory Loss

7.8.3.1 Memory

Physiology

Memory can be defined as the ability by which information is acquired, stored, retained and subsequently retrieved. Memory embraces a number of recognisable functions that are mediated by different regions of the brain. In general terms, memory is based on the duration of memory retention. It can be categorised into sensory memory and two types of memory stores, short term and long term. Sensory memory has limited capacity to receive information corresponding to about 0.250 s in the visual mode and 1–2 s in the auditory mode [235] after the item is perceived. Short-term memory (or primary memory or working memory) has a duration between 15 and 30 s [236] and there is only a brief retention and retrieval of information. However information can be retained for longer by repeated going over [237] (rehearsed as in repeating a telephone number silently or aloud until dialling is over), and it can go into long-term storage or become lost. An alternate model to short-term memory is working memory which provides a temporary storage and for processing of information necessary for complex cognitive tasks [238].

In long-term memory (secondary memory) unlike short-term memory, there is the ability to hold on to information for longer periods of time. There are two types of long-term memory: declarative (or explicit) memory and non-declarative (or implicit) [239, 240]. In declarative memory, all the memories can be recognised consciously and is a memory for facts such as dates, names and events [241]. There are two subtypes, episodic and semantic. Two helpful differentiations can be made about the working of long-term memory. One is the memory for an event or 'episode' that is memorisation of information within a spatiotemporal environment. It is declarative and is relevant for both recent and remote events. The other subtype is memory for language and knowledge (semantic memory) [242] that is memory for words and facts. Non-declarative (or implicit) memory is undeclared memories, once learned habits that are contained in procedures and activities such as driving a car. Procedural memory is depicted by changes in performance as a result of prior experience, and there are three subclasses, namely, motor (skill learning), perceptual (priming) [241] and cognitive [243]. Procedural memory is involved in learning and retaining skill or procedure, for example, as to how to ride a bicycle [235].

Many of the events in the distant past is referred to as remote memory. The remote (long-term) memory buffer stores information and contains a vast array of personal experiences and knowledge which may last from months to a lifetime [235]. Both short- and long-term memory embrace three processes, namely, encoding (registration), storage and retrieval. The first step in explicit declarative material is the encoding or registration which is an effortful process. The next step storage (retention or consolidation) is the creation of a permanent record of the encoded information. The third step retrieval (recall or decoding) is by which this information is accessed and brought back to consciousness.

It has been proposed that the short-term memory and long-term memory are dissociated and represent separate systems [244]. Supporting evidence for this is that patients with classic amnesic syndrome with damage to temporal lobes and hippocampi have difficulty in learning and remembering new material [247] but have normal short-term memory. Other investigators have recognised an opposite pattern of deficit in patients with damage to the perisylvian area of the left cerebral hemisphere with apparent normal long-term memory but limited digit span [248].

Neuroanatomic correlates

Table 7.4 shows the memory subtypes localised to different anatomical sites. An interplay between the medial temporal lobes including the hippocampus and the neocortical sites is required for consolidation of the long-term memories [249]. The basal forebrain has widespread connections to the medial temporal lobe and projects widely to the frontal, parietal and temporal cortices [250]. The medial temporal lobe including the hippocampus and midline diencephalon and the connections

Table 7.4 Memory subtypes and neuroanatomic substrates

Type	Subtype	Neural substrate
Sensory memory		Brain stem arousal systems sensory cortex, frontal lobes
Primary (short term)	Working memory	Frontal cortex and parietal lobe
Secondary (long term)		
(i) Explicit memory (declarative)	Episodic Semantic	Hippocampus and medial temporal lobes
(ii) Implicit (non-declarative)	Procedural skills, lexical priming, learning	Cerebellum, basal ganglia and frontal cortex

Information sources: Kandel [240], Poldrack and Gabrielli [241], Budson [245], Schacter and Tulvig [246]

between these regions and the projection sites of long-term storage in the neocortex have been identified as important structures in declarative memory [251]. The processes of registration, retention and retrieval have different neuroanatomic substrates [235]. The different forms of non-declarative memory rely upon the cerebellum, basal ganglia and cerebral cortex [241]. It is useful for clinical purposes to divide memory into registration (capacity to add new information), retention (retain information) and recall (to retrieve and recognise and appreciate awareness or familiarity of object, individual or others that has been experienced before).

Age-related changes

Memory decline occurs in more than 40 % of individuals over the age of 60 years although the exact prevalence is not clear [252]. With ageing, the different memory systems are affected differently. The short-term forgetfulness in older persons is attributed to ageing effects resulting in difficulty in forming associations as rapidly as in younger patients [253]. Working memory, episodic memory and prospective memory decline largely, whereas procedural memory and some prospective memory show few age-related changes [254]. There is an age-related decline in retrieval and encoding of recent memory. When explicit and implicit memory were examined in both old and younger patients , the ability to recall verbal and visual materials was found to decline with age [255]. With increasing age, the speed of retrieval is slowed so is working memory and the encoding and retrieval of newly acquired information [256]. Memory for knowledge (semantic memory) is not affected in older adults provided information is frequently used [254], but there is a decline in the ability to retrieve highly specific information such as names.

Box 7.13. Key Points. Age-Related Memory Changes

- About 40 % of individuals over the age of 60 years show memory decline [252].
- The short-term forgetfulness in older persons is attributed to ageing effects [253].
- Working memory, episodic memory and prospective memory decline [254].

- Procedural memory and some prospective memory show few age-related changes [254].
- With increasing age, the speed of retrieval is slowed [256].
- There is a decline in the ability to retrieve highly specific information such as names.
- Memory for knowledge (semantic memory) is not affected in older adults [254].

7.8.3.2 Memory Loss

Pathophysiology

Temporary or permanent global memory loss is referred to as amnesia or amnestic syndrome in which memory and learning are impaired with grossly normal cognition in an alert person [257]. This syndrome includes several aspects – anterograde amnesia (inability to acquire and retain new information) – and may reflect limbic and neurochemical dysfunction [258] and retrograde amnesia (inability to recall information and events experienced prior to the disorder and confabulation (a tendency to fabricate or produce false memories). There are two types of confabulation, one is 'provoked' which a normal response to poor memory and the other 'spontaneous' which reflects incoherent and context-free retrieval and is associated with severe frontal lobe pathology [258]. Memory disturbances has been associated not only with Alzheimer's disease (AD) but also with cerebrovascular disease, metabolic diseases, toxic effects of medication and depression, among others:

(i) Dementia and Alzheimer's disease

Complaints of poor memory or forgetfulness may be an early symptom of Alzheimer's disease (AD). The most frequent complaint is impaired memory for recent information and events [235]. One of the first signs of dementia is a marked deficit in episodic memory [259]. In AD memory is not only an early symptom but is a foremost feature throughout its course and varies with the stage of the disease. Memory impairment in AD is global in nature but declarative (episodic and semantic) memory is affected first. The actual encoding of explicit declarative memory is the primary memory deficit which rests primarily on the integrity of the hippocampal region [260]. Episodic memory involves retrieval of information that is encoded at a particular time in a particular place such as list of words and photographs of faces encountered in the laboratory [261]. Procedural memory is conserved in AD. Perceptual skill learning such as mirror reading [262], reading skill [263] and motor skill learning [262, 264] are preserved.

(ii) Korsakoff Syndrome (Amnestic or dymnesic syndrome)

Korsakoff syndrome is a chronic disorder characterised by memory deficit for recent memory learning new skills. There is no intellectual impairment. Gaps in the memory are often filled by confabulation. It often follows an acute neurological syndrome known as Wernicke's encephalopathy and the chronic disorder is sometimes known as Wernicke-Korsakoff syndrome; the main features being confusion, ataxia, memory deficit and ophthalmoplegia. It does not however always follow Wernicke's encephalopathy [265].

Episodic memory is severely affected and the learning of new semantic memories is variably affected [266]. Implicit aspects of memory including response to primary and procedural memory are preserved [266, 267]. The neuropathological lesions include neuronal loss, microhaemorrhages and gliosis in the paraventricular and periaqueductal grey matter [266]. The memory dysfunction is largely due to lesions in the mammillary bodies, mammillothalamic tract and anterior thalamus. Alcohol is the most frequent cause and acts through thiamine deficiency [266]. Other examples of thiamine deficiency are severe dietary deficiency and gastric carcinoma.

(iii) Cerebrovascular syndrome

Thalamic ischaemic lesions are known to cause memory impairment [268, 269]. Confusion and memory loss have been reported after capsular genu infarction and believed to be due to thalamocortical disconnection [270]. It had been reported that anterior thalamic nuclei damage results in a more consistent memory loss than does dorsomedial nuclear damage [271]. Procedural memory is unaffected, but autobiographic recollections and newly acquired information tends to be disorganised [268]. In another patient with left anterior thalamic infarct, antegrade amnesia persisted for more than a year [272].

(iv) Depression

Individuals with mild depression often present with memory loss and may be more obvious than abnormal mood, sleep disorder or depressive thought content. Severe depression may be mistaken for dementia. Depressed mood is generally associated with diminished ability to think or concentrate and are often misinterpreted as memory disturbances by the patient. In one study 51 % of the patients referred with memory complaints were found to have significantly depressed mood and no subjective evidence of memory difficulties [273]. In another study decline in memory function ratings was related to affective states rather than to poor performance on tests for memory [274].

(v) Chronic subdural haematoma

The older people are at increased risk due to the fragility of bridging cerebral veins and cerebral atrophy [275]. There is history of trauma in 75 % of the cases [275]. The head injury may be trivial. It is common in the elderly and in alcoholics. Other risk factors include anticoagulant and antiplatelet therapy, age coagulopathy and thrombocytopenia [276]. The symptoms in chronic subdural haematoma may often be delayed for several weeks and the diagnosis overlooked because of thc time lapse. Headache and amnesia may be missed if there is confusion.

(vi) Transient global amnesia
Transient global amnesia (TGA) is an episode of transient memory loss which cannot be attributed to such conditions as a stroke, transient ischaemic attack, atypical type of migraine or epilepsy. It occurs suddenly and usually lasts for few hours and improves over the next 12–24 h [277]. It usually occurs in the elderly who otherwise are healthy. The precipitant factors are physical and emotional stress, swimming in cold water and sexual intercourse, among others. Apart from severe anterograde amnesia, retrograde amnesia typically covered at least two decades [277].

(vii) Head Injury
The severity and duration of the amnesia will very much depend on the severity of the head injury. It may take a few days to a few weeks before the short-term memory recovers, and in most patients recovery is complete. The retrograde amnesia gradually gets shorter until it is just minutes before the injury.

(viii) Psychogenic (functional) amnesia
Psychogenic amnesia is characterised by transient or episodic anterograde and/or retrograde memory loss with non-discernible neurological disorder [278]. Several terms have been used to describe these patients, 'psychogenic', 'functional', 'dissociative' and 'medically unexplained amnesia', among others [278, 280]. Functional amnesia is the preferred term by some and more acceptable to patients [281] but dissociative amnesia is favoured by others [282]. In functional amnesia, there is sudden onset of memory loss especially confined to personal life [279, 280] characterised by severe retrograde amnesia [277]. Psychogenic amnesia is often triggered by environmentally induced stressful life events [279, 280]. The episodes persisted from several weeks to a couple of years or more [277]. It has to be distinguished from transient global amnesia (TGA) where the patient during the episode has severe anterograde amnesia and retrograde amnesia that characteristically involved at least two decades [277].

Box 7.14. Key Points. Memory Loss in the Elderly

- Working memory, episodic memory and prospective memory decline largely with age [254].
- Procedural memory and some perceptual memory show few changes [254].
- Memory for knowledge (semantic memory) is not affected [254].
- With age, there is a decline in the ability to retrieve highly specific information such as name language [256].
- Amnestic syndrome includes several aspects – anterograde amnesia (inability to acquire and retain new information) – and may reflect limbic and neurochemical dysfunction retrograde amnesia (inability to recall information and events experienced prior to the disorder and confabulation) [258].

- Korsakoff syndrome includes several aspects: anterograde memory, retrograde memory and confabulation.
- Memory disorders can be associated not only with Alzheimer's disease but also with cerebrovascular disease, metabolic diseases, toxic effects of medication and depression, among others.
- Transient global amnesia (TGA) where the patient during the episode has severe anterograde amnesia and retrograde amnesia that characteristically involved at least two decades [277].
- In functional amnesia (psychogenic), there is sudden onset of memory loss especially confined to personal life events characterised by severe retrograde amnesia) [277].

7.8.4 Chronic Pain in the Elderly

Introduction
The International Association for the Study of Pain defined pain as 'an unpleasant sensory and emotional experience associated with actual or potential tissue damage or described in terms of such damage' [283]. Chronic pain has been defined as 'pain that persists beyond the usual course of an acute disease to heal or beyond a reasonable time for an injury to heal' [284]. The prevalence of pain increases with age to about 70 years [285] but it is not a normal part of ageing. As age advances, frailty and chronic diseases associated with pain will increase [286]. Up to 80 % of older people in long-term residential facilities and between 25 and 50 % of community dwellers have chronic pain [285, 287]. Between 25 and 40 % of elderly cancer patients studied have daily pain [288]. Central post-stroke pain (CPSP) affects between 2 and 6 % of stroke patients, i.e. there is an annual incidence between 2000 and 6000 in the United Kingdom. It is reported that approximately 30,000 survivors of stroke in the United States are affected by the so-called thalamic pain [289]. Andersen et al. [290] indicated an incidence of 6 % among unselected stroke patients. The chronic pain in the elderly, unlike that in younger adults, are more complex and often not likely to be reversible. The severity of the sensory components is only one aspect of the problem and there is often a significant emotional input to the clinical syndrome [291]. As the patients age, the pain intensity usually diminishes. There are issues of psychological implications such as anxiety, anger, denial, loss of self-esteem and depression, and these have a negative effect on health and quality of life in the elderly [286].

Neurophysiology
The neurophysiology of pain can be divided into four phases, namely, transduction, transmission, perception and modulation. In transduction the afferent nerve endings

engage in translating noxious stimuli into nociceptive impulses [292]. At the free nerve endings of the primary nerve are the afferent nociceptors. These nociceptors are distributed throughout the body.

Transmission is the way the pain impulse is transferred from the peripheral to the central nervous system. The nociceptors have a cell body in the dorsal root ganglia, and their axons are of two general types. One is with thinly myelinated fibres (A-delta) and the other small diameter nonmyelinated C-fibres [293]. In the normal tissue, they are silent in the absence of tissue injury. The axons synapse to the second-order neurons in the dorsal horn of the spinal cord, and some project through the ventral root. The nociceptors have several different receptors on their surfaces, and they include, bradykinin, histamine, opiate, GABA, substance P and serotonin [294] which modulate the sensitivity to stimulation.

The grey matter of the spinal cord is divided into ten laminae [295, 296] and the dorsal part constituting the laminae I to V, and these deal with the incoming fibres. The major spinal pathways for pain cross over to the anterolateral spinal quadrant to form the spinothalamic tract. The thalamic nuclei project to somatosensory area of the cortex and to the limbic and frontal lobes. The somatosensory cortex is involved in the localisation, identification, and the limbic and frontal lobes are responsible for the emotional aspects, suffering and anxiety [297].

Perception is the awareness, and both the cortex and limbic system are involved in the conscious awareness of pain. It has been surmised that in the elderly, pain perception may be different [286].

Modulation. Many of the pain signals transmitted through the dorsal horn do not reach consciousness. The modulatory system is quite different from the sensory system and is diffusely organised, highly interconnected and appears to act as a unit [298]. This network and its pain suppressing action are organised at three levels of the neuraxis: the spinal cord, medulla and midbrain [298]. Pain signals pass through the dorsal horn via the ascending pathway to the periaqueductal grey matter, and the immediate control theory is focused on descending pathway which passes to the raphe nucleus in the upper medulla and then back to the dorsal horn via the reticulospinal fibres inhibiting pain signalling (Fig. 7.6). Neurotransmitters involved in these pathways include endogenous opiates (enkephalins, beta-endorphins, dynorphins), serotonin and norepinephrine [283]. Activation of the neurons in the midbrain periaqueductal grey matter excites neurons in the rostral medulla, some of which contain serotonin. The medullary neurons in turn project to and specifically inhibit the firing of trigeminal and spinal pain – transmission neurons [299]. Another system that modulates pain apart from the gating of transmission is the endogenous opioid system which consists of three groups of endogenous compounds, the enkephalins, endorphins and dynorphin which bind to the opioid receptors [293].

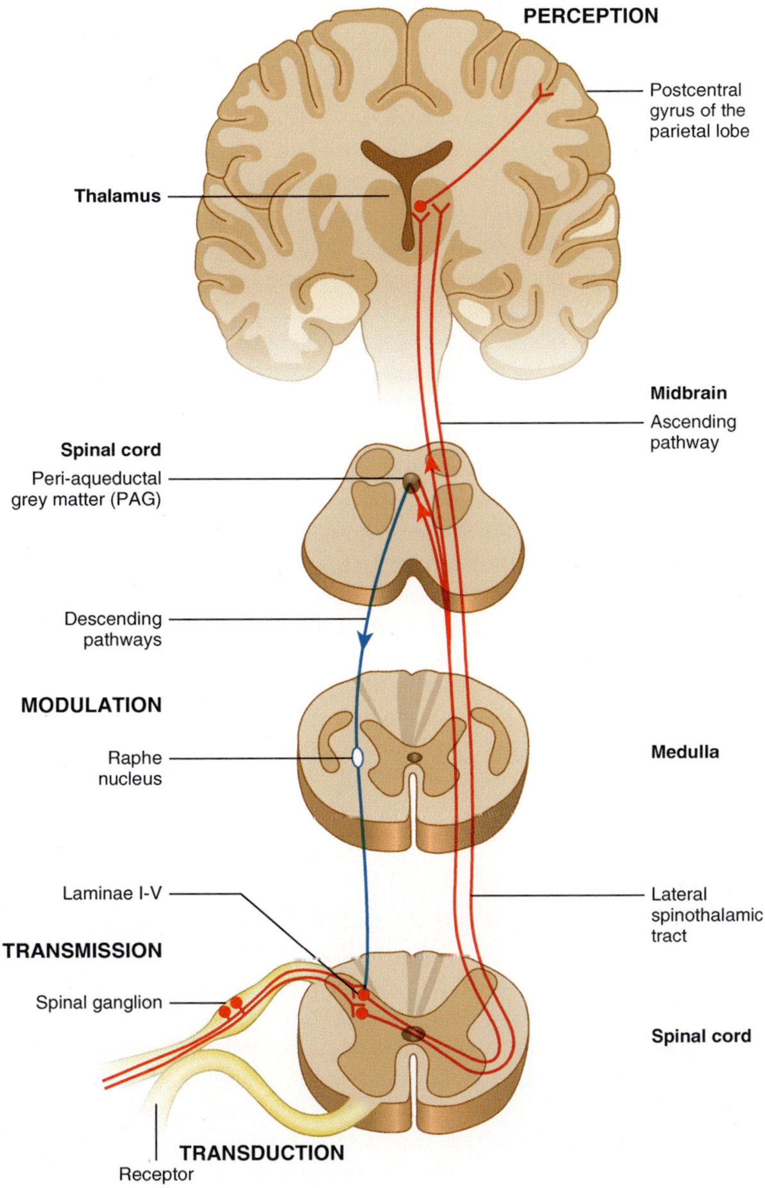

Fig. 7.6 Pain pathways

Pathophysiology

In the elderly pain can be categorised pathophysiologically as either nociceptic or neuropathic [286]. Nociceptive pain results from chemical, mechanical or thermal stimulation of the nociceptors (peripheral sensory receptors) in the muscles and joints; nociceptors can become sensitive to a variety of chemical factors present at the time of injury such as substance P, serotonin, bradykinin and histamine, among others [294, 297]. Neuropathic pain is caused by damage to the peripheral nerves (peripheral neuropathy, phantom limb, spinal cord or brain (central pain syndrome, e.g. stroke)) and occurs more frequently in older people. In the elderly post-herpetic neuralgia and diabetic neuropathy are common examples of neuropathic pain [286]. Chronic pain may sometimes consist of mixed pathologies with a combination of nociceptive and neuropathic mechanisms. This type is sometimes classified as non-specific pain [300]. Spinal cord disorders as in spinal canal stenosis are an example [301].

In 1906 Dejerine and Roussy [302] described the thalamic pain syndrome which carried their name. Subsequently it was shown that the syndrome can occur with extrathalamic lesions. For these reasons, the term, thalamic pain syndrome, has been replaced by 'central stroke pain'. The central stroke pain in most instances develops within a week post-stroke in 36 % of patients. The frequency is 14 % after thalamic lesions and 24 % after geniculothalamic artery territory stroke [303].

Box 7.15. Key Points. Chronic Pain

- Chronic pain in the elderly is complex and often not likely to be reversible.
- Pain can be divided into four phases, namely, transduction, transmission, perception and modulation.
- In the elderly pain can be categorised pathophysiologically as either nociceptic or neuropathic [292, 293].
- Nociceptive pain results from chemical, mechanical or thermal stimulation of the nociceptors [294, 297].
- Neuropathic pain is caused by damage to the peripheral nerves [286].
- At the free nerve endings of the primary nerves are the afferent nociceptors.
- The nociceptors have several different receptors on their surfaces [294].
- Chronic pain sometimes consists of mixed pathologies with combination of nociceptive and neuropathic mechanisms [300].
- Many of the pain signals transmitted through the dorsal horn do not reach consciousness.
- Central stroke pain affects between 2 and 6 % of stroke patients and occurs in thalamic and extrathalamic lesions [290, 303].

7.8.5 Gait Disorders in the Elderly

Introduction

Gait disorders in the elderly may arise from a single or a combination of neurological and musculoskeletal factors. They may interact with physiological-related changes which increase with age and are part of normal ageing. Ageing however is not necessarily accompanied by disordered gait for some elderly maintain a normal gait into their 90s [304]. 8 to 10 % of non-institutionalised older adults and 60 % of nursing home residents reported having difficulty in walking and required assistance of another person or special equipment to walk [305–307]. Abnormal gait is seen in 35 % of people over the age of 70 years [308], and gait changes are seen in the majority of people over the age of 85 years [309].

Pathophysiology

Neurological and musculoskeletal factors together with physiological changes with ageing contribute to gait changes in the elderly. Age-related changes include sensory impairment, visual, auditory and tactile. The pattern of movement, or gait is the control of posture and balance on movement and at rest. Postural stability or balance is maintained by continued adjustments to sensory outputs, visual, vestibular and somatosensory [310] which tend to decline with age. Loss of visual acuity, peripheral vision, depth perception and contrast sensitivity occurs with ageing [311]. Proprioceptive loss includes the threshold to movement and impaired sense of vibration in the legs leads to increased postural sway [312] The vestibular system is also affected by ageing.

With ageing, there is decreased muscle bulk, flexibility and strength together with loss of vision and hearing. The major changes in gait are in the reduction in the overall step/stride length and velocity. There is also decreased rotation and more flat-footed landing and less vigorous push off [313–315]. Other workers however have found no differences with step length, stride length and velocity [316]. When healthy young women were compared with elderly women, the stride length, step length, velocity and range of ankle motion had lower values in the elderly [317]. Similar studies between healthy young men and older men showed no significant differences between them but for stride length [316]. When gender were compared, the free-speed cadence was faster for women than for both young and older men. According to Hageman [318], the gait characteristics of older healthy adults are an adaptation towards safe walking rather than an abnormality or disability. Thus, there is no accepted standard of normal gait in the elderly [319].

What has been described as 'senile gait disorder' [320] is characterised as a gait pattern with broad base, small steps, diminished arm swing, stooped posture, flexion at the hip and knees, uncertainty, stiffness in turning, occasional difficulty in initiating steps and performing tandem gait and a tendency to fall. Many of the older adults with senile gait disorder have cognitive impairment [321], and others are mildly demented [322]. It is likely that senile gait disorder is of multifactorial aetiology, and it now believed that these changes are early manifestations of subclinical disease [323].

Nutt et al. [324] drew attention to gait disorders termed higher-level gait disorder that are not explained by basic sensorimotor deficits in comparison to lower-level and middle-level disorders. Basically the abnormal gait is motor programming failure [325]. Five types have been described, namely, frontal gait disorder, frontal disequilibrium, subcortical disequilibrium, isolated gait ignition failure and cautious gait [324]. The middle level are largely from basal ganglia disorders (Parkinson's disease), cerebrovascular disease (hemiparesis, paraparesis associated with UMN signs) and spinal cord lesions leading to spastic paraparesis with sensory level and cerebellar [309]. The lower level includes weakness of muscles involving the motor neurons (LMN spinal muscular atrophy; UMN + LMN amyotrophic lateral sclerosis, UMN primary lateral sclerosis), the peripheral nerves (peripheral neuropathy, radiculopathy, plexopathy), the neuromuscular junction (myasthenia) and primary muscle disorders (dystrophies, myopathies) [309].

Box 7.16. Key Points. Gait Disorders in the Elderly

- Ageing is not necessarily accompanied by disordered gait for some elderly maintain normal gait into their 90s [304].
- With ageing, there is decreased muscle bulk, flexibility and strength together with loss of vision and hearing [311].
- The major changes in gait are in the reduction of overall step/stride length and velocity [313–315].

Types of gait disorder:

I. Frontal gait disorder – short steps, loss of balance, freezing but with a wider base and upright posture unlike in parkinsonism
II. Spastic gait – short, shuffling, stiff-legged with slight flexion at the hips and in extreme form scissoring
III. Cerebellar ataxia – wide based and staggering
IV. Sensory ataxia – high steppage and imbalance
V. Extrapyramidal gait – shuffling, narrow based, difficulty in starting and turning
VI. Antalgic gait – adopts a limp with very short stance phase
VII. Trendelenburg gait – weight shift on the affected side

Multiple Choice Questions

1. The following changes occurring in the central nervous system with ageing are true, EXCEPT:
   A. With ageing, there is overall decline in brain weight and volume, the decline increasing with age, more so over the age of 70 years.
   B. Age-related changes in the white matter (leukoaraiosis) occurs as zones of high density.
   C. As age advances, there is an increasing diminution in the number of motor neurons in the spinal cord.
   D. As age advances, it is the quality of sleep rather than the quantity that changes.
2. The following in Parkinson's disease are true EXCEPT:
   A. Degeneration of the dopaminergic cells in the substantia nigra results in the dysfunction of the striatonigral-thalamic outflow.
   B. Dopamine that is not bound to the postsynaptic receptors and inactivated by binding to the autoreceptors are also inactivated by enzymes monoamine oxidase type B(MAO-B) and catechol-O-methyltransferase (COMT).
   C. The intraneuronal enzymes required for dopamine synthesis are diminished.
   D. It is a pyramidal disorder.
3. The following are true in the pathophysiology of Parkinson's disease (PD), EXCEPT:
   A. The striatonigral pathway plays a regulatory role in the system of positive and negative pathways that serve to modulate feedback from the thalamus to the motor cortex.
   B. Alpha-synuclein is a presynaptic neuronal protein linked genetically and neuropathologically with PD and other neurodegenerative disorders.
   C. The lack of dopamine leads to excitation of the direct pathway and inhibition of the indirect pathway and increased inhibition of the ventrolateral nucleus of the thalamus.
   D. Age influences both the development and progression of PD.
4. The following are true of multisystem atrophy (MSA), EXCEPT:
   A. MSA can cause combinations of parkinsonism, autonomic, pyramidal and cerebellar symptoms.
   B. Presently if parkinsonian features predominate, it is referred to as MSA-A and accounts for two-thirds of the cases.
   C. In MSA there is an aggregation of filamentous alpha-synuclein in the neurons in several regions.
   D. Most patients were initially considered to have Parkinson's disease, and even at death one-third still carry that diagnosis.
5. The following are true of amyotrophic lateral sclerosis (ALS), EXCEPT:
   A. Amyotrophic lateral sclerosis (ALS) is characterised by a progressive degeneration and death of the anterior horn cells, corticospinal tracts and/or bulbar motor nuclei.
   B. There is an association between frontotemporal dementia (FTD) and ALS.

C. Most cases with both are characterised by neuronal inclusions immunoreactive for ubiquitin and tau.
D. About 10 % of the familial cases of ALS result from a specific genetic defect which gives rise to mutation of the gene Cu/Zn, superoxide dismutase 1 (SOD1).

6. The following physiological definitions of nerve degeneration are true, EXCEPT:
   A. Axonal degeneration results in axonal damage starting in the distal portion of the axon and proceeding proximally towards the cell body, with breakdown of the myelin sheath.
   B. Wallerian degeneration results in degeneration of the axon and myelin sheath, and changes also occur in the neuronal body.
   C. Neuronal degeneration is caused by damage to the motor or sensory cell bodies followed by degeneration of their peripheral and central processes.
   D. Segmental demyelination results from unifocal injury to the myelin sheath with preservation of the underlying axon.
7. The following pathophysiological mechanisms in Guillain-Barre syndrome are true, EXPECT:
   A. The autoimmune response is directed against the axon.
   B. The pathophysiology of the syndrome was recently determined with the presence of anti-GQ1b antibodies.
   C. The Miller-Fisher subtype is particularly associated with antibodies to GQ1b.
   D. GBS is reclassified based on different electrodiagnostic criteria into acute inflammatory demyelinating polyradiculoneuropathy (AIDP), acute motor and sensory axonal neuropathy (AMSAN) and acute motor axonal neuropathy (AMAN).
8. The following physiological mechanisms in myasthenia gravis (MG) are true, EXCEPT:
   A. The autoantibodies in MG are either directed to the muscle nicotine acetylcholine receptor (AChR) or to the muscle-specific tyrosine kinase (MuSK).
   B. In MG there is a reduction in the number of functional AChRs, and several mechanisms have been proposed as to the mechanism for AChR impairment.
   C. Titin and ryanodine receptor antibodies are seen in 95 % of thymic MG and in 50 % of late-onset MG and is associated with severe disease.
   D. Antibodies against LRP4 were found in some patients who had antibodies directed against AChR or MuSK.
9. The following pathological changes that occur after cerebral infarction are true, EXCEPT:
   A. The thrombogenic cascade is triggered as the result of endothelial injury.
   B. The vasogenic oedema occurs over hours to days and is reversible.
   C. An ischaemic infarct can undergo haemorrhagic conversion or transformation.
   D. Parenchymatous haemorrhage differs from haemorrhagic infarction in that it extends beyond the vascular territory, is symptomatic and often exerts mass effect.

10. The following events occurring in cerebral haemorrhage are true, EXCEPT:
    A. Many of the haemorrhages continue to expand over several hours after the onset of symptoms.
    B. Inflammation caused by thrombin and end products of coagulation causes most of the brain injury and swelling.
    C. The expansion is likely to be due to oedema which accumulates in the extracellular space.
    D. The late-onset oedema which persists for several weeks after the initial haemorrhage is the result of disruption of the blood-brain barrier, lysis of red cells and formation of free radicals and direct cytotoxicity.
11. The following are true of narcolepsy, EXCEPT:
    A. Narcolepsy is uncontrollable episodes of falling asleep during day time.
    B. Cateplexy, sleep waking, hypnagogic and hypnopompic hallucinations are associated with narcolepsy.
    C. It is associated with restless leg syndrome.
    D. When it occurs in late life, it is usually associated with diseases such as Parkinson's disease.
12. The following in relation to non-rapid eye movement (NREM) parasomnia are true EXCEPT:
    A. Sleep walking
    B. Bruxism
    C. Uncontrollable episodes of falling asleep during day time
    D. Restless leg syndrome
13. The following are true, EXCEPT:
    A. Sleep walking occurs during non-REM sleep.
    B. Individuals with narcolepsy enter sleep directly into REM sleep instead of entering through non-REM.
    C. A complete sleep cycle takes 30–45 min.
    D. During REM sleep, muscle tone decreases, and breathing becomes rapid, irregular and shallow.
14. A 72-year-old man was seen in the out-patient accompanied by his son. He lives alone and according to the son, his father has become forgetful and unsteady on his feet and has had a few falls over the past 3 months. When specifically asked whether his father has had any trauma to his head, he said that his father did knock his head on a post several months earlier. Furthermore the father had complained of headaches on the right side of his head. Physical examination revealed he was alert but had evidence of cognitive impairment and subtle weakness on the left arm and leg. Apart from this, the neurological examination was unremarkable. Which of the following is the most likely diagnosis?
    A. Vascular dementia
    B. Chronic subdural haematoma
    C. Brain tumour
    D. Normal pressure hydrocephalus

15. A 65-year-old woman was seen in the emergency department complaining of severe throbbing headache over the right temporal and occipital regions for the past 3 days. She further complained of tiredness, fatigue and joint pains, and the scalp was extremely tender when she brushed her hair. Chewing food caused pain in the jaws. She denied any visual disturbances. Physical examination revealed tenderness over the affected scalp. The right temporal artery was not painful on palpation and was thickened. Which of the following is the most likely diagnosis?
    A. Herpes ophthalmicus
    B. Carotid artery dissection
    C. Giant cell arteritis
    D. Trigeminal neuralgia
16. A 70-year-old man was seen in the neurological clinic with headaches over the past 2 months. That morning he had developed sudden weakness of the left of his body. The pain was over the right side of his head throbbing in character and was mild at the beginning but now more severe and lasting longer. The headache is worse on lying down and on coughing, sneezing or bending over. There was no history of head trauma. He had been vomiting as of late. Examination of the nervous system revealed a sixth nerve deficit and weakness of the left arm and leg. The optic fundi showed early papilloedema. Examination of the systems was normal. Which of the following is the most likely diagnosis?
    A. Cerebral infarction/haemorrhage
    B. Primary brain tumour
    C. Metastatic tumour
    D. Benign intracranial hypertension (pseudotumour cerebri)
17. The following are true of headaches in the elderly, EXCEPT:
    A. Temporal arteritis occurs over the age of 50 years.
    B. Hypnic headaches tend to start before the age of 50 years.
    C. In the elderly 2 % of migraine, headaches begin after the age of 50 years.
    D. Tension headaches occur at any age.
18. A 68-year-old man sustained head injuries following a motor vehicle accident. He was unable to recall events prior to the accident. Which of the following is consistent with his condition?
    A. Retrograde amnesia
    B. Anterograde amnesia
    C. Transient global amnesia
    D. Dissociate amnesia
19. A 72-year-old man was seen in the emergency department accompanied by his daughter. According to her, he was in good health, but that morning, he had suddenly became confused and sat on chair staring into space and seemed muddled. In about 4 h, he returned to normal but could not remember what had happened. What is the likely diagnosis?

A. Transient ischaemic attack
B. Transient global amnesia
C. Partial seizure
D. Acute confusional state

20. The following are true of chronic pain in the elderly, EXCEPT:
    A. As the patients age, the pain intensity usually increases.
    B. The chronic pain in the elderly unlike that in younger adults are more complex and often not likely to be reversible.
    C. In the elderly pain can be categorised pathophysiologically as either nociceptic or neuropathic.
    D. The prevalence of pain increases with age to about 70 years [3], but it is a normal part of ageing.
21. The following are true in relation to the pathophysiology of pain, EXCEPT:
    A. The nociceptors have several different receptors on their surfaces which modulate the sensitivity to stimulation.
    B. The major spinal pathways for pain crosses over to the anterolateral spinal quadrant to form the spinothalamic tract.
    C. Another system that modulates pain apart from the gating of transmission is the endogenous opioid system.
    D. The thalamic pain syndrome occurs with thalamic lesions.
22. In relation to gait disorders in the elderly, the following are true, EXCEPT:
    A. The major changes in gait in the elderly are the reduction of overall step/stride and velocity.
    B. Frontal gait disorder is characterised by short steps, loss of balance, freezing and stooping posture.
    C. Myelopathy from cervical spondylosis is a common cause of gait disorder in the elderly.
    D. In normal pressure hydrocephalus, the clinical triad consists of gait disorder, incontinence and cognitive impairment.

Extended Matching Questions

1. Gait
    A. Scissor gait
    B. Drunken gait
    C. Steppage gait
    D. Hemiparetic gait
    E. Antalgic gait
    F. Frontal gait disorder
    G. Waddling gait
    H. *Marche a petit pas*
    I. Trendelenburg gait
    J. Spastic gait

The following have in common a gait disorder. Chose the most likely type of gait from the list above. Each option can be used only once.

1. A 60-year-old man developed sudden pain in his low back while trying to lift a heavy object. The pain radiated down the back of the left leg. He adopted a limp with very short stance phase on walking.
2. A 65-year-old man with known cancer complained of difficulty in walking over a week. There was weakness with increase in tone in both lower limbs right more than left. The reflexes were brisk and plantar extensor with diminution in sensation with sensory level at the level of the umbilicus. He was stiff-legged with slight flexion at the hips.
3. A 70-year-old man has been slowing down over the past 6 months or more. He had a rest tremor in the right hand with rigidity and bradykinesia. He had difficulty in turning and starting, and gait was narrow based.
4. A 72-year-old woman in an nursing care facility had difficulty in rising from the chair and walking. She had weakness of the pelvic girdle muscles. Her serum calcium was low and the alkaline phosphatase raised.
5. A 70-year-old man was seen with difficulty in walking. On examination his left arm was flexed at the elbow and at the wrist. The flexors were weak in the leg and extended with slight cross over.

2. Theme: Memory loss
   A. Alzheimer's disease
   B. Korsakoff syndrome
   C. Depression
   D. Anterior thalamic nuclei damage
   E. Transient global amnesia
   F. Dissociative amnesia

   The following patients have in common memory loss. Chose the most likely diagnosis from the list above once more than once or not at all.

   A. A 65-year-old man with a history of heavy and long-term alcohol use is seen in the out-patient clinic because of his inability to walk or stand without support. He frequently denied that anything was wrong with him. He lacked insight. His short-term memory was impaired compared to other intellectual functions. Neurological examination revealed he had a tremor, ocular abnormalities and a markedly ataxic gait.
   B. A 62-year-old bank executive has been under severe stress. One morning he left home for work, but did not turn up at the bank. His car was found abandoned several kilometers away from where he lived. Few weeks later, someone had recognised him in another town. He was subsequently evaluated by a doctor. He was distressed and could not say who he was nor was able to recall about his past life.
   C. A 75-year-old woman accompanied by her daughter attended the surgery. According to the daughter, her mother has failing memory. She has become forgetful over the last 18 months. Her quality of domestic chores is beginning

to decline. Her house is untidy, food is left in the refrigerator, and there is a deterioration in her personal hygiene.

D. A 72-year-old man was seen in the emergency department accompanied by his daughter. According to her, he was in good health, but that morning he had suddenly became confused and sat on chair staring into space and seemed muddled. In about 4 h, he returned to normal, but could not remember what had happened.

Answers to MCQs

1=B; 2=D; 3=C; 4=B; 5=C; 6=D; 7=A; 8=D; 9=B; 10=C; 11=C; 12=C; 13=C; 14=B; 15=C; 16=B; 17=B; 18=A; 19=B; 20=D; 21=D; 22=B.

Answers to EMQs

EMQ 1. 1=E;2=J; 3=H; 4=G; 5=D.
EMQ 2. 1=B; 2=F; 3+A; 4=E.

References

Anatomical and Physiological Changes with Ageing

1. Aderton BH. Ageing of the brain. Mech Ageing Dev. 2002;123(7):811–7 (abstract).
2. Peters R. Ageing and the brain. Postgrad Med J. 2006;82(964):84–8.
3. Scahill R, Frost C, Jenkins R, Whitwel JL, Rossr MN, Fox NC. A longitudinal study of brain volume changes in normal ageing using serial registered magnetic resonance imaging. Arch Neurol. 2003;60:989–94.
4. Aderton BH. Changes in the ageing brain in health and disease. Philos Trans R Soc Lond B Biol Sci. 1997;352(1363):1781–9.
5. Raz N, Rodrique KN. Differential aging of the brain: patterns cognitive correlates and modifiers. Neurosci Biobehav Rev. 2006;30:730–48.
6. Troller J, Valenzuela M. Brain ageing in the new millennium. Aust N Z J Psychiatry. 2001;35:788–805.
7. Raz N, Rodrique KM, Acker D. Hypertension and the brain: vulnerability of prefrontal regions and executive functions. Behav Neurosci. 2003;17:1169–80.
8. Artero S, Tiemeier H, Prins ND, Sabatier R, Breteler MM, Ritchie K, et al. Neuroanatomical localisation and clinical correlates of white matter lesions in the elderly. J Neurol Neurosurg Psychiatry. 2004;75:1304–8.
9. Lexell J. Evidence for nervous system degeneration with advancing age. J Nutr. 1997;127(5): 10115–35.
10. Tomlinson BE, Irving D. The number of limb motor neurons in the human lumbosacral cord throughout life. J Neurol Sci. 1977;34:213–9.

11. Kawamura Y, O'Brien PC, Okazaki H, Duyck PJ. Lumber motor neurones of man. II. Numbers and diameter distributions of large and intermediate-diameter cytons in motor neuron columns of spinal cord of man. J Neuropathol Exp Neurol. 1997;36:860–70.
12. Esiri MM. Aging and the brain. J Pathol. 2007;211:181–7.
13. Knight J, Nigam Y. Exploring the anatomy and physiology of aging. Part 5. Nurs Times. 2008;104(35):18–9.
14. Verdu E, Ceballos D, Villches JJ, Navarro X. Influence of aging on peripheral nerve function and regeneration. J Peripher Nerv Syst. 2000;5(4):191–208 (abstract).
15. Vaughan DW. Effects of advancing age on peripheral nerve regeneration. J Comp Neurol. 1992;323(2):219–37 (abstract).
16. Kuhl DE, Koeppe RA, Minoshima S, Synder SE, Ficaro EP, Foster NL, et al. In vivo mapping of cerebral acetylcholine activity in aging and Alzheimer's disease. Neurology. 1999;52:691–9.
17. Wang Y, Chan GL, Holden JE, Dobko T, Mak E, Schulzer M, et al. Age dependent decline of dopamine D1 receptors in human brain: a PET study. Synapse. 1998;31(1):56–61.
18. Van Dyck CH, Malison RT, Seibyl JP, Larnele M, Klumpp H, Zoghbi SS, et al. Age related decline in cerebral serotonin transporting availability with [(1230I] beta-CIT SPECT. Neurobiol Aging. 2000;21(4):497–501 (abstract).
19. Spurduso WW. Physical dimensions of aging. Champaigns: Human Kinetics; 1995.
20. Edwards BA, O'Driscoll DM, Ali A, Jordan AS, Trinder J, Malhotra A, et al. Aging and sleep: physiology and pathophysiology. Semin Respir Crit Care Med. 2010;31(5):618–33 (abstract).

Parkinson's Disease, Secondary Parkinsonism and Parkinson Plus Syndromes

21. Dickson DW. Parkinson's disease and parkinsonism: neuropathology. In: Cold Spring Harbor Perspectives in Medicine. Cold Spring Laboratory Press; 2012. doi:10.1101/cshperspective.a000258. (abstract).
22. Chan DK, Cordato D, Karr M, Ong B, Lei H, Liu J, et al. Prevalence of Parkinson's disease in Sydney. Acta Neurol Scand. 2005;111:7–11.
23. McCann SJ, Lecouteur DG, Green AC, Bretne C, Johnson AG, Chan D, et al. The epidemiology of Parkinson's disease in an Australian population. Neuroepidemiology. 1998;17:310–7.
24. Van Den Eeden SK, Tanner CM, Bernstein AL, Fross RD, Leimpeter A, Bloch DM, et al. Incidence of Parkinson's disease: variation by age, gender and race/ethnicity. Am J Epidemiol. 2003;157(11):1015–22 (abstract).
25. Tanner CM. Occupational and environmental causes of parkinsonism. Occup Med. 1992;7:503–13.
26. Braak H, Del Tredici K, Ruib U, de Vos RA, Jansen Steur EN, Brack E, et al. Staging of brain pathology related to sporadic Parkinson's disease. Neurobiol Aging. 2003;24:197–211.
27. Lang AE. The progression of Parkinson disease: a hypothesis. Neurology. 2007;68:948–52 (abstract).
28. Smith Y, Bevan MD, Shink E, Bolam JP. Microcircuitry of direct and indirect pathways of the basal ganglia. Neuroscience. 1998;86(2):353–97 (abstract).
29. Lotharius J, Brundin P. Pathogenesis of Parkinson's disease: dopamine vesicles and a – synuclein. Nat Rev Neurosci. 2002;3:932–42 (abstract).
30. Dauer W, Przedborski S. Parkinson's disease. Neuron. 2003;39(6):889–909 (abstract).
31. Glasson BI, Lee VM-Y. Parkin and molecular pathways of Parkinson's disease. Neuron. 2001;31(6):885–8 (abstract).
32. Braak H, Braak E, Yilmazer D, Schultz C, De Vos RA, Jansen EN, et al. Nigral and extranigral pathology in Parkinson's disease. J Neural Transm. 1995;46(Suppl):15–31 (abstract).
33. Stefanis L. α-Synuclein in Parkinson's disease. Cold Spring Harb Perspect Med. 2012;2:a009399 (abstract).

34. Recchia A, Debetto P, Negro A, Guidolin D, Skaper SD, Giusti P. α-Synuclein and Parkinson's disease. FASEB J. 2004;18:617–26 (abstract).
35. Goedert M. Filamentous nerve cell inclusions in neurodegenerative diseases: taupathies and alpha-synucleinopathies. Philos Trans R Soc Lond B Biol Sci. 1999;354(1386):1101–18 (abstract).
36. Chua CE, Tang BL. Alpha-synuclein and Parkinson's disease: the first road block. J Cell Mol Med. 2006;10(4):837–46 (abstract).
37. Hindle JV. Ageing neurodegeneration and Parkinson's disease. Age Ageing. 2010;39(2):156–61 (abstract).
38. Levy G. The relationship of Parkinson disease with aging. Arch Neurol. 2007;64(9):1242–8 (abstract).
39. Rivlin-Etzion M, Marmor O, Heimer G, Raz A, Nini A, Bergman H. Basal ganglia oscillations and pathophysiology of movement disorders. Curr Opin Neurobiol. 2006;16(6):629–37 (abstract).
40. Bergman H, Deuschl G. Pathophysiology of Parkinson's disease: from clinical neurology to basic neuroscience and back. Mov Disord. 2002;17 Suppl 3:S28–40 (abstract).
41. Weinberger M, Hutchison WD, Lozano AM, Hodale M, Dostrovsky JO. Increased gamma oscillatory activity in the subthalmic nucleus during tremor in Parkinson's disease patients. J Neurophysiol. 2009;101(2):789–802.
42. Bergman H, Wichmann T, Karmon R, De Long MR. The primate subthalamic nucleus. II. Neuronal activity in the MPTP model of parkinsonism. J Neurophysiol. 1994;72: 507–20.
43. Deuschi G, Raethjen J, Baron R, Lindemann M, Wilms H, Krack P, et al. The pathophysiology of Parkinsonian tremor: a review. J Neurol. 2000;247 Suppl 5:V33–48 (abstract).
44. Zaidel A, Arkadir D, Israel Z, Bergman H. Akineto-rigid vs tremor syndromes in Parkinsonism. Curr Opin Neurol. 2009;22(4):387–93 (abstract).

Multisystem Atrophy (MSA)

45. Quinn NP, Marsden CD. The motor disorder of multiple system atrophy. J Neurol Neurosurg Psychiatry. 1993;56:1239–42.
46. Jellinger KA. Pathogenesis of multisystem atrophy. Recent Developments. Int J Neurol Neurother 2015;2:1.
47. Quinn NP, Wenning G. Multiple system atrophy. Br J Hosp Med. 1994;51:492–4.
48. Stefanova N, Biicke P, Duerr S, Wenning GK. Multiple system atrophy: an update. Lancet Neurol. 2009;8(12):1172–8 (abstract).
49. Bower JH, Maragamore DM, McDonnell SK, Rocca WA. Incidence of progressive supranuclear paralysis and multiple system atrophy in Olmsted County, Minnesota. Neurology. 1997; 49:1284–8.
50. Jamora RD, Gupta A, Tan AK, Tan LC. Clinical characteristics of patients with multiple system atrophy in Singapore. Ann Acad Med Singapore. 2005;34(9):553–7 (abstract).
51. Papp MI, Kahn JE, Lantos G. Cytoplasmic inclusions in the central nervous system of patients with multisystem atrophy(striato nigral degeneration; olivo-cerebellar atrophy and Shy-Drager syndrome). J Neurol Sci. 1989;94:79–100.
52. Wakabayashi K, Takahashi H. Cellular pathology in multiple system atrophy. Neuropathology. 2006;26(4):338–45.
53. Yoshida M. Multiple system atrophy: alpha-synuclein and neuronal degeneration. Neuropathology. 2007;27(5):484–93 (abstract).
54. Delacourte A. Multiple System Disease (MSA). 2009. www.alzheimer-europe.org. Accessed 5.6.2012.

Motor Neurone Disease

55. Logroscino G, Tragnor BJ, Hardiman O. Descriptive epidemiology of amyothrophic lateral sclerosis: new evidence and unsolved issues. J Neurol Neurosurg Psychiatry. 2008;79:6–11.
56. Rocha JA, Reis S, Simeo F, Fonseca J, Mendes Ribeiro J. Diagnostic investigation and multidisciplinary management in motor neurone disease. J Neurol. 2005;252(12):1435–47 (abstract).
57. Gordon PH. Amyotrophic lateral sclerosis; pathophysiological, diagnosis and management. CNS Drugs. 2011;4(5):1–15 (abstract).
58. Mackenziel RA, Bigio ZH, Ince PG, Geser F, Neumann M, Cairns NJ, et al. TDP-43 distinguishes sporadic amytrophic lateral sclerosis from amyotrophic lateral sclerosis with SODI mutations. Ann Neurol. 2007;61:427–43.
59. Siddique T, Nijhawan D, Hentati A. Familial amyotrophic lateral sclerosis. J Neural Transm Suppl. 1997;49:219–33 (abstract).
60. Munch C, Ludolph AC. Pharmacological treatment of amyothrophic lateral sclerosis. Neurol Neurochir Pol. 2001;35(suppl):41–50 (abstract).
61. Gurney ME, Cutting FB, Zhai P, Andrus PK, Hall ED. Pathogenic mechanisms in familial amyotrophic lateral sclerosis due to mutation of Cu, Zn superoxide dismutase. Pathol Biol (Paris). 1996;44(1):51–6 (abstract).
62. Gordon PH, Cheng B, Katz IB, Pinto M, Hayys AP, Mitsumoto H, et al. The natural history of primary lateral sclerosis. Neurology. 2006;66(5):647–53 (abstract).

Peripheral Neuropathy

63. Verghese J, BiariPL GC, Schaumburg HH, Herskovitz S. Peripheral neuropathy in young-old and old-old patients. Muscle Nerve. 2001;24:1476–81.
64. Shields RW Jr. Peripheral neuropathy. Cleveland clinic. Center for Continuing Education. http://www.clevelandclinicmeded.com/medicalpubs/diseasemanagement/neurology/per. Accessed on 2 Apr 2014.
65. Agamanolis DP. Peripheral nerve pathology. In: Neuropathology, Chapter 12. http://neuropathologyweb.org/chapter12/chapter12Neuropathy.html. Retrieved on 19 Feb 2015.
66. Poncelet AN. An algorithm for the evaluation of peripheral neuropathy. Am Fam Physician. 1998;57(4):755–64.
67. Kumar NB. Neurological aspects of cobalamin (B12) deficiency. Handb Clin Neurol. 2014;120:915–26 (abstract).
68. Wynn M, Wynn A. The danger of B12 deficiency in the elderly. Nutr Health. 1998;12:215–26.
69. Sewell RA. Excerpt from nutritional neuropathy. http://www.emedicine.com/neuro/byname/nutritional-neuropathy.htm.
70. Chin RL. Neuropathology and the gastrointestinal system. http://www.neuropathy.org/site/DocServer/nutritional. GI-RussellCMD.pdf?docID=1601.
71. Walsh JC, McLeod JG. Alcohol neurophysiological electrophysiological and pathological study. J Neuro Sci. 1970;10:457–69.
72. Camdessanche JP, Antoine JC, Honnorat J, Vial C, Petiot P, Convers P, et al. Paraneoplastic peripheral neuropathy associated with anti –Hu antibodies. A clinical and electrophysiological study pf 20 patients. Brain. 2002;125(Pt1):166–75 (abstract).
73. Graus F, Dalmau J. Paraneoplastic neuropathies. Curr Opin Neurol. 2013;26(5):489–95 (abstract).
74. Lin CS-Y, Krishnan AV, Lee M-J, Zaga MI, You H-L, Yang CC, et al. Nerve function and dysfunction in acute intermittent porphyria. Brain. 2008;131:2510–9.
75. Bolton CF. Sepsis and the systemic inflammatory response syndrome: neuromuscular syndrome. Crit Care Med. 1996;24:1408–16.

76. Bolton CF, Gilbert JJ, Hahn AF, Sibbald WJ. Polyneuropathy in critically ill patients. J Neurol Neurosurg Psychiatry. 1984;47:1223–31.
77. Berger AR, Schaumburg HH, Lowe ES. Human toxic neuropathy due to industrial agents. http://www.neuropathy.org/site/DueServer/Toxin-Induced_Neuropathies.pdf?dociD=1603. Retrieved on 7 Apr 2014.
78. Ludolph AC, Spencer PS. Toxic neuropathies and their treatment. Baillieres Clin Neurol. 1995;4(3):505–27.
79. Kuwabara S. Guillain-Barre' syndrome: epidemiology, pathophysiology and management. Drugs. 2004;64(6):597–610 (abstract).
80. Hughes RA, Comblath DR. Guillain-Barre syndrome. Lancet. 2005;366(9497):1653–66 (abstract).
81. Vucic S, Kierman MC, Comblath DR. Guillain-Barre syndrome: an update. J Clin Neurosci. 2009;16(6):733–41 (abstract).
82. Newswanger DL, Warren CR. Guillain-Barre syndrome. Am Fam Physician. 2004. http://www.aafp.org/afp/20040515/2405.html.
83. Hahn AF. Guillain-Barre syndrome. Lancet. 1998;352:635–41.
84. Odaka M, Yuki N, Hiurata K. Anti-GQib IgG antibody syndrome: clinical and immunological range. J Neurol Neurosurg Psychiatry. 2001;70(1):50–5 (abstract).
85. Kaplan JE, Schoenberger LB, Hurwitz ES, Katona P. Gullain Barre syndrome in the United States 1978–1981. Neurology. 1983;33:633–7.
86. Arnason BGW. Acute inflammatory demyelinating polyradiculopathies. In: Dyck PJ, Thomas PK, Lambert EH, Bunce R, editors. Peripheral neuropathy. Philadelphia: WB Saunders; 1984. p. 2050–99.
87. Winner SJ, Grimley EJ. Age specific incidence of Guillain-Barre' syndrome in Oxfordshire. Q J Med. 1990;77(3):1297–304.
88. Aloor M. The epidemiology of Guillain-Barre syndrome. Ann Neurol. 1900;27(supp): 57–80.
89. Thomas PK, Ochoa J. Symptomatology and differential diagnosis of peripheral neuropathy. In: Dyck PJ, Thomas PK, editors. Peripheral neuropathy. Philadelphia: Saunders; 1993. p. 749–74.
90. Odaka M, Yuki N. Variants and differential diagnosis of Guillain-Barre syndrome. Expert Rev Neurol. 2002;2(6):877–89 (abstract).
91. Hughes RA, Hadden RD, Gregson NA, Smith KJ. Pathogenesis of Guillain-Barre syndrome. J Neuroimunol. 1999;100(1–2):74–97 (abstract).
92. Ho TW, Mishu B, Li CY, Cornblath DR, Griffin JW, Asbury AK, et al. Guillain Barre Syndrome in norther China, relationship to Campylobacter jejuni infection and anti-glycolipid antibodies. Brain. 1988;118:597–605.
93. Rees JH, Sondain SE, Gregson N, Hughes RA. Campylobacter jejuni infection in Guillain-Barre syndrome. NEJM. 1995;333:1374–9.
94. Igawara K, Kuwabara S, Mori M, Hattori T, Koga M, Yuki N. Axonal Guillain-Barre syndrome: relation to antiganglioside antibodies and Campylobacter infection in Japan. Ann Neurol. 2000;48:62–3.
95. Azulay JP, Verschueren A, Attarian S, Pouget J. Guillain-Barre syndrome and its frontiers. Rev Neurol (Paris). 2002;158(12Pt2):S21–6 (abstract).
96. Kimoto K, Koga M, Odaku M, Hirata K, Takahashi M, Li J, et al. Relationship of bacterial strains to clinical syndromes of Camphylobacter associated neuropathies. Neurology. 2006;67(10):637–43.
97. Winer JB. An update in Guillain-Barre syndrome. Autoimmune Dis. 2014;2014:793024. doi:10.1155/2014/793024. Epub. 2014 Jan 6 (abstract).
98. Uncini A, Kuwabara S. Electrodiagnostic criteria for Guillain-Barre syndrome: a critical revision and the need for an update. Clin Neurophysiol. 2012;123(8):1487–95 (abstract).

Disorders of Neuromuscular Transmission

99. Gomez AM, Van Ben Broeck J, Vrolix K, Janssen JP, Lemmens MA, Van Der Esch E, et al. Antibody effector mechanisms in myasthenia gravis-pathogenesis at the neuromuscular junction. Autoimmunity. 2010;43(5–6):353–70 (abstract).
100. Robertson NP, Denns J, Compston DA. Myasthenia gravis: a population based epidemiological study in Cambridgeshire, England. J Neurol Nurosurg Psychiatry. 1998;65:492–6.
101. Slesak G, Mclins A, Gerneth T, Sommer N, Weissert R, Dichans J. Late onset myasthenia gravis: almost one third of all cases present in the elderly population: follow-up of 113 patients diagnosed after age of 60. Ann NY Acad Sci. 1998;841:777–80.
102. Trouth JA, Dabi A, Solieman N, Kurukumbi M, Kalyanam J. Myasthenia gravis: a review. Autoimmune Dis. 2012;2012:874680. doi:10.1155/2012/874680. Epub 2012 Oct 31. (abstract).
103. Phillips LH, Torner JC. Epidemiologic evidence for a changing natural history of myasthenia gravis. Neurology. 1996;47(5):1233–8.
104. Thanvi BR, Lo TC. Update on myasthenia. Postgrad Med J. 2004;80:690–700.
105. Vincent A, Clover L, Buckley C, Evans JG, Rothwell PM. Evidence of underdiagnosis of myasthenia gravis in older people. J Neurol Neurosurg Psychiatry. 2003;74(8): 1105–8.
106. Aarli JA. Myasthenia gravis in the elderly: is it different. Ann NY Acad Sci. 2008;1132:238–43 (abstract).
107. Aragones JM, Bolibar I, Bonfill X, Bufill E, Mummany A, Alonsof F. Myasthenia gravis: a higher than expected incidence in the elderly. Neurology. 2003;60(6):1024–6.
108. Montero-Odasso M. Dysphonia as first symptom of late onset myasthenia gravis. J Gen Intern Med. 2006;21:C4–6.
109. Aarli JA. Late-onset myasthenia gravis: changing scene. Arch Neurol. 1999;56:25–7.
110. Simpson JF, Westerberg MR, Magee KR. Myasthenis gravis: an analysis of 295 cases. Acta Neurol Scand. 1996;42 Suppl 23:1–27.
111. Shah AK. Excerpt from myasthenis gravis. eMedicine –myasthenia gravis. http://www.emediine.com/neuro/byname/myasthenia-gravis.htm.
112. Koneczay I, Cossins J, Vincent A. The role of muscle specific tyrosine kinase (MuSK) and mystery of MuSK myasthenia gravis. J Anatomy. 2014;224:21–35.
113. Berman SH, Sanders DB. Assessment of neyromuscular tansmissions. In: eMedicine. Neurology. Lorenzo N, editor. 2007.
114. Zhang B, Luo S, Wong O, Suzuki T, Xiong W, Mei L. LRP4 serves as a coreceptor of agrin. Neuron. 2008;60:285–97.
115. De Chiara TM, Bowen DC, Valenzuela DM, Simmons MV, Poneymiron WT, Thomas S, et al. The receptor tyrosine kinase MuSK is required for neuromuscular junction formation in vivo. Cell. 1996;85:501–12.
116. Kim N, Stiegler AL, Cameron TO, Hallock PT, Gomez AM, Huang JH, et al. LRP4 is a receptor to agrin and forms a complex with MuSK. Cell. 2008;135:334–42.
117. Mantegazza R, Bonanno S, Camera G, Antozzi A. Current and emerging therapies for the treatment of myasthenia gravis. Neuropsychiatr Dis treat. 2011;7:151–60.
118. Reddel SW. Treatment of myasthenis gravis. Aust Pres. 2007;30(6):160.
119. Lennon VA. Experimental auto-immune myasthenia gravis induced by immunization with solubilized acetyl choline. Hum Pathol. 1978;9(5):541–51.
120. Vincent A, McConville J, Farrugia ME, Newsom-Davis J. Seronegative myasthenia gravis. Semin Neurol. 2004;24:125–33.
121. Suzuki S, Utsugisawa K, Nagane Y, Satoh T, Kuwana S, Suzuki N, et al. Clinical and immunological differences between early and late-onset myasthenia gravis in Japan. J Neuroimmunol. 2011;230(1–2):148–52 (abstract).
122. Hoch W, McConvilk JH, Holms S, Newsom-Davis J, Melms A, Vincent A. Autoantibodies to the receptor tyrosine kinase MuSK in patients with myasthenis gravis without acetylcholine receptor antibodies. Nat Med. 2001;7:365–8.

123. Skeie GO, Aarli JA, Gilhus NE. Titin and ryanodine receptor antibodies in myasthenia gravis. Acta Neurol Scand. 2006;183(Suppl):19–23 (abstract).
124. Romi F. Thymoma in myasthenia gravis: from diagnosis to treatment. Autoimmue Dis. 2011;2011:474512. doi:10.4061/2011/474512. Epub 2011 Aug 10 (abstract).
125. Higuchi O, Hamuro J, Motomura M, Yamanashi Y. Autoantibodies to low sensitivity lipoprotein receptor related protein 4 in myasthenia gravis. Ann Neurol. 2011;69:418–22.
126. Cossins J, Bohya K, Zoltowska K, Koneczny I, Maxwell S, Jacobson L, et al. The search for new antigenic targets in myasthenia gravis. Ann NY Acad Sci. 2012;1275:123–8.
127. Drachman DB. Myasthenia gravis. N Engl J Med. 1994;330(25):1797–810.
128. Chaudhuri A. Myasthenic crises. QJM. 2014;102(2):97–107.
129. Wikipedia. Myasthenia gravis. http://en.wilkipedia.org/wiki/Myasthenia_gravis#Pathophysiology. Retrieved 7 Apr 2014.
130. Gunji K, Skolnick C, Bednarczuk T, Benes S, Ackrell BA, Cochran B, et al. Eye muscle antibodies in patients with ocular myasthenia gravis: possible mechanism for eye muscle inflammation in acetylcholine receptor antibody-negative patients. Clin Immunol Immunopathol. 1998;87(3):276–81 (abstract).
131. Wang W, Hen YP, Wei DN. The clinical characteristics of early-onset versus late-onset types of myasthenia gravis. Zhonghua Nei Ke Za Zhi. 2011;50(6):496–8 (abstract).
132. Writz PN, Nijnuis MG, Sotodeh M, Willems LN, Brahim JJ, Putter H, et al. The epidemiology of myasthenia gravis. Lambert-Eaton myasthenia gravis and their associated tumours in the northern part of the province of South Holland. J Neurol. 2003;250(6):698–701.
133. Gilhus NE. Lambert-Eaton myasthenia gravis: pathophysiology diagnosis and therapy. Autoimmune Dis. 2011;2011:973808. doi:10.4061/2011/973808.
134. Mahadeva B, Phillips LH, Juel VC. Autoimmune disorders of the neuromuscular transmission. Semin Neurol. 2008;28(2):212–27 (abstract).
135. Eymard B. Autoimmune myasthenia and Lambert-Eaton myasthenic syndrome. Pathophysiologic concepts. Ann Med Interne (Paris). 1989;140(6):462–6 (abstract).
136. Lisy L. Immunopathogenesis of myasthenia gravis and Lambert-Eaton syndrome. Bratisl Lek Listy. 1997;98(4):217–20 (abstract).
137. Lang B, Vincent A. Autoantibodies to ion channels at the neuromuscular junction. Autoimmun Rev. 2003;2(2):94 (abstract).
138. Lin RC, Scheller RH. Mechanism in synaptic vesicle exocytosis. Ann Rev Cell Div Biol. 2000;16:19–49.

Stroke

139. Bramford J, Sandercock P, Dennis M, Warlow C, Jones L, McPherson K, et al. A prospective study of acute cerebrovascular disease in the community, the Oxfordshire Community Stroke Project 1981-86-1: methodology, demography and incidence increase of first ever stroke. J Neurol Neurosurg Psychiatry. 1988;51:1373–80.
140. Brown RD, Whisnsant JP, Sicks D, O'Fallow WM, Wickers DO. Stroke incidence, prevalence and survival: recent trends in Rochester Minnesota through 1989. Stroke. 1996;27:373–80.
141. Di Carlo A, Launer LJ, Breteler MMB, Fratiglioni L, Lobo A, Marinez-Lage J, et al. Frequency of stroke in Europe: a collaborative study of population based cohorts. ILSA working Group and the Neurological Diseases in the Elderly Research Group: Italian Longitudinal Study on Ageing. Neurology. 2000;54(11 (Suppl 5)):S34–7.
142. Boyle Jr EM, Lille ST, Allaire E, Clowess AW, Verrier ED. Endothelial cell injury in cardiovascularsurgery: atherosclerosis. Ann Thorac Surg. 1997;63(3):885–94 (abstract).
143. Reiner Z, Tedeschi-Reiner E. New information on pathophysiology of atherosclerosis. Lijec Vjesn. 2001;123(1–2):26–31 (abstract).

144. Davies MJ. Arterial Thrombosis and Acute Coronary Syndromes. In Acute Coronary Syndrome. J Amer Coll Cardiol, 1999.
145. Lammie GA. Pathology of small vessel stroke. Br Med Bull. 2000;56(2):206–306.
146. Fisher CM. Pathological observation in hypetension and cerebralhaemorrhage. J Neuropathol Exp Neurol. 1971;30:536–50.
147. Brott T, Broderick J, Kothari R, Barsam W, Tomsick T, Sauerbeck L, et al. Early haemorrhagic growth in patients with intracerebral haemorrhage. Stroke. 1997;28:1–5.
148. Qureshi AI, Tuhrim S, Broderick JB, Batjer HH, Hondo H, Hanley DF, et al. Spontaneous intracerebral haemorrhage. N Engl J Med. 2001;344(19):1450–60.
149. Chakravathy A, Shivane A. Pathology of intracerebral haemorrhage. ACNR. 2008;8:20–1.
150. Butcher KS, Baird T, MacGregor I, Desmod P, Tress B, Davis S. Perihaematomal oedema in primary cerebral haemorrhage is plasma derived. Stroke. 2004;35:1879–85.
151. Smith EE, Greenberg SM. Clinical diagnosis of cerebral amyloid angiopathy: validation of the Boston Criteria. Curr Atheroscler Rep. 2003;5:260–6.

Insomnia and Related Sleep Disorders in the Elderly

152. Groulx B. Management of sleep disorders in the elderly. Ther Update. 1999;7(4):3–8.
153. American Psychiatric Association. Diagnostic and statistical manual of mental disorders. In: Text revision. 4th ed. Washington, DC: American Psychiatric Association, Inc; 2000.
154. Avidan AY. Insomnia in the geriatric patient. Clin Cornerstone. 2003;5(3):51–60 (abstract).
155. Ancoli-Israel S. Insomnia in the elderly: a review for the primary care practitioner. Sleep. 2000;23 Suppl 1:S23–30 (abstract).
156. Bain KT. Management of chronic insomnia in elderly persons. Am J Geriatr Pharmacother. 2006;4(2):168–92 (abstract).
157. McCall WV. Sleep in the elderly: burden diagnosis and treatment. J Clin Psychiatry. 2004;6(1):9–20.
158. Mazza M, Della Marca G, De Risio S, Mennuni GF, Mazza S. Sleep disorders in the elderly. Clin Ther. 2004;155(9):391–4 (abstract).
159. Bombois S, Derambure P, Pasquier F, Monaca C. Sleep disorders in aging and dementia. J Nutr Health Aging. 2010;14(3):212–7 (abstract).
160. Jensen E, Dehlin O, Hagberg B, Samuelson G, Svensson T. Insomnia in an 80-year old population: relationship to medical, psychological and social factors. J Sleep Res. 1998;7: 83–189.
161. Maggi S, Langlois JA, Minicuci N, Grigoletto F, Pavan M, Foley DJ, et al. Sleep complaints in a community-dwelling older persons, prevalence, associated factors and reported causes. J Am Geriatr Soc. 1998;46:161–8.
162. Karacan I, Thornby JI, Anch M. Prevalence of sleep disturbance in a primarily urban Florida county. Soc Sci Med. 1976;27:239–44.
163. Quera-Salva MA, Borderies P, Moreau J, Cugy D. The efficacy of zolpidem during and after shift from BZD hypnotics in elderly chronic insomniac patients. Sleep Res. 1991;20A:370.
164. Miles LE, Dement WC. Sleep and aging. Sleep. 1980;3:119–220.
165. Iber C, Ancoli-Israel S, Chesson A, Quan SF. AASM manual for the scoring of sleep and associated events. Westchester Ill: American Academy of Sleep Medicine; 2007.
166. Carskdon MA, Dement WC. Normal human sleep. An overview. In: Kryger MH, Roth TT, Dement WC, editors. Principles and practice of sleep medicine. 4th ed. Philadelphia: Elsevier Saunders; 2005. p. 13–22.
167. Kryger MH, Roth T, Dement WC, editors. Principles and practice of sleep medicine. 4th ed. Philadelphia: Elsevier Saunders; 2005.
168. Stevens MS. Normal sleep, sleep physiology and sleep deprivation. http://emedicine.mediscape.com/article/1188226-overview. Updated 5 Dec 2011. Accessed 27 Mar 2013.

169. Townsend-Roccichelli J, Sanford JT, Vandewaa E. Managing sleep disorders in the elderly. Nurse Prac Am J Primary Health Care. 2010;35(5):30–7.
170. Waterhouse J, Fukuda Y, Morita T. Daily rhythms of the sleep-wake cycle. J Physiol Anthropol. 2012;31:5. doi:10.1186/1880-6805-31-5 (abstract).
171. Beullens J. Sleep disorders in elderly, the sleep apnea syndrome in particular: are they cause of insomnia? A review of literature. Tijdschr Gerontol Geriatr. 1999;30(6):256–63 (abstract).
172. Prinz PN, Vitiello MV, Raskind MA, Thorphy MJ. Geriatric: sleep disorders and aging. New Eng J Med. 1990;323:320–6.
173. Culebras A. 1994. El sucho au la vegezau La medicine.
174. Derment W, Richardson G, Prinz P, Carskadon M, Kripke D, Czeisler C, et al. The changes of sleep and wakefulness with age. New York: In CE Finch and EL Schneidei eds. The Biology of Aging van Nostrand Reinhold; 1985. p. 692–717.
175. Ancoli-Israel S. Epidemiology of sleep disorders. Clin Geriatr Med. 1989;5:347–62.
176. Lewis SA. Sleep patterns during afternoon naps in the young and elderly. Br J Psychiatry. 1969;115:107–8.
177. Carskadon MA, van den Hoed J, Dement WC. Sleep and daytime sleepiness in the elderly. J Geriatr Psychiatry. 1980;13:135–51.
178. Martin J, Shochat T, Ancoli-Israel S. Assessment and treatment of sleep disturbances in older adults. Clin Psychol Rev. 2000;20:783–805.
179. Prinz PN, Vitielo MV, Smallwood RG, Schoene RB, Halter JB. Plasma norepinephrine in normal young and aged men relationship with sleep. J Gerontol. 1984;39:561–7.
180. Matheson JK. Sleep disorders in the elderly. Med Health/Rhode Island. 2008;91(5): 144–6.
181. Allen RP, Picchietti D, Hening WA, Trenkwalder C, Waters AS, Montplaisi J, et al. Restless leg syndrome: diagnostic criteria, special considerations, and epidemiology workshop at the National Institutes of Health. Sleep Med. 2003;4(2):101–19.
182. Cox Health. Restless leg syndrome and periodic leg movements disease. http://www.cox-health.com. Accessed 6 Feb 2014.
183. Hornyak M, Feige B, Riemann D, Voderholzer U. Periodic leg movements in sleep and periodic limb movement disorder: prevalence, clinical significance and treatment. Sleep Med Rev. 2006;10(3):169–77 (abstract).
184. Uddin UBMS, Jarmi T. REM sleep behaviour disorder. eMedicine Neurology. 2007. website: http://emedicine.medscape.com/article/1188651-overview.
185. International classification of sleep disorders, revised diagnostic and coding manual. Rochester. Minn: Am Sleep Dis Assoc. 1997;177–80
186. Tachibana N. REM sleep behaviour disorder in Parkinson's disease. J Neurol. 2007;254:8–14 (abstract).
187. Carskdon MA, Rechtschaffen A. Monitoring and staging human sleep. In: Kryger MH, Roth TT, Dement WC, editors. Principles and practice of sleep medicine. 4th ed. Philadelphia: Elsevier Saunders; 2005. p. 1359–77.
188. Rye DB, Dihenia B, Weissman JD, Epstein C, Bliwise DL. Presentation of narcolepsy after 40. Neurology. 1998;50:459–65.
189. Attaruian H. Narcolepsy in the older adult. In: Goswami M, Pando-Perumal SR, Thorpy NJ, editors. Narcolepsy: a clinical guide. New York: Humana Press; 2009. p. 69–76.

Headaches

190. Waters WE. The pontypridd headache survey. Headache. 1974;14:81–90.
191. Cook NR, Evans DA, Funkenstein HH, Scherr PA, Ostfeld AM, Taylor JO, et al. Correlates of headache in a population-based cohort of the elderly. Arch Neurol. 1989;46(12):1338–44.

192. Solomon GD, Kunkel RS, Frame J. Demographics of headaches in elderly patients. Headache. 1990;30:273.
193. Hale WE, Perkins LL, May FE, Marks RG, Stewart RB, et al. Symptom prevalence in the elderly: an evaluation of age, sex, disease and medication. J Am Geriatr Soc. 1986;3495:333.
194. Biondi DM, Saper JR. Geriatric headache: how to make the diagnosis and manage pain. Geriatrics. 2000;55(12):40, 43–5.48–50 (abstract).
195. Reinisch VM, Schankin CJ, Felbinger J, Sostak P, Straube A. Headache in the elderly. Schmerz. 2008;22 Suppl 1:22–30 (abstract).
196. Prencipe AM, Casini AR, Ferretti C, Santini M, Pezzella F, Scaldaferri N, et al. Prevalence of headache in an elderly population: attack frequency, disability and use of medication. J Neurol Neurosurg Psychiatry. 2001;70:377–81.
197. Tanganetti P. Secondary headaches in the elderly. Neuro Sci. 2010;31(Suppl 1):S73–6. doi:10.1007/s10072-010-02776 (abstract).
198. Headache Classification Committee of the International Headache Society Classification. Classification and diagnostic criteria for headache disorders, cranial neuralgias, facial pain. Cephalalgia. 1988;8 Suppl 7:1.
199. Lipton RB, Bigal ME, Steiner TJ, Siberstein SD, Olesen J. Classification of primary headaches. Neurology. 2004;63(3):427–35 (abstract).
200. Gobel H, Heinze A. Headache and facial pain in the elderly. Schmerz. 2007;21(6):561–9 (abstract).
201. Silberstein SD, Lipton RB. Chronic daily headaches including transformed migraine, chronic tension headache and medications overuse. In: Silberstein SD, Lipton RB, Dalessio DJ, editors. Wolff's Headache and other head pain. New York: Oxford University Press; 2001. p. 247–82.
202. Hershey LA, Bednarczyk EM. Treatment of headache in the elderly. Curr Treat Options Neurol. 2013;15(1):56–62 (abstract).
203. Silberstein SD. Chronic daily headaches. J Am Osteopath Assoc. 2005;105(4 Suppl):23S–9.
204. Goadsby PJ, Boes C. New daily persistent headaches. J Neurol Neurosurg Psychiatry. 2002;72:ii6–9. doi:10.1136/jnnp.72suppl_21.6.
205. Lipton RB, Pfeffer D, Newman LC, Solomon S. Headaches in the elderly. J Pain Symptom Manage. 1993;8:87–97.
206. Selby GW, Lance JW. Observations on 500 cases of migraine and allied vascular headache. J Neurol Neurosurg Psychiatry. 1960;23:23–32.
207. Wilkinson M. Clinical features of migraine. In: Vinken PJ, Bruyn GW, Klawans HL, et al., editors. Headache. New York: Elsevier; 1986. p. 117–83.
208. Manusov EG. Late-life accompaniments: a case presentation and literature review. J Fam Pract. 1987;24(6):591–4 (abstract).
209. Edmeads J. Headaches in older people. Postgrad Med. 1997;101(5):91–4.
210. Hanky GJ. Stroke. Edinburgh: Churchill Livingston; 2002.
211. Raskin NH. The hypnic headache syndrome. Headache. 1988;28(8):534–6.
212. Evers S, Goadsby PJ. Hypnic headache. Pract Neurol. 2005;8:144–9 (abstract).
213. Newman LC, Lipton RB, Solomon S. The hypnic headache syndrome: a benign headache disorder of the elderly. Neurology. 1990;190(12):1904–5.
214. Obermann M, Holle D. Hypnic headache. Expect Rev Neurother. 2010;10(4):1391–7 (abstract).
215. Evans RW. Diagnostic testing for the evaluation of headaches. Neurol Clin. 1996;14(1):1–26 (abstract).
216. Greig NH, Ries LG, Yancik R, Rapoport SI. Increasing incidence of primary malignant tumours in the elderly. J Natl Cancer Inst. 1990;82:1621–4.
217. Crawford J, Cohen HJ. Relationship of cancer and aging. Clin Geriatr Med. 1987;3:419–32.
218. Legler JM, Reis LA, Smith MA, Warren JL, Heinman EF, Kaplan RS, et al. Cancer surveillance series (corrected) brain and other central nervous system cancers. Recent trends in incidence and mortality. J Natl Cancer Inst. 1999;91:1382–92.

219. Nayak L, Iwamoto FM. Primary brain tumours in the elderly. Curr Neurol Neurosci Rep. 2010;10(4):252–8 (abstract).
220. Cancer Control. Brain tumours in the older person. Medscape. 2000;7(6). http://www.Medscape.com/viewarticle./409013_9. Accessed 17 Nov 2013.
221. Purdy RA, Kirby S. Headaches and brain tumours. Neurol Clin. 2004;22(1):39–53 (abstract).
222. Edmeads J, et al. Headaches in cerebrovascular disease. In: Vinken PJ, Bruyn GW, Klawans HL, editors. Hand-book of clinical neurology: headache. 7th ed. New York: Elsevier; 1986. p. 273–90.
223. Forsyth PA, Posner JB. Headaches in patients with brain tumours: a study of 111 patients. Neurology. 1993;43(9):1678–83.
224. Alexander M, Wagner EH, Buchner DM, Cain KC, Lason EB. Do surgical brainlesions present as isolated dementia? A population based study. J Am Geriatr Soc. 1995;43:138–43 (abstract).
225. Tagle P, Mery F, Torreilbe G, Del Villar S, Carmona H, Campos M, et al. Chronic haematoma: a disease of the elderly. Rev Med Clin. 2003;131(2):177–82.
226. Asghar M, Adhiyaman V, Greenway MW, Bhowmich BK, Bates A. Chronic subdural haematoma in the elderly –a North Wales experience. J R Soc Med. 2002;95(6):290–2 (abstract).
227. Jones S, Kafetz K. A prospective study of chronic subdural haematoma in elderly patients. Age Aging. 1999;28(6):519–21 (abstract).
228. Adhiyaman V, Asghar M, Ganeshram RN, Bhowmicl BK. Chronic subdural haematoma in the elderly. Postgrad Med J. 2002;78(916):71–5 (abstract).
229. Domingo P, Pomar V, de Benito N, Coll P. The spectrum of acute bacterial meningitis in elderly patients. BMC Infect Dis. 2013;13:108. doi:10.1186/1471-2334-13-108.
230. Gorse GJ, Thrupp LP, Nadelman KL, Wyle FA, Hawkins G, Cesario TC, et al. Bacterial meningitis in the elderly. Arch Intern Med. 1984;144:1603–7.
231. Wenger JD, Hightower AW, Facklam RR, Gaventa S, Brome CV. Bacterial meningitis 1986: report of multistate surveillance study. J Infect Dis. 1990;162:1316–23.
232. Laguna-Del-Estal P, Garcia Madero R, Gil-Navarro M, Garcia-Zubiri C, Agud Fernandez AM. Acute bacterial meningitis in older people. Rev Clin Esp. 2010;210(2):57–64 (abstract).
233. Hussein AS, Shafran SD. Acute bacterial meningitis in adults: a 12 year review. Medicine (Baltimore). 2000;79(6):360–8.
234. Wersfelt M, van de Beek D, Soanjaard L, Reitsma JB, Gans J. Community acquired bacterial meningitis in older people. J Am Geriatr Soc. 2006;54(10):1500–7 (abstract).

Memory and Memory Loss

235. Erickson KR. Amnestic disorders. Pathophysiology and patterns of memory dysfunction. West J Med. 1990;152(2):159–66.
236. Atkinson RC, Shiffrin RM. The control process of short term memory. Institute of Mathematical Studies in the Social Services. Stanford California: Stanford University; 1971.
237. McLeod S. Short term memory. Retrieved form: http://www.simplypsychology.org/short-term-memory-html.
238. Baddeley A. Working memory. Science. 1992;255(5044):556–9. abstract.
239. Anderson JR. Language memory and thought. Mahwah NJ: Erlbaum; 1976.
240. Kandal ER. The biology of memory: a forty year perspective. J Neurosci. 2009;29(41):12748–56.
241. Poldrack RA, Gabrieli JD. Functional anatomy of long-term memory. J Clin Neurophysiol. 1997;14(4):294–310 (abstract).
242. Squire LR, Zola SM. Episodic memory, semantic memory and amnesia. Hippocampus. 1998;8(30):205–11.

243. Squire LR. Declarative and non-declarative memory: multiple brain systems supporting learning and memories. J Cogn Neurosci. 1992;4:232–43.
244. Baddeley AD. The psychology of memory. In: Baddeley AD, Kopelman MD, Wilson BA, editors. The essential handbook of memory disorders for clinicians. Chichester: John Wiley &Sons Ltd; 2004.
245. Budson AE. Understanding memory dysfunction. Neurologist. 2009;15(2):71–9 (abstract).
246. Schacter DL, Tulvig E. What are the memory systems of 1994? In: Sachacter DL, Tulvig E, editors. Memory systems 1994 (pp. 1–38). Cambridge: MIT Press; 1957. p. 7–38.
247. Milner B. Amnesia following operation on temporal lobes. In: Whitty CWM, Zangwill OL, editors. Amnesia. London: Butterworth; 1966.
248. Shallice T, Warrington EK as quoted by Baddeley AD.
249. Small SA. Age-related memory decline. Current concepts and future directions. JAMA Neurol. 2001;58(3):360–4.
250. Mesulam MM, Mufson BJ, Levey AI, Wainer BH. Cholinergic innervation of cortex by basal forebrain: cytochemistry and cotical connections of the septal area diagonal band nuclei, nucleus basalis (substantia innonunta), and hypothalamus in rhesus monkey. J Comp Neurol. 1983;214:170–97.
251. Zola-Morgan S, Squire LR. Neuroanatomy of memory. Ann Rev Neurosci. 1993;16:547–63.
252. Hanniuen T, Korristo K, Reinikainen KJ, Helkali E-C, Soininen H, Mykkanen L, et al. Prevalence of ageing associated cognitive decline in an elderly population. Age Aging. 1996;25:201–5.
253. Fisk JE, Warr PB. Associative learning and short term forgetting as a function of age perceptual speed and central executive functioning. J Gerontol Psychol Sci. 1998;54B:P112–21.
254. Luo L, Craik FIM. Aging and memory: a cognitive approach. La Revue canadienne de psychiatrie. 2008;53(6):346.
255. Schugens MM, Daum I, Spindler BN. Differential effects of aging on explicit and implicit memory. Aging Neuropsychol Cogn. 1997;4:33–44.
256. Huktsch DF, Dixon RA. Learning and memory in ageing. In: Birren JE, Schaie KW, editors. Handbook of the psychology of aging. New York: Academic; 1990. p. 258–74.
257. Victor M, Adamds RD, Collins GH. The Wernicke-Korsakoff syndrome. Philadelphia: FA Davis; 1971.
258. Kopelman MD. Amnesia: organic and psychogenic. Br J Psychiatr. 1987;150:428–42.
259. Blackman L. Memory functioning in dementia. Amsterdam: North Holland; 1992.
260. Libon KJ, Bogdanoff B, Cloud BS, Skalina S, Giovannetti T, Gitlin HL, et al. Declarative and procedural learning, qualitative measures of the hippocampus and subcortical white matter alterations in Alzheimer's disease and ischaemic vascular dementia. J Clin Exp Neuropsychiatry. 1998;20(1):30–4.
261. Tulvig E. Memory functioning in dementia. Amsterdam: North Holland; 1992.
262. Deweer R, Ergis AM, Fosati P, Pillon B, Bller F, Agid Y, et al. Explicit memory procedural learning and lexical priming in Alzheimer's disease. Cortex. 1994;30:113–26.
263. Ikeda M, Tanabe H, Kazui H, Komoni K, Nishimura A. Procedural memory in mild to moderate Alzheimer's disease. Ann Psychiatry. 1995;5:23–9.
264. Eslinger PJ, Damasio AR. Preserved motor learning in Alzheimer's disease: implications for anatomy and behaviour. J Neurosci. 1986;6(10):3006–9 (abstract).
265. Smith I, Hillmar A. Management of alcoholic Korsakoff syndrome. Adv Psychiatr Treat. 1999;5:271–8.
266. Kopelman MD, Thomson AD, Guerrini I, Marshall J. The Korsakoff syndrome: clinical aspects. Psychol Treat Alcohol Alcoholism. 2009;44(2):148–54.
267. Fama R, Pfefferbaum A, Sullivan SP. Visuoperceptual learning in alcoholic Korsakoff syndrome. Alcohol Clin Exp Res. 2006;30:680–7.
268. Clarke S, Assal G, Bogousslavsky J, Regli F, Townsen DW, Leenders KL, et al. Pure amnesia after unilateral left polar thalamic infarct topographic and sequential neuropsycholoical and metabolic (PET) correlations. J Neurol Neurosurg Psychiatry. 1994;57:27–34 (abstract).

269. Nagaratnam N, Ghougassian D, Mudridge V. Syndrome of downward gaze paralysis amnesia and hypersomnolence. Postgrad Med J. 1989;65:840–2.
270. Tatemichi TK, Desmond DW, Mayeux R. Dementia after stroke: baseline, frequency, risks and clinical features in a hospitalized cohort. Neurology. 1992;42:1185–93 (abstract).
271. Tatemichi TK, Desmond DW, Prohovnik I, Cross DT, Gropen TI, Mohr JP. Confusion and memory loss from capsular genu infartction: a thalamocortical disconnection syndrome? Neurology. 1992;42:1966–79 (abstract).
272. Tsuboi Y, Kojima S, Mori M, Nakai R, Fujita K. Prolonged antegrade amnesia due to anterior thalamic infarct, and SPECT findings. No To Shinkei. 1997;49(1):77 (abstract).
273. Bolla-Wilson K, Bleecher MI. Memory complaints: dementia or depression? Gerontologist. 1986;26:142.
274. Larrabee GJ, Levin HS. Verbal, visual and remote memory performance on a normal elderly sample. Presented at the 12th Annual Meeting of the International Neuropsychological Society. Houston; 1984.
275. Karnath B. Subdural haematoma. Presentation and management of older adults. Geriatrics. 2004;58:18–23.
276. Chen JCT, Levy ML. Causes epidemiology and risk factors of chronic subdural haematoma. Neurosurg Clin North Am. 2000;11(3):399–406.
277. Kritchevsky M, Zouzounis J, Squire LR. Transient global amnesia and functional retrograde amnesia: contrasting examples of episodic memory loss. Philos Trans R Soc Lond B Biol Sci. 1997;352(1362):1747–54 (abstract).
278. McKay GC, Kopelman MD. Psychogenic Amnesia: when memory complaints are medically unexplained. Adv Psychiatr Treat. 2009;15:152–8.
279. Markowitsch HJ. Psychogenic amnesia. Neuroimage. 2003;20 Suppl 1:S132–8 (abstract).
280. Brandt J, Van Gorp WG. Functional ("psychogenic") amnesia. Semin Neurol. 2006;26(3):331–40 (abstract).
281. Stone J, Carson A, Sharpe M. Functional symptoms in neurology assessment. J Neurol Neurosurg Psychiatry. 2005;76:13–21.
282. World Health Organisation.The ICD-10 classification of Mental and Behavioural Disorders. Clinical Descriptions & Diagnostic Guidelines,WHO.1992.

Chronic Pain

283. Chronic pain network. The pathophysiology of pain. http://www.chronicpainnetwork.com/pathophysiologypain.aspx?text=1. Accessed on 16 Nov 2008.
284. Wall RT. Pharmacological treatment of pain in the elderly. Management of chronic pain in the elderly. Aust J Hosp Pharm. 1998;28:361–7.
285. Crook J, Rideout E, Brown G. The prevalence of pain complaints in a general population. Pain. 1984;18:299–314.
286. Cavalieri TA. Managing pain in geriatric patients. J Am Osteopath Assoc. 2007;107 Suppl 4:ES10–6.
287. Ferrell BA, Ferrell BR, Osterwell D. Pain in the nursing home. J Am Geriatr Soc. 1990;38:409–14.
288. Kaye AD, Baluch A, Scott JT. Pain management in the elderly population: a review. Ochsner J. 2010;10(3):179–87.
289. Segatore M. Understanding central post-stroke pain. J Neurosci Nurs. 1996;28(1):28–35.
290. Andersen G, Vestergaard K, Ingeman-Neilsen M, Jensen TS. Incidence of central post stroke pain. Pain. 1995;61:187–93.
291. Lynch D. Geriatric pain. In: Raj PP, editor. Practical management of pain. 3rd ed. St Louis: Mosby; 2000. p. 270–1.
292. EDU.org. Pathophysiology of pain. https://www.painduorg/tools/pathpyhsiology_pain_asp. Accessed 6 Mar 2015.

293. Patel NB. Chap. 3. Physiology of pain. In: Kopf A, Patel NB, editors. Guide to pain management in low –resources settings. Seattle: IASP; 2010. p. 13–7.
294. Macres M, Richeimer SH, Duran PJ. Understanding neuropathic pain. http://www.helpforpain.com/articles/understand-neuropathic-pain/understanding.htm. Accessed 18 Feb 2015.
295. Nogradi A, Vrbova G. Anatomy and physiology of the spinal cord. Madame Curie Bioscience Database (internet). http://www.ncbi.nim.gov/books/NSK5229/. Retrieved 18 Feb 2015.
296. Dafny N. Anatomy of the spinal cord. Neuroscience. Chap. 3 Section 2. http://www.neuroscience.uth.tms.edu/s2/chapter03.html. Accessed 18 Feb 2015.
297. Thamburaj AV. Physiology & management of pain. Global Spine Network. http://www.globalsoinal.net.physiology_of_pain.html. Accessed on 16 Nov 2008.
298. Fields HL, Heinricher MM. Anatomy and physiology of nociceptive modulatory system. Philos Trans R Soc Lond B Biol Sci. 1985;308:361–74.
299. Basbaum AI, Fields HL. Endogenous pain control mechanisms: review and hypothesis. Ann Neurol. 1978;4(5):451–62 (abstract).
300. AGS Panel on Persistent Pain in Older Persons. The management of persistent pain in older persons. J Am Geiatr Soc. 2002;50:5205–24.
301. Helme RD, Katz B. Management of chronic pain. Med J Aust. 1993;158:478–81.
302. Dejerine J, Rossy G. Le syndrome douloureux thalamique. Rev Neurol (Paris). 1906;14:521–32.
303. Nasreddine ZS, Saver JL. Pain after thalamic stroke: right diencephalic predominance and clinical features in 1980 patients. Neurology. 1997;48:1196–9.

Gait Disorders

304. Bloem BR, Gussekloo J, Lagaay AM, van Beek W, Wintzen AR, Rs RA, et al. Investigation of gait in elderly subjects over 88 years of age. J Geriatr Psychiatry Neurol. 1992;5:78–84.
305. Dawson D, Hendershot G, Fulton J. Aging in the eighties: functional limitations of individuals age 65 and over. National Center for Health Statistics Advance Data.
306. Leon J, Lair T. Functional status of the noninstitutionalised elderly: estimates of ADL and IADL difficulties (DHHS Publication No. (OPHS) 90–3462). National Medical Expenditure survey Research Findings Agency for Health Care Policy and Research, Rockville: Public Health Service; 1990 (as quoted by Alexander, 2007).
307. Lair T, Lefkowitz D. Mental health and functional status of residents of nursing and personal care homes. (DHHS publication No. (PHS) 90–3470). National Medical Expenditure Survey Research Findings, Agency for Health Care Policy and Research. Rockville: Public Health Service; 1990.
308. Verghese J, LeValley A, Hall CB, Katz MJ, Ambrose AE, Lipton EB. Epidemiology of gait disorders in community –residing older adults. J Am Geriatr Soc. 2006;54(2):255–61.
309. Camiciolli R, Rosano C. Understanding gait in aging: finding the way forward: Part I. Website Edition April/May 2012: The Movement Disorder SocietyMDS. http://www.movementdisorders.org/monthly_edition/2012/04/understanding_gait_in_. Accessed 18 July 2013.
310. Lee D, Lishman R. Vision in movement and balance. New Sci. 1975;9:59–61.
311. Spirduso WW. Physical dimensions of aging. Champaign: Human Kinetics; 1995.
312. Brockelhurst JC, Robertson D, James-Groin P. Clinical correlates of sway in old age-sensory modalities. Age Aging. 1982;11:1–10.
313. Murray MP, Kory RC, Clarkson BH. Walking patterns in healthy old men. J Gerontol. 1969;24(2):169–78.
314. Winter DA, Patla AE, Frank JS, Walt SE. Biomechanical walking changes in the fit and healthy elders. Phys Ther. 1980;70:740–7.

315. Judge JO, Ounuu S, Davis RB. Effects of age in the biomechanics and physiology of gait. Clin Geriatr Med. 1996;12(4):659–78.
316. Blanke DJ, Hageman PA. Comparison of gait of young men and elderly men. Phys Ther. 1989;69:2.
317. Hageman PA, Blanke DJ. Comparison of gait of young women and elderly women. Phys Ther. 1986;66:9–11.
318. Hageman PA. Gait characteristics in healthy elderly: a literature review. Section of geriatrics. Am Physiol Therapy Assoc. 1995;18:2–5.
319. Alexander NB. Gait disorders in older adults. Clin Geriatrics. http://www.clinicalgeriatrics.com/article/1231.
320. Koller WC, Wilson RS, Glatt SL, Huckman MS, Fox JR. Senile gait. Correlation with computed tomographic scans. Ann Neurol. 1983;13:343–4.
321. Hogan DB, Bermann DB, Fox RA, Hubley-Kozey CL, Turnbull G, Wall J. Idiopathic gait disorders in the elderly. Clin Rehab. 1987;1:17–22.
322. Eible RJ, Hughes L, Higgins C. The syndrome of senile gait. J Neurol. 1992;239:71–5.
323. Bloem BR, Gussekloo J, Lagaay AM, Remarque EJ, Haan J, Westendorp RG. Idiopathic gait disorders are signs of subclinical disease. J Am Geriatr Soc. 2000;48(9):1098–101 (abstract).
324. Nutt JG, Marsden CD, Thompson PD. Human walking and higher –level gait disorders, particularly in the elderly. Neurology. 1993;43(2):268–79.
325. Liston R, Mickelboruogh J, Bene J, Tallis R. A new classification of higher level gait disorders in patients with cerebral multi-infarct states. Age Ageing. 2003;32:252–8.

Skin Disorders in the Elderly

8

8.1 Anatomy and Physiological Changes with Ageing

The outermost layer of the skin is the epidermis composed of keratinocytes, Langerhans cells, melanocytes and Merkel cells. Beneath the epidermis is the basement membrane, a multilayered structure. Below this is the dermis, an area of supportive connective tissue and embodies hair roots, sweat glands, blood vessels, nerve cells and fibres and lymph vessels. Beneath the dermis is the subcutis, a loose connective tissue layer. There are two types of ageing of the skin. One is intrinsic, attributable to the passage of time, and the other extrinsic caused by environmental factors such as chronic exposure to sunlight (photoageing). The former moves at a genetically determined pace [1]. With ageing structural and functional changes occur [1] in all the structures of the skin. The epidermis, dermis and the subcutaneous layers become thinned out [2], the keratinocytes shrink and there is a decrease in the number of melanocytes, Langerhans cells [3] and Merkel cells. There is a reduction in the fibroblasts [2] as well as nerve endings, blood vessels and exocrine sweat glands [3]. With ageing there are atrophy of the vasculature and deterioration of the supporting dermis [4], and these changes result in thinner and transparent skin and loss of elasticity. The skin becomes dry with tendency to itch, inability to sweat [2], loss of hair follicles [3] and greying of hair. There is also a reduction of immune cells in the skin compromising immune response [5–7].

With normal ageing process, a number of extrinsic factors act to prematurely age the skin. Chronic sun exposure over the years causes changes to the skin. About 80 % of facial ageing is due to sun exposure [8]. They are most noticeable in fair-skinned people. Wrinkling, dryness, coarseness, telangiectasia, irregular pigmentation, blotchy complexion and actinic keratoses are some of the indicators of photoageing. Reduction in the number of melanosomes synthesised results in reduced pigmentation [3]. The extent and severity of these changes will depend on the duration and intensity of exposure to the sun and also on the colour of the skin.

N. Nagaratnam et al., *Diseases in the Elderly: Age-Related Changes and Pathophysiology*, DOI 10.1007/978-3-319-25787-7_8

Box 8.1. Key Points. Anatomy and Physiological Skin Changes with Ageing

- The epidermis is composed of keratinocytes, Langerhans cells, melanocytes and Merkel cells [2, 3].
- There are two types of ageing of the skin. One is intrinsic, attributable to the passage of time, and the other extrinsic caused by environmental factors such as chronic exposure to sunlight (photoageing).
- With ageing structural and functional changes occur in all the structures of the skin, epidermis, dermis and the subcutaneous layers [1].
- There is also a reduction of immune cells in the skin compromising immune response [5–7].

8.2 Common Skin Disorders in the Elderly

Introduction

Pruritic eruptions are common in the elderly especially in those in their 70s and 80s [9]. The frequency of the dermatological diseases shows a variation depending on the age, gender and season [10]. Melanoma is the fourth common cancer and is due to an uncontrolled growth of the pigmented cells, the melanocytes. Australia has the highest incidence rate of melanoma and represents 10 % of all cancers with nearly 9600 cases annually and 1200 deaths each year [11]. The incidence of malignant melanoma increases with age and is the sixth most common cancer in the United States [12, 13]. Lentigo maligna melanoma subtype is more common in men over the age of 65 and has been shown with increasing incidence over a 10-year period [14]. In both community-dwelling elderly and nursing home residents, seborrhoeic keratosis and xerosis had the highest prevalence exceeding over 75 %, but in the dermatologic clinic the presenting conditions were actinic keratosis, fungal infections and xerosis each not exceeding 25 %[15]. The major types of the keratinocytic cancers are the basal cell carcinoma (BCC), squamous cell carcinoma (SCC) and melanoma; an exposure to sun UV radiation is the most important environmental risk factor for all three types [16].

Pathophysiology

There is loss of resistance to environmental and mechanical trauma with intrinsic ageing. There is a decline in several functions of the skin, including barrier efficacy, immune responsiveness [9] wound healing [2], sensory perception and DNA repair and greater risk of neoplastic growth [17]. Skin diseases in the elderly are more often than not the effects of sun damage or vascular disease [18]. Ultraviolet radiation (UV) from the sun is the main environmental cause for premature ageing of the skin (photoageing) [19, 20]. Repeated exposure to the sun's rays will lead to breakdown of the collagen and impair formation of new collagen, and the photoaged skin is characterised by overgrowth of abnormal elastic fibres and reduced collagen in the dermis [21]. UV radiation induces delayed UV-responsive genes, among them

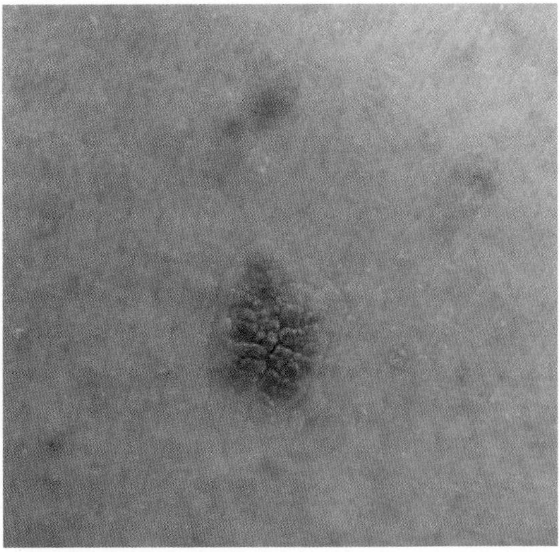

Fig. 8.1 Seborrhoeic keratosis – manifests as verrucous plaques, greasy to touch and a warty appearance (Reproduced with permission from Dr Derrick Davies, Orange Dermatology)

the matrix metalloproteinases [21], which degrade the collagenous extracellular matrix of the connective tissue [20], a hallmark of ageing and carcinogenesis [21]. Recently, it has been shown that with UV-induced skin damage and the process of photoageing, the neutrophils are initially the main infiltrating cell type in the dermis, and these infiltrating cells are the main source for such enzymes as elastase and matrix metalloproteinases [22].

Clinically, the sun-exposed skin loses its elasticity and has disrupted elastin and decreased glycosaminoglycans; as a result it becomes thin, breaks easily, bruises, increases irritability and itches [23]. Long and continued exposure in those who live in sun-intense regions will develop actinic keratoses. The number of melanocytes decreases by about 10–20 % per decade and declines in the development of new melanocytic nevi resulting in pigmentary changes in the skin with ageing [24]. Melanin pigmentation of the skin absorbs UV light, and this protects the skin cells from injurious effects of UV exposure [25].

Seborrhoeic keratosis is usually seen in patients over the age of 50 and most Caucasians are affected sooner or later [26]. The areas involved are generally those exposed to sunlight such as the regions of the face, neck and trunk (Fig. 8.1).

Actinic or solar keratosis is usually seen after the age of 65 and results from continued exposure to solar radiation. They are common after the age of 45 years in the Caucasian Australians [27]. Many of the lesions regress, but a few, estimated at about 1 % [21] to 12 % [28], may progress to squamous cell carcinoma within 10–25 years [29]. A high frequency of p53 mutation has been reported in actinic keratosis [30] (Fig. 8.2).

The most frequently occurring skin cancers are the basal cell carcinoma, squamous cell carcinoma and melanoma [31, 32]. Exposure of the skin to UV radiation over years increases the risk of the development of skin cancers, but it may take

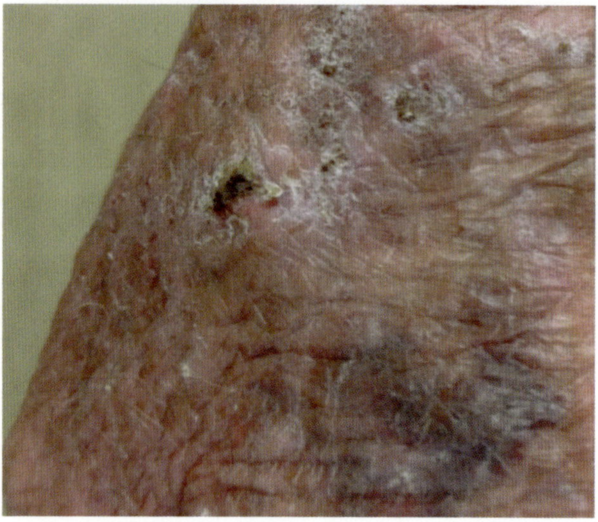

Fig. 8.2 Actinic/solar keratosis – scaly papules grey to dark brown in colour and easily palpated (Reproduced with permission from Dr Derrick Davies, Orange Dermatology)

several years after exposure before malignancy occurs [33]. UV light induces DNA damage of the keratinocytes and the damaged cells are removed by apoptosis [34] which is under the control of p53, a suppressor gene [31, 32]. Extensive exposure to UV light leads to resistant DNA-damaged cells to apoptosis. UV-inducing mutations in p53 gene have been detected in majority of skin cancers [30]. In skin cancers the pathways that regulate cell cycling and apoptosis are degraded [35], for example, mutation in the hedgehog pathway-related genes especially PTCH1 in basal cell carcinoma [33]. Fas-L is another proapoptotic molecule involved in the removal of sunburn cells [31, 32].

Basal cell carcinoma is a common malignant skin condition. It has been reported that 50 % of Caucasian Australians will develop basal cell carcinoma before the age of 70 years [21 and is most common in older adults. Exposure to the sun is the major risk factor [36]. Other signs include a nodule varying in colour red, pink or white and translucent or an area resembling a scar. They enlarge slowly and are usually found on the sun-exposed areas of the head and neck in fair-skinned individuals. They rarely metastasise [27] (Fig. 8.3a).

Squamous cell carcinoma is another common tumour of the skin. It usually occurs in the same fair-skinned individuals as basal cell cancer in the chronically sun-exposed areas but occasionally in sites of previous ulceration like chronic venous ulcers or other skin damage like radiodermatitis. It is the most common type of skin cancer in dark-skinned people (Fig. 8.2b).

Bowen's disease is squamous cell carcinoma in situ with a high frequency of p53 mutation [30]. It is a disease of the elderly and the mean age at diagnosis is in the sixth decade [37]. It can occur anywhere on the skin or mucous membranes. There is a 3–5 % risk of developing invasive squamous carcinoma [38]. Internal malignancies are often associated with multiple lesions and need close follow-up (Fig. 8.4).

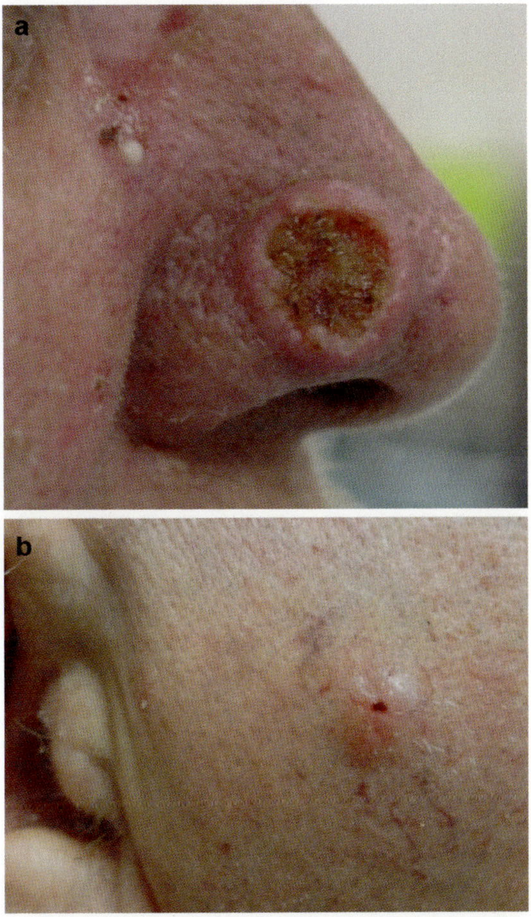

Fig. 8.3 (**a**) Squamous cell carcinoma – red plaques, scaly hyperkeratotic with irregular borders and ulcerated (Reproduced with permission from Dr Derrick Davies, Orange Dermatology). (**b**) Basal cell carcinoma – firm pearly appearance, telangiectasia on the surface and rolled borders (Reproduced with permission from Dr Derrick Davies, Orange Dermatology)

Lentigo appears as a slowly enlarging macule with irregular borders. It is an in situ melanoma of chronically sun-damaged skin. It has to be distinguished from solar lentigo which is smaller with regular borders and homogenous in colour.

Melanoma is an aggressive and highly metastatic cancer [39]. During the past decade melanoma has been considered to be a spectrum of melanocytic malignancies characterised by mutations in several kinases such as BRAF, NRAS and KIT [40]; BRAF mutation is present in two-thirds of cutaneous melanomas [39, 41]. About 40–60 % of patients have activating BRAF mutation in their melanotic cancer [42]. The most common mutation is V600E followed by V600K [43]. The remaining have NRAS mutations [41] and they tend to have thicker tumours and a higher mitotic rate [44]. Tumours that do not have BRAS or NRAS are referred to as wild type for BRAF and NRAS [44]. These mutations occur in the mitogen-activated protein kinase (MAPK) pathway [41] and are a common site for genetic deviations in melanoma.

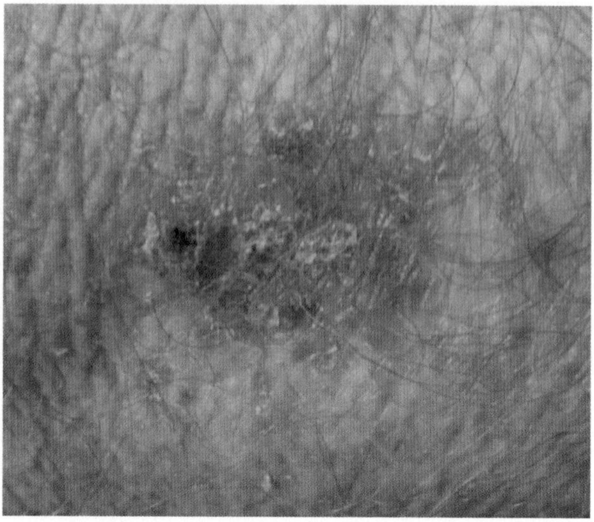

Fig. 8.4 Bowen's disease – red scaly plaque with well-defined margins (Reproduced with permission from Dr Derrick Davies, Orange Dermatology)

The common subtypes of melanoma are (i) lentigo maligna (Hutchinson's freckles), (ii) lentigo maligna melanoma, (iii) nodular melanoma and (iv) superficial spreading melanoma. Lentigo maligna is a premalignant pigmented macular lesion with an irregular border (Fig. 8.5a, b). In a study of 610 patients with malignant melanoma, 237 patients were above the age of 75 years; it had been shown that malignant melanoma was more common in men and the clinical and pathological expression was different to that of their younger counterparts [45]. The investigators found that the melanoma in the elderly patients presented with thicker melanomas, and this was attributed to delayed diagnosis and a higher mitotic rate but with fewer sentinel lymph node metastases [45]. There was an incidence of head and neck involvement set down to cumulative photodamage [45] and starting in the pigment cells, melanocytes, of the skin. The lesions are brown or black in colour and usually asymmetrical.

In the elderly the common dermatoses seen are xerosis, pruritus, eczematous dermatitis, stasis dermatitis [4, 46] and fungal and viral infections [9, 10]. The immune response is affected by the decrease in the Langerhans cells with ageing [47]. Immunosenescence leads to similar levels of occurrence of autoimmune skin disorders such as bullous pemphigoid, paraneoplastic pemphigus and pemphigus vulgaris and in older women lichen sclerosus and potential reactivation of the zoster virus [4]. These autoimmune skin disorders result from either the production of antibodies that react with the host tissue or to autoreactivity of the immune effector T cells [48]. Autoimmunity to hemidesmosomal proteins present in the basement membrane of stratified squamous epithelia results in bullous pemphigoid, and paraneoplastic pemphigus results from autoimmunity to multiple desmosomal antigens [49]. Dermatomyositis is an autoimmune systemic disorder [48] which manifests with cutaneous eruptions and inflammatory myopathy [48, 50]. In the elderly dermatomyositis is associated with underlying malignancies and commonly associated with malignancies from the colon, breast, lung and uterus [50]. Lichens sclerosus has an increased risk of squamous cell carcinoma in the elderly [48].

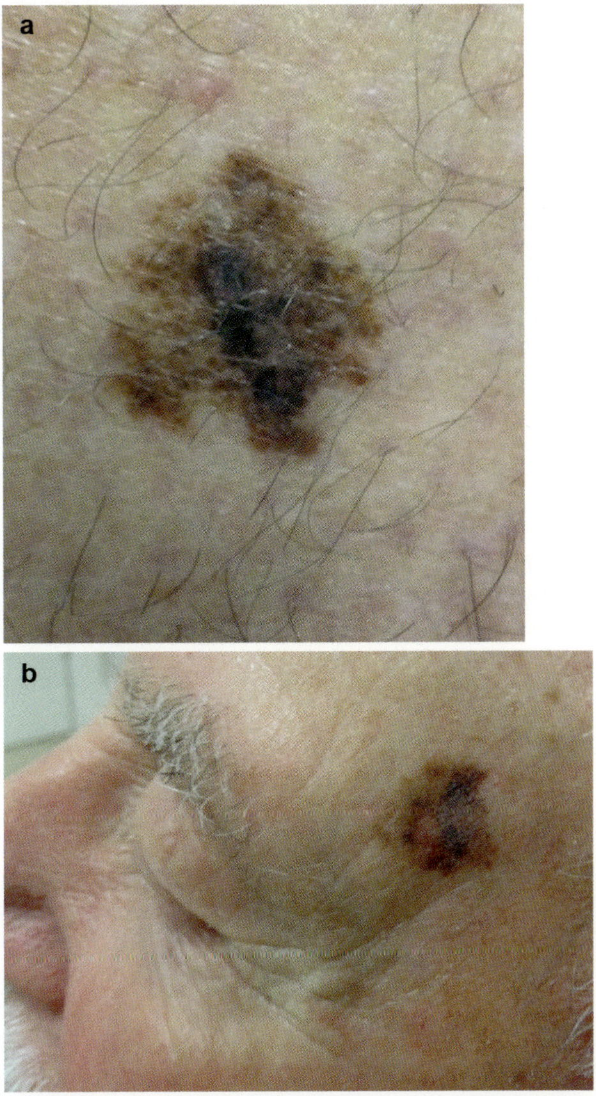

Fig. 8.5 (**a**) Lentigo maligna melanoma (Reproduced with permission from Dr Derrick Davies, Orange Dermatology). (**b**) Lentigo maligna – enlarging macule with irregular borders (Reproduced with permission from Dr Derrick Davies, Orange Dermatology)

Box 8.2. Key Points. Common Skin Disorders in the Elderly [4, 7]

- There is loss of resistance to environmental and mechanical trauma with intrinsic ageing.
- Ultraviolet radiation (UV) from the sun is the main environmental cause for premature ageing of the skin (photoageing) [19, 20].
- Basal cell carcinoma and squamous cell carcinoma are common malignant skin conditions.
- Bowen's disease is squamous cell carcinoma in situ with a high frequency of p53 mutation [30].

- Melanocytic malignancies are characterised by mutations in several kinases such as BRAF, NRAS and KIT [40].
- The common clinicopathological subtypes of melanoma are (i) lentigo maligna (Hutchinson's freckles), (ii) lentigo maligna melanoma, (iii) nodular melanoma and (iv) superficial spreading melanoma.
- Skin diseases in the elderly are more often than not the effects of sun damage or vascular disease.
- The immune response is affected by the decrease in the Langerhans cells with ageing. Immunosenescence leads to similar levels of occurrence of autoimmune skin disorders such as bullous pemphigoid, paraneoplastic pemphigus and pemphigus vulgaris [4, 47].

8.3 Pruritus in the Elderly

Introduction
Itching or pruritus is a desire to scratch and is often considered to be synonymous though the term pruritus is generally taken as itching without any apparent diagnostic skin lesions. It is common among the elderly over the age of 65 and its incidence increases with advancing age.

Pathophysiology
In the last few years, our understanding of the basic effects of pruritus has changed in the light of modern concepts of physiology. It is necessary for those treating pruritus to have a clear understanding of the pathophysiology of pruritus [51]. It is now known that the epidermis especially the keratinocytes with associated ramifications of fine intra-epidermal C-neuron filaments constitutes the itch receptor [52]. The C-neuroterminals and the spatially related dermal mast cells play an important role in the pathophysiology of pruritus. The tissue redundant cells such as the keratinocytes, mast cells and cells of inflammatory infiltrate in the skin interact with the sensory nerve endings [53]. This interaction results in the release of multiple pruritogenic mediators. Several mediators and receptors have been identified including histamine [41], serotonin, acetylcholine [54], prostaglandins [55], neuropeptides such as substance P and cytokines such as interleukin-3 [56], among others.

Histamine [56] and other mast cell mediators such the tumour necrosis factor-alpha and cytokines are important mediators of itching in inflammatory skin diseases and stimulate the sensation of itch. Mast cell tryptase may be an important mediator in itch by activation of proteinase-activated receptor 2 in the sensory nerves [57]. The neuropeptide, substance P that is released as a result, causes pruritus and also evokes further mast cell activity. The opioids have both peripheral and central itch-producing activity [57]. Pruritus may be the result of an imbalance between opioid action on central u and k receptors, one increasing and the other decreasing the itch [58].

The mediators activate the cutaneous network of free nerve endings in the dermal-epidermal junction leading to itch [59]. The sensation of itch is carried by unmyelinated C-fibres and myelinated Ad nerve fibres [60] to the ipsilateral dorsal root ganglion to the dorsal horn of the spinal cord across the anterior commissure to the spinothalamic tract terminating in various brain centres including the cortex and thalamus [61–63]. The itch signals are conveyed by a specific subclass of lamina-1 spinothalamic tract neurons to an 'itch matrix' in the brain with a left hemispheric dominance. The substantia gelatinosa in the posterior horn of the grey matter of the spinal cord acts as a 'gated mechanism' to regulate the 'itch traffic'. Scratching activates the inhibitory neuronal circuits in the substantia nigra [58].

The elderly are potentially vulnerable to pruritic disorders and this is largely due to physiological changes in the skin associated with ageing. The immune response in the elderly is defective [9], and there are impaired function of the skin as a barrier [9], loss of hydration, loss of collagen and impaired circulation to the skin [64] and altered pigmentation [65].

Multiple Choice Questions

1. The following are true relating to age-related changes in the skin, EXCEPT:
   A. About 80 % of facial ageing is due to sun exposure.
   B. There is an increased number of melanosomes synthesised resulting in increased pigmentation.
   C. There is a reduction of immune cells in the skin compromising immune response.
   D. There is impaired circulation to the skin with ageing.
2. The following are true of primary dermatological disorders, EXCEPT:
   A. Actinic keratosis is usually seen after the age of 65 years.
   B. Most Caucasians are affected sooner or later by seborrhoeic keratosis.
   C. Basal cell carcinoma metastasises early.
   D. In Bowen's disease, there is a 3–5 % risk of developing invasive squamous cell carcinoma.
3. The following are true of pruritus in the elderly, EXCEPT:
   A. The keratinocytes with associated ramifications of fine C-neuron filaments constitute the 'itch receptor'.
   B. Physiological changes in the skin due to ageing make the elderly potentially vulnerable to pruritic disorders.
   C. The sensation of itch is carried by myelinated C-fibres and unmyelinated Ad nerve fibres.
   D. Histamine and other mast cell mediators are important mediators of itching in inflammatory skin disorders.

Answers to MCQs

1=B; 2=C; 3=C.

References

1. Farage MA, Miller KW, Elsner P, Maibach HI. Characteristics of aging skin. Adv Wound Care (New Rochelle). 2013;2(1):5–10 (abstract).
2. Lifshitz OH. The ageing skin. Cleveland Clinic for continuing education. Accessed 29 Oct 2013.
3. Montagna W, Carlisle K. Structural changes in aging skin. Br J Dermatol. 1990;122 Suppl 35:61–70.
4. Farage MA, Miller KW, Berardesca E, Maibach HI. Clinical implications of aging skin: cutaneous disorders in the elderly. Am J Clin Dermatol. 2009;10(2):73–86 (abstract).
5. Kligman AM, Balin AK. Aging of human skin. In: Balin AK, Kligman AM, editors. Aging of the skin. New York: Ravin Press; 1989.
6. Ullrich SE. Mechanisms underlying ultraviolet induced immune suppression. Mutat Res. 2005;571(1–2):185–205.
7. Yaar M, Gilchrest BL. Skin aging. Postulated mechanisms and consequent changes in structure and function. Clin Geriatr Med. 2001;17:617.
8. Uitto J. Understanding premature skin ageing. N Engl J Med. 1997;337(20):1463–5.
9. Berger TG, Steinhoff M. Pruritus in elderly patients-eruptions of senescence. Semin Cutan Med Surg. 2011;30:113–7.
10. Yalcin B, Tamer E, Toy GG, Oztaz P, Hayran M, Alli N. The prevalence of skin diseases in the elderly: analysis of 4099 geriatric patients. Int J Dermatol. 2006;45(6):672–6 (abstract).
11. Cancer Council Australia. http://www.cancer.org.au/aboutcancer/cancer types/melanoma.htm
12. Jemal A, Siegel R, Xu J, Ward E. Cancer statistics 2010. CA Cancer J Clin. 2010;60: 277–300.
13. Lasithiotakis KG, Petrakis IE, Garbe C. Cutaneous melanoma in the elderly: epidemiology prognosis and treatment. Melanoma Res. 2010;20:163–70.
14. Swetter SM, Boldrick JC, Jung SY, Egbert BM, Harvell JD. Increasing incidence of lentigo maligna melanoma subtypes: northern California and national trends 1990-2000. J Invest Dermatol. 2005;125:685–91.
15. Smith DR, Leggat P. Prevalence of skin disease among the elderly in different clinical environments. Australas J Ageing. 2005;24(2):71–6.
16. El- Ghassassi F, Baan R, Straif K, Grosse Y, Secretan B, Bouvard V, et al. A review of human carcinogens-part D: radiation. Lancet Oncol. 2009;10:751–2.
17. Omar MH. Common skin disorders in the elderly. SA Fam Pract. 2006;48:29–34.
18. Webster GF. Common skin disorders in the elderly. Clin Cornerstone. 2001;4:39–44.
19. Fisher GJ, Voorhees JJ. Molecular mechanisms of photoaging and its prevention by retinoic acid: ultraviolet irradiation induces MAP kinase signal transduction cascades that induce Ap-1 –regulated matrix metalloproteinases that degrade human skin in vivo. J Investig Dermatol Symp Proc. 1998;3(1):61–8 (abstract).
20. Fisher GJY. The pathophysiology of photoaging of the skin. Cutis. 2005;75(2 Suppl):5–8 (abstract).
21. Brenneisen P, Sies H, Scharffetter-Kochanek K. Ultraviolet-B irradiation and matrix metalloproteinases: from induction via signalling to initial events. Ann N Y Acad Sci. 2002;973:31–43 (abstract).
22. Rijken F, Kiekens RCM, van den Worm E, Lee PL, van Weeldeen H, et al. Pathophysiology of photoaging of human skin: focus on neutrophils. Photochem Photobiol Sci. 2006;3:184–9 (abstract).
23. Webster GF. Common skin disorders in the elderly. Am Fam Physician. 1993;47(6):1445–50.
24. Scheinfeld NS. Skin disorders in older adults: age-related pigmentary changes. Consultant http://www.consultant360.com/content/skin-disorders-older-adults-agr-related-pigment. Retrieved 31 Mar 2015.
25. Balakrishnan KP, Narayanaswamy U. Botanicals as sun creams: their role in the prevention of photoaging and skin cancer. Int J Res Cosmetic Sc. 2011;1(1):1–12.

26. Luong KVQ, Nguyen LTH. The roles of vitamin D in seborrhoeic keratosis: possible genetic a cellular signalling mechanisms. Int J Cosmetic Science. 2013. doi:10.1111/ics.12080. (abstract).
27. Shumack SP. Non-surgical treatments for skin cancer. Aust Prescr. 2011;34:6–7.
28. Graham JH. Selected precancerous skin and mucocutaneous lesions. In: Neoplasm of skin and malignant melanoma. Chicago: Book Medical Publishers; 1976. p. 69.
29. Lebowhl M. Actinic keratosis epidemiology and progression to squamous cell carcinoma. Br J Dermatol. 2003;149(Suppl 66):31–3.
30. Tomas D. Apoptosis, UV-radiation, precancerous and skin tumours. Acta Med Croatica. 2009;63 Suppl 2:53–8 (abstract).
31. Erb P, Ji J, Kump E, Mielgo A, Wernli M. Apoptosis and pathogenesis of melanoma and non-melanoma skin cancer. Adv Exp Med Biol. 2008;624:283–95 (abstract).
32. Massari LP, Kastelan M, Gruber F. Epidermal malignant tumours: pathogenesis influence of UV light and apoptosis. Coll Antropol. 2007;31 Suppl 1:83–5 (abstract).
33. Rass K, Reichrath J. UV damage and DNA repair in malignant melanoma and nonmelanoma skin cancer. Adv Exp Med Biol. 2008;624:162–78 (abstract).
34. Erb P, Ji J, Wernli M, Kump E, Glaser A, Buchner SA. Role of apoptosis in basal cell and squamous cell carcinoma. Immunol Lett. 2005;100(1):68–72 (abstract).
35. De Gruijl FR, van Kranen HJ, Mullenders LH. UV-induced DNA damage, repair, mutations and oncogenic pathways in skin cancer. J Photochem Photobiol B. 2001;63(1–3):19–27 (abstract).
36. Uminski A. New systemic treatment options for advanced basal cell carcinoma. Cancer Forum. 2012;36(3):138–141.
37. Lee MM, Wick MM. Bowen's disease. CA Cancer J Clin. 1990;40(4):237–42.
38. Neubert T, Lehmann P. Bowen's disease-a review of newer treatment. Ther Clin Risk Manag. 2008;4(5):1085–95.
39. Lin K, Baritaki S, Militello L, Malaponte G, Bevelacqua Y, Bonavide B. The role of B-RAF Mutations in Melanoma and the Induction of EMT via Dysregulation of the NF-kB/Snail/RKIP/PTEN Circuit. Genes Cancer. 2010;1(5):409–20.
40. Goldringer SM, Murer C, Sieger P, Dummer R. Targeted therapy in melanoma-the role of BRAF, RAS and KIT mutations. Eur J Cancer Suppl. 2013;11(2).92–6.
41. Saldanha G, Potter L, Dafomo P, Pringle JH. Cutaneous melanoma subtypes show different BRAF and NRAS mutation frequencies. Clin Cancer Res. 2006;12(15):4499–505 (abstract).
42. Flaherty KT, Puzanov I, Kim KB, Ribas A, McArthur GA, Sosman JA, et al. Inhibition of mutated activated BRAF in metastatic melanoma. N Engl J Med. 2010;363:809–19.
43. Menzies AM, Haydu LE, Visintin L, Carlino MS, Howele JR, Thompson JF, et al. Distinguishing clinicopathological features of patients with V6000E and V600K BRAF-mutant metastatic melanoma. Clin Cancer Res. 2012;18:3242–9.
44. Kelleher FC, McArthur GA. Targeting NRAS in melanoma. Cancer J. 2012;18(2):132–6 (abstract).
45. Macdonald JB, Dueck AC, Gray RJ, Wasif N, Swanson DL, Sekulic A, et al. Malignant melanoma in the elderly: different regional disease and poorer diagnosis. J Cancer. 2011;2:538–43.
46. Beacham BE. Common dermatoses in the elderly. Am Fam Physician. 1993;47(6):1445–50 (abstract).
47. Yaar M, Gilchrest BA. Skin aging: postulated mechanisms and consequent changes in structure and function. Clin Geriatr Med. 2001;17:617.
48. Loo WJ, Burrows NP. Management of autoimmune skin disorders in the elderly. Drugs Aging. 2004;21(12):767–77 (abstract).
49. Mutasim DF. Autoimmune bullous dermatoses in the elderly: an update on pathophysiology diagnosis and management. Drugs Aging. 2010;27(1):1–19 (abstract).
50. Scheinfeld NS. Skin disorders in older adults: papulosquamous and bullous diseases, Part 2. Consultant. 2011; 168. http://www.consultant360.com/content/skin-disorderes-older-adults-papulosquamous-a. Retrieved 28 Mar 2015.

51. Greaves MW. Recent trends in pathophysiology and current management of itch. Ann Acad Med Singapore. 2007;31:788–92.
52. Inoue K, Koizumi S, Fuzuwara S, Denda S, Inoue K, Denda M, et al. Functional vanilloid receptors in cultured normal human epidermal keratinocytes. Biochem Biophys Res Commun. 2002;291:128–9.
53. Stander S, Raap U, Weisshaar E, Schmelz M, Mettang T, Handwerker H, et al. Pathogenesis of pruritus. J Dtsch Dermatol Ges. 2011;9(6):456–63 (abstract).
54. Rukweid R, Lischetzki G, McGlove F, Heyer G, Schmelz M. Mast cell mediators other than histamine induce pruritus in atopic dermatitis patients. A dermal microdialysis study. Br J Dermatol. 2000;42:1114–20.
55. Greaves MW, McDonald-Gibson W. Itch: role of prostaglandins. Br Med J. 1973;3:608–9.
56. Raap U, Sttander S, Metz M. Pathophysiology of itch and new treatments. Curr Opin Allergy Clin Immunol. 2011;11(5):420–7 (abstract).
57. Yosipovitch G, Fleischer A. Itch associated with skin disease: advances in pathophysiology and emerging therapies. Am J Dermatopathol. 2003;4(19):617–22.
58. Greaves MW, Wall PB. Pathophysiology of itching. Lancet. 1996;348:938–40.
59. Burns DA. Itching-physiology, causes, management. Curr Paediatr. 1991;1(3):142–4.
60. Potenzier C, Undem BJ. Basic mechanisms of itch. Clin Exp Allergy. 2012;42(1):8–9 (abstract).
61. Stander S, Setinhoff M, Schmeltz M. Neurophysiology of pruritus. Arch Dermatol. 2003; 139:1463–6.
62. Shanley K. Pathophysiology of pruritus. Vet Clin North Am Small Anim Pract. 1988;18: 971–81.
63. Bernhard J. Itch & pruritus. What are they, how should itches be classified. Dermatol Ther. 2005;18:288–91.
64. Reich A, Stander S, Szepietowski J. Pruritus on the elderly. Clin Dermatol. 2011;29:15–23.
65. Waller JM, Monbach HI. Age and skin structure and function: a quantitative approach II Protein, glycosaminoglycan, water and lipid content and structure. Skin Res Technol. 2006; 12(3):145–54.

9 Endocrine Disorders

9.1 Anatomical and Physiological Changes with Ageing: Endocrine System

9.1.1 Pancreatic Endocrine Function

The islets of Langerhans contain four major types of secretory cells; cells A and B secrete glucagons and insulin, respectively and have major actions on glucose metabolism. D cells and PP or F cells secrete somastatin and pancreatic polypeptide which exert modulating actions on insulin and glucagon secretion. With ageing, few morphological changes have been reported in the endocrine pancreas which include a degree of atrophy, fatty infiltration and fibrosis [1] and the presence of amyloid material and lipofuscin granules.

Several hormones participate in the regulation of carbohydrate metabolism. Apart from those mentioned, other hormones that affect carbohydrate metabolism are the thyroid hormone, glucocorticoids, growth hormone and epinephrine. In the elderly one of the hallmarks of ageing process is the reduction in the whole body carbohydrate metabolism [2]. There is a progressive impairment of glucose tolerance with advancing age [3–5], independent of obesity and sex [6]. This progressive decline in glucose tolerance occurs from the third decade through to the ninth decade [2]. Some workers found a rise of approximately 1 mg/dl per decade in the fasting glucose levels [7]. Others have found no significant change with age on fasting levels in men although there is a small significant positive correlation in women [8]. The balance between insulin secretion and tissue sensitivity to insulin constitutes a major component of glucose homeostasis. The age-related decline in glucose handling seems to result from insulin resistance rather than an impairment of insulin secretion [9]. Only 2–3 % of the glucose uptake is by the adipose tissue which is relatively inert, and the primary uptake is by the muscle [10]. Possible explanations for this age-related insulin resistance include various factors such as fat mass, fat distribution, dietary composition, physical activity and the capacity of glucose uptake [9, 11].

N. Nagaratnam et al., *Diseases in the Elderly: Age-Related Changes and Pathophysiology*, DOI 10.1007/978-3-319-25787-7_9

9.1.2 Thyroid Gland

A number of morphological and functional changes are associated with ageing in the thyroid. With ageing, the thyroid gland undergoes changes in its structure. The number and size of the follicles and the colloid content decrease. Furthermore it becomes nodular with age. There is lymphocytic infiltration and fibrosis of the connective tissue on histological examination.

With normal ageing, the thyroid metabolism and production change and secretion of T3 and TSH is reduced [12]. Although T4 production declines with advancing age [13], the concentration of total and free T4 remains unchanged [14] and this is not a primary thyroid failure but rather a physiological compensation for decreased tissue requirement of the hormone. Furthermore the degradation of T4 is also reduced in the elderly [13] as the clearance of T4 by the liver decreases with age and is offset by the decline in its secretion by the thyroid so that the serum levels remain relatively constant. Serum T3 concentration demonstrates an age-dependent decline [14] because of both reduced secretion and peripheral conversion from T4. However, serum levels of thyroid hormones change very little with age. TSH changes during healthy ageing are equivocal, normal [15, 16] or may be slightly decreased [14].

There is an elevation of thyroid antibodies with ageing, but this increase appears to be related to age-associated diseases rather than to ageing per se [16]. Studies have shown that there is decrease in lean body mass with normal ageing meaning that the body needs less thyroid hormone balancing it with thyroid's reduced output [17]. Many believe that hypothyroidism is a normal part of ageing because of the many age-related physiological changes that occur in the normal thyroid gland, which contribute to an increased risk of hypothyroidism seen with ageing [17]. The increased prevalence of subclinical hypothyroidism is due to an age-dependent increase in anti-thyroglobulin and antithyroperoxidase antibodies [18, 19]. In the elderly thyroid function tests may be influenced by illness, malnutrition and medication [12].

9.1.3 Parathyroid Gland

Several studies have shown an increase in the level of parathyroid hormone (PTH) with age and is due to diminishing calcium absorption and serum 25-hydroxy vitamin D levels and diminishing renal function [20]. This increase in response has been implicated in osteoporosis and bone loss [21]. In contrast to PTH, calcitonin levels seem to decrease with age [22].

Box 9.1. Key Points. Anatomical and Physiological Changes

Pancreatic

- Few morphological changes – a degree of atrophy, fatty infiltration and fibrous and presence of amyloid and lipofuscin granules [1].
- There is a whole body reduction in carbohydrate metabolism with ageing [2].

- There is progressive impairment of glucose tolerance with advancing age [2].
- The age-related decline in glucose handling results from insulin resistance rather than impairment of insulin secretion [9].
- Insulin resistance – various factors include fat mass, fat distribution, dietary component, physical activity and capacity for glucose uptake [9, 11].

Thyroid

- Number and size of follicles and colloid content decrease.
- Becomes nodular with age with lymphocytic infiltration and fibrous [72].
- The metabolism and production change with secretion of T3, and TSH is reduced [14].
- T4 production declines with advancing age, but concentration of total and free T4 remains unchanged [72].
- Degradation of T4 is also reduced.
- There is an elevation of thyroid antibodies with age [12].
- In the elderly thyroid function tests may be influenced by illness, malnutrition and medication [20].

Parathyroid

- Increase in the level of PTH with age [22].
- Calcitonin levels seem to decrease with age.

9.2 Diabetes Mellitus in the Elderly

Introduction

Diabetes mellitus is a metabolic disorder characterised by chronic hyperglycaemia and disorders of carbohydrate, protein and fat metabolism as a result of either insulin deficiency or to insensitivity of its receptors or combination of both. Worldwide, diabetes mellitus (DM) affects 10–20 % of the elderly in the age groups 65–74 years and about 40 % of the elderly over the age of 80 years [23]. In the industrialised countries, the greatest increases in the total number of cases of diabetes are among the elderly people [24]. This is because of not only the increase in the ageing population, but there is an absolute increase in the prevalence of DM in the elderly people [25]. About 13 % of adults over the age of 70 years have DM, and 11 % of adults between 65 and 74 years remain undiagnosed [26]. About 800,000 Australians have diabetes mellitus [27]. The epidemiology of diabetes in the elderly is not well understood. A Canadian study found DM to be common among elderly people, but the incidence declines among the very old [28]. The prevalence of diagnosed cases of type 2 DM rises with age from 1.4 % between the ages of 25–41 years to over 10 % over the age of 65 years [29]. With the adoption of the new diagnostic criteria and people living longer, the prevalence of DM is likely to increase.

Pathophysiology

The hormones that regulate glucose metabolism include insulin, amylin derived from the beta cells and glucagon from the alpha cells of the pancreas. The other hormones include Glucagon-like peptide-1 (GLP-1), glucose-dependent insulinotropic peptide (GIP) derived from the L cell of the intestine and cortisol, growth hormone and epinephrine [30]. Insulin reduces blood sugar by allowing the glucose to enter muscle and fat cells and controls the conversion of glucose into glycogen (glycogenesis) for storage in the liver and muscle cells. It is released into the blood in response to the rising blood sugar levels after a meal. High glucose levels result when insulin deficiency leads to uninhibited gluconeogenesis and prevent the use and storage of circulating glucose. Insufficient insulin, defective insulin, insulin resistance or insensitivity will impede the glucose being absorbed by those cells that require it nor will it be stored properly in the muscle and liver resulting in high levels of blood glucose.

With ageing, independent of obesity and sex, there is a progressive impairment of glucose tolerance in the nondiabetic individual with advancing years [31], and this is more related to insulin resistance rather than to decreased insulin secretion although the latter is controversial [32]. The age-related insulin resistance has been attributed to a number of factors such as dietary and physical activity and decreased capacity of glucose uptake system, among others [32, 33]. Type 1 diabetes may be due to an autoimmune destruction of the beta cells or idiopathic. Immune-mediated diabetes most commonly occurs in childhood and adolescents, but it can occur at any age even in the 8 and 9th decades of life [34].

Type 2. Multiple genes and environmental factors play an important role in type 2 diabetes and contribute to the development of insulin resistance in the liver and muscle as well as to beta-cell failure [35, 36]. Insulin resistance is considered to play an essential role in the pathogenesis of the disease [37]. Environmental risk factors include those that are modifiable such as obesity and physical activity and non-modifiable such as genetic factors, older age, race/ethnicity and positive family history. The risk of developing this form of diabetes increases with age, obesity and lack of physical activity [34]. Most of these patients are obese. In the obese elderly patient, there is no impairment in glucose-induced insulin release as evidenced by a normal second phase insulin secretion [38] in contrast to that seen in lean elderly diabetic [38]. The primary impairment in the obese elderly patient is insulin resistance, and in the lean elderly patient, it is impaired glucose-induced insulin release [39]. Autoimmune changes normally attributed to younger type 1 diabetes is seen in the lean elderly diabetic patients. Insulin deficiency and islet cell antibodies are increasingly seen in the lean elderly diabetics [38, 40]. It important to know that both type 1 (insulin dependent) and type 2 (non-insulin dependent) diabetes occur in the elderly [39]. Diabetes individuals with insulin resistance usually have a relative (rather than an absolute) insulin deficiency.

Diabetic ketoacidosis (DKA) and hyperosmolar hyperglycaemic state (HHS) are two most serious acute decompensations of diabetes mellitus due to various degrees of insulin deficiency and elevations of counterregulatory hormones. DKA is characterised by hyperglycaemia and ketoacidosis [41], and precipitating cause is either infection or insulin omission. HHS is characterised by hyperglycaemia, osmotic diuresis, dehydration [42] and little or no ketosis, and precipitating causes are undiagnosed diabetes, infection and substance abuse. The absolute or relative deficiency in insulin levels leads to altered metabolism of protein, carbohydrate and fat and varying degrees of osmotic diuresis, dehydration, ketosis and acidosis. In DKA the lack of insulin combined with increased catecholamines results in accelerated lipolysis and thus production of excess fatty acids giving rise to beta-oxidation and ketogenesis [43]. In HHS there is an osmotic shift of water into the intravascular compartment resulting from the hyperosmolarity caused by the hyperglycaemia resulting in severe dehydration.

Long-standing diabetes is associated with damage and dysfunction of large (macrovascular) and small (microvascular) blood vessels resulting in damage to the various organs. Several hypotheses have been advanced, and the postulated mechanisms are hyperglycaemia, advanced glycosylation products and activation of cytokines. Hyperglycaemia leads to increased levels of intracellular glucose which may cause variety of metabolic disturbances inside the vascular cells. The inimical effects are identified through multiple pathways: (i) The extra glucose shunted into the *polyol pathway* is converted into sorbitol and fructose through the enzyme aldose reductase [44]. Accumulations of sorbitol and fructose leads to reduced nerve myoinositol, decreased membrane N+/K+ -ATPase activity and impaired axonal transport eventually to structural breakdown in the tissues involved [44]. (ii) High levels of intracellular glucose activate the enzyme protein kinase C which alters cell function [45]. *Protein kinase C pathway* is believed to play an important role in the development of diabetic complications in that it has been shown that an inhibitor of protein kinase C is able to correct renal and retinal dysfunction in experimental diabetic animals [46]. Protein kinase inhibition increases expression of transforming growth factor-beta (TGF-beta) which is a potent prosclerotic cytokine [47]. (iii) In diabetes the advanced glycation end products (AGEs) are considerably increased as compared with the normal brought about by hyperglycaemia which activates the *nonenzymatic glycation reaction* and thereby disturbs the biological function of various proteins and alters interactions of matrix and other cells and with the AGE receptors [48]. (iv) High glucose levels activate the *hexosamine pathway* which through a product of the pathway, N-acetyl-glucosamine causes a permanent modification of proteins and transcription factors [48]. Oxidative stress is increased in diabetes [44, 49] and it is reported that oxidative stress may injure endothelial function that may be related to diabetic complications [50]. In the nerve cell oxidative stress increases vasoconstriction causing ischaemia furthering nerve cell injury and death [44].

Pathological changes in the microvasculature with capillary basement thickening and endothelial hypoperfusion result in diminished oxygen and hypoxia. Microvascular dysfunction occurs early in diabetes and parallels the progression of neural dysfunction [51]. According to the autoimmune theory, there are immunological alterations of the endocapillary cells. Laminins have the ability to self-polymerise and are vital for the formation of basement membranes [52]. Laminin theory postulates that there is a lack of normal expression of the laminin beta 2 gene and may contribute to diabetic neuropathy.

Many diabetics develop some form of nerve damage known as diabetic neuropathy. The prevalence of diabetic neuropathy varies from 28.5 % [53] up to 50 % [54] to 60 % [55]. In the hyperglycaemic state, there is an increase in the enzymes aldose reductase and sorbitol dehydrogenase which converts the intracellular glucose to sorbitol and fructose [44]. Increase in sorbitol and fructose inhibits the synthesis of nerve cell myoinositol which is required for normal motor nerve conduction, and furthermore there is increase in oxidative stress in the nerve cell resulting in nerve cell injury and death due to vasoconstriction and ischaemia [44]. More recently there has been considerable interest in the vascular and neurotrophic hypotheses, oxidative stress and possible role of autoimmunity which has led to new approaches for therapeutic intervention [56].

Box 9.2. Key Points. Diabetes Mellitus

- The hormones that regulate glucose metabolism include insulin, amylin and glucagon. Other hormones include GLP-1, glucose-dependent insulinotropic peptide (GIP) cortisol, growth hormone and epinephrine [3].
- Lowered glucose levels result in both reduced release of insulin and increased conversion of glycogen to glucose.
- With ageing, independent of obesity and sex, there is a progressive impairment of glucose tolerance in a nondiabetic individual, and this is more related to insulin resistance rather than to decreased insulin secretion [31].
- Immune-mediated diabetes can occur at any age even in the 8 and 9th decades of life [34].
- Multiple genes and environmental factors play an important role in type 2 diabetes [35, 36].
- Long-standing diabetes is associated with damage and dysfunction of large (macrovascular) and small (microvascular) blood vessels resulting in damage to various organs.
- Hyperglycaemia leads to increase levels of intracellular glucose which may cause results of metabolic disturbances inside vascular cells.
- Microvascular dysfunction occurs early in diabetes and parallels progression of neural dysfunction [56].

9.3 Thyroid Disease in the Older Patient

Introduction

The thyroid gland gives rise to either excessive or decreased secretion of thyroxine or is non-functional and do not cause any disturbance of the thyroid hormone output. A prevalence of 14 % in older Australian population had been reported based on abnormal TSH levels, history of thyroid disease or current use of thyroxine [57]. Thyroid disease is relatively common in older Australian women and may be underdiagnosed. A 5.6 % prevalence of abnormal TSH was reported in women and increased with age [57]. Several epidemiological studies have revealed a higher prevalence of thyroid disease in women than in men particularly hypothyroidism and an age-related increase in hypothyroidism from less than 15 % in women aged 50 years to double the number in women 75 years or older [58, 59]. There is an increased prevalence of subclinical hypothyroidism with increasing age [60, 61] especially in females over the age of 60 years [58]. Thyroid abnormalities are relatively common in the general population but has important clinical implications in the elderly because of the co-existing co-morbidities and increased risk of heart disease and hypercholesterolaemia [62, 63]. In the elderly the presence of clinically significant disease in geriatric institutions is between 2 and 5 %[64].

Physiology

The thyroid gland is composed of two lateral lobes and an isthmus and weighs about 15–20 g. A number of ingredients are necessary for thyroid hormone synthesis, namely, iodide, thyroid peroxidase, thyroglobulin and hydrogen peroxide [65, 66]. Thyroid-stimulating hormone (TSH) is the major regulator of thyroid gland growth and function. T4 and T3 regulate metabolism and protein synthesis and increase oxygen consumption and are important for growth and development [67]. All the reactions necessary for intrathyroidal formation of T4 and T3 are under the control of the TSH. The control of TSH synthesis is complex. The hypothalamic thyrotropin-releasing hormone (TRH) is transported to the thyrotropin of the anterior pituitary gland which causes the release of TSH [68]. Inhibition of TRH and TSH results from a negative feedback exerted by the circulating T3 [68].

The follicular cells of the thyroid in response to TSH release thyroglobulin [67]. Iodine is required for the formation of the thyroid hormones and is derived from ingested food and water. Iodine is converted to inorganic iodide after absorption and then concentrated in the thyroid gland. The inorganic iodide is converted to organic iodine by the enzyme thyroid peroxidase and in the presence of hydrogen peroxide which is an important substrate for thyroid peroxidase [69]. It incorporates the organic iodine into tyrosine molecules in thyroglobulin, a glycoprotein in the colloid within the thyroid follicle. Hydrogen peroxide generation is a rate-limiting step in thyroid hormone synthesis [69]. The iodination of the tyrosines occurs at either one (monoiodotyrosine) or two (diiodotyrosine) sites. Both are then coupled by an enzymatic reaction into one molecule of each which would yield T3 and two molecules of diiodotyrosine would yield T4. The reaction producing T4 is the major one for the T4/T3 ratio and in the thyroglobulin it is about 13:1. About 80 % of the total plasma T3 production is extrathyroidically converted to T3, only 20 % is secreted by the thyroid gland [70]. Most T3 is produced by deiodination of T4 in the peripheral tissues. After coupling the nascent thyroid hormones remain bound to thyroglobulin in the colloid follicles. The unbound active fraction is only 0.04 % of total T4 and 0.4 % of the total T3 [68]. The major portion (80 %) of the T4 is transported by the thyroid binding protein (TBG). T4 is also bound by transthyretin (TTR) and to a lesser extent by the thyroxine binding pre-albumin and albumin [68]. T3 is largely bound to TBG and to a minor degree to albumin.

Pathophysiology
Thyroid dysfunction is common in the elderly and takes the form of clinical and subclinical hypo- and hyperthyroidism, nodules and thyroid cancer [71]. With normal ageing, the thyroid gland undergoes changes, and consequently T4 production declines with advancing age [72], but the serum T4 (total and free) concentration remains unchanged [73] for this is a physiological compensation for decreased tissue requirement of the hormone. Most of the T4 in the blood is attached to a protein, the thyroid binding globulin. Less than 1 % is free, and free thyroxine affects thyroid function in the body but not the bound. Most of the T3 in is attached to the thyroid-binding globulin, and less than 1 % is free. Serum levels of the thyroid hormones change very little with age. Many elderly patients have abnormal TSH levels without changes in serum thyroid hormone levels [74], conditions termed subclinical hypothyroidism and subclinical hyperthyroidism [75]. In the elderly autoimmune thyroiditis is the most common cause of hypothyroidism [76]. The rate of aggressive forms of thyroid cancer is higher in older than in younger patients [76] and more aggressive in men than in women [77].

9.3.1 Hypothyroidism

Introduction
Hypothyroidism is defined as a group of signs and symptoms resulting from thyroid hormone deficiency. In the over 70 years, the TSH level of >4.5 U/L was found in 14 %[78]. The prevalence rises with age. Women are more commonly afflicted than men. In elderly females, the prevalence of subclinical and hypothyroidism varies in different population ranging between 1 and 17.5 %[79].

Pathophysiology
Hypothyroidism in many has a autoimmune basis (Hashimoto's disease) [73, 76, 80] and finally results in fibrosis, shrinkage and destruction of the thyroid acini. Hypothyroidism occurring as irreversible thyroid failure is due to idiopathic hypothyroidism, from autoimmune damage to the thyroid gland (Hashimoto's disease), surgical removal of the gland (Graves' disease or patients with multinodular goitre or thyroid cancer) [73, 80], irradiation, infrequently iodine-induced hypothyroidism and treatment with radio-iodine and antithyroid drugs. Medications such as amiodarone, lithium and cytokine blockers diminish secretion of thyroid hormones [81, 82]. Proton-pump inhibitors, antacids, oestrogens, phenobarbital and rifampicin can alter T4 absorption, metabolism of T4 and T3 and their transport in the serum [75]. Drugs such as dopamine, opiates and glucocorticoids decrease TSH levels [81, 83]. More than 95 % of cases are due to primary hypothyroidism and have been reported to be between 2 and 6 % in England and the United States [84]. Secondary hypothyroidism is due to pituitary and hypothalamic lesions.

Idiopathic hypothyroidism in adults is generally thought to be the result of undiagnosed Hashimoto's disease for in many antithyroid antibodies are detected in the serum. Hashimoto's disease is one of a number of interrelated conditions comprising autoimmune thyroid disease (AITD), others being Graves' disease and postpartum thyroiditis among others [85], and occurs in about 5–10 % of middle-aged and elderly women [85]. The hallmark of AITD is the presence of antibodies to thyroid peroxidase (TPO), thyroglobulin and thyroid-stimulating hormone receptor (TSH-R) [86]. Hashimoto's disease is an inflammatory disorder and includes goitrous and atrophic variants. Antibodies appear in the serum of patients with the disease: (i) anti-microsomal antibody and (ii) inhibitory antibodies which bind to the TSH receptors. The frequency of serum antibodies and evidence of Hashimoto's disease rises with advancing age especially in women and hence the likelihood of developing hypothyroidism after subtotal thyroidectomy as age increases. In the elderly with Hashimoto's disease, the goitre size is smaller, hypothyroidism is more common and Graves' disease less common [87].

9.3.1.1 Subclinical Hypothyroidism

Subclinical hypothyroidism is characterised by mild elevation of serum TSH level with normal free thyroid hormone concentrations. Its prevalence varies from 4 to 10 % in women especially in the elderly and about 3 % in men [88–90]. Post-thyroid ablation and Hashimoto's thyroiditis are common causes of subclinical hypothyroidism. The patients are usually asymptomatic with no clinical signs or symptoms [91].

9.3.2 Hyperthyroidism

Introduction

Hyperthyroidism is characterised by symptoms and signs resulting from an excess production of thyroid hormones by an overactive thyroid. The prevalence of hyperthyroidism changes very little with age. The causes of hyperthyroidism in the elderly are due to toxic nodular goitres, iodine-induced thyrotoxicosis, excessive thyroxine replacement therapy, Graves' disease and subacute thyroiditis and rarely a metastatic thyroid follicular carcinoma, a primary TSH-producing pituitary lesion or excessive TSH production caused by pituitary resistance to thyroid hormones. Large multinodular goitre (Plummer's disease) accounts for an increasing proportion of cases of hyperthyroidism in middle-aged and elder persons [92]. Graves' disease is the next most common disorder causing hyperthyroidism. Hyperthyroidism is usually due to diffuse hyperplasia and occurs most commonly in a condition known as Graves' disease. Sometimes the hyperplasia is confined to one or two nodules in an otherwise inactive multinodular goitre, or hyperplasia is confined to a single benign thyroid adenoma. In Graves' disease, an autoimmune disorder leads to the production of an antibody to the receptor in the thyroid follicular cells and acts like the TSH itself stimulating the thyroid cell. In the case of adenomas, the responsible area is autonomous, and it produces and secretes excessive thyroid hormone even though the serum TSH is suppressed. In subacute thyroiditis, the damaged follicles release T3 and T4 and thyroglobulin into the circulation.

9.3.2.1 Subclinical Hyperthyroidism

About 1–2 % of the elderly population has subclinical hyperthyroidism [90] manifesting as suppressed TSH levels with free T3 in the reference range and often with some nodular changes [93]. Those caused by large nodular goitre have a prevalence of up to 20 %[88]. The causes are similar to hyperthyroidism, and in addition thyroid suppression therapy is a frequent cause in the elderly [94, 95]. The adverse consequences of subclinical hyperthyroidism need intervention if reversible biochemical abnormalities due to overreplacement with thyroxine, transient subacute thyroiditis, and transient iodine-induced thyrotoxicosis have been excluded [93]. This state is associated with moderately increased frequency of atrial fibrillation in the elderly [89, 96] and increased likelihood of osteoporosis [89, 97]. In older patients age >65 years or in the presence of co-morbidities such as atrial fibrillation or osteoporosis, treatment is mandatory [98].

9.3.3 Cancer of Thyroid

Introduction
The incidence in the over 65 years age group appears to be increasing, and between 2.5 and 12 % of differentiated cancer of the thyroid occur in this group [99, 100].

Pathophysiology
Cancer of the thyroid takes four forms, papillary, follicular, anaplastic and medullary. Each has its own characteristics. About 90 % of thyroid cancers originate from the follicular cells, and some develop from the parafollicular cells or C cells. Papillary thyroid cancer (PTC) is the most common endocrine malignant cancer in older individuals and follicular(FTC) the next common and second least aggressive thyroid cancer [101]. The mutated Braf gene is related to advanced age and is an independent predicting factor of poor outcome [102]. Thyroid tumours are highly vascular, and vascular endothelial growth factor (VEGF) and associated VEGF-specific receptor tyrosine kinase have been incriminated in neovascularisation of the tumour [103]. Several signalling pathways are involved in contributing to cell cycle progression, proliferation, metabolism, tumorigenesis and angiogenesis [104] and the major ones being RAS/RAF/MEK/ERK pathway and the P13K/Akt/mTOR signalling pathways [103] (Table 9.1).

Box 9.3. Key Points. Thyroid Disease in Older Patients

- Thyroid dysfunction is common in elderly and takes the form of clinical and subclinical hypo- and hyperthyroidism, nodules and cancer [71].
- T4 production declines with advancing age, but serum T4 (total and free) concentration remains unchanged [72, 73].
- Many elderly have abnormal TSH levels without changes in serum thyroid hormone levels, conditions termed subclinical hypothyroidism and subclinical hyperthyroidism [74, 77].
- Thyroid tumours are highly vascular, and the vascular endothelial growth factor (VEGF) and associated VEGF-specific receptor tyrosine kinase have been incriminated in neovascularisation of the tumour [103].

Table 9.1 Cancers of the thyroid

Type	Incidence, age gender	Mode of growth	Pattern of spread	Prognosis	Treatment
1. Papillary	80–86 %, young	More malignant in women May be TSH dependent	Via lymphatics Regional nodes Metastasise late	Best 80–90 % 10-year survival 4.51 %	Thyroidectomy Hormone therapy Radio-I2 therapy
2. Follicular	9–10 %, elderly	Lateral aberrant thyroid rests – occult Metastases	Metastasise earlier Blood stream to lung/bone	More aggressive 80–90 % 10-year survival 4.50 %	Thyroidectomy Radio-I2 therapy
3. Anaplastic	1–2 %, elderly	Grow very rapidly Painful	Involve local tissues Bulkiness in neck	7 % at 5 years	Thyroidectomy Chemotherapy Radiation
4. Medullary	2–10 %	Secretes calcitonin Familial (autosomal amyloid dominant), sporadic	Lymphatic/ blood	Worse than 1 stream and 2 4.28%	Surgery

Information sources: Health Encyclopedia [105]; Medicine.net.com [106]; University of Virginia, Health System;@Survival Statistics [107]

9.4 Hyperparathyroidism

9.4.1 Primary Hyperparathyroidism

Introduction

The incidence of primary hyperparathyroidism (PHPT) is approximately 1 in 1000 people [108]. Majority of cases are made up of women; the female/male ratio is 3:1 [109]. In the general population, the prevalence was established to be 1 in 1000 [110]. Hyperparathyroidism is characterised by an increase in the level of parathyroid hormone in the blood. Hyperparathyroidism increases with age and is higher in postmenopausal women. Epidemiological studies performed in Rochester, Minnesota, showed an apparent decline in the incidence of PHPT from 75 to approximately 20/10,000 during the last decade [111]. This progressive decline is said to be suggestive of a change in the epidemiology of the disease [112].

Pathophysiology

Systemic calcium ($Ca2^{+}$) is regulated by the parathyroid hormone, and it is through the G protein-coupled receptor that the parathyroid chief cells sense changes in the circulating Ca(o)2+ [113, 114]. In primary hyperparathyroidism (PHTH), Ca(o)2+ is reset at a higher level [113], and this is likely due to increases in the parathyroid mass [113, 115]. Primary hyperparathyroidism is characterised by an increase in the parathyroid hormone secretion occurring as a result of an abnormality in one or more parathyroid glands. A single parathyroid adenoma accounts for 89 % of the cases [116] and double adenoma in 4 % and hyperplasia of all four glands in 6 % and cancer in 2 % [115, 117]. The fundamental biochemical parameter is persistent hypercalcaemia. Familial forms occur in about 1 % and in association with other endocrine tumours. Several mutations have been shown to play a role in the familial forms and include menin gene for MEN type 1, RET for MEN type 2a, and parafibromin gene for PHPT – jaw tumour and carcinoma [118]. In familial hypercalciuric hypercalcaemia, there is an inherited inactivation of the 120 kDa calcium sensing receptor [119]. Another sensing calcium protein is 550 kDa expressed on calcium binding sites on it external domain [119]. Its function is not only for calcium sensitive binding but for the uptake of steroid hormones such as 25-OH-vitamin D3 and retinol [119]. Patients with PHPT have an increased bone turnover and decreased BMD associated with low vitamin D states and high plasma 1,25(OH)(2) D [120]. Excess of PTH increases bone turnover leading to irreversible loss of cortical bone due to increased endocortical resorption [121] even in mild and asymptomatic cases [122].

9.4.2 Secondary Hyperparathyroidism

Introduction
In secondary hyperparathyroidism (SHPT), the abnormality in the parathyroid glands is induced by a sustained hypocalcaemic stimulus and usually associated with parathyroid hyperplasia [123].

Pathophysiology
It usually results from chronic renal failure [124] or occasionally malabsorption states, osteomalacia, dietary calcium deficiency and vitamin D deficiency [123]. The last two often co-exist in the elderly. Hyperphosphataemia due to impaired renal tubular absorption together with decreased absorption of calcium from inability to convert 25-OH cholecalciferol to 1,25-dihydroxycholecalciferol results in hypocalcaemia [123]. As a result, PTH secretion increases resulting in parathyroid chief cell hyperplasia [125]. More recently it has been demonstrated that fibroblast growth factor 23 (FGF-23) has an important role in the regulation of phosphate-vitamin D homeostasis [126]. Secondary hyperparathyroidism is said to result from the increase in FGF-23 concentration in chronic kidney disease [126]. SHPT occurs early in chronic kidney disease, and about 90 % of the patients with CKD develop secondary hyperparathyroidism by the time haemodialysis is begun [127]. Bisphosphonates such as alendronate and risedronate are widely used to treat osteoporosis and Paget's disease which commonly cause secondary hyperparathyroidism. Untreated SHPT due to chronic renal failure leads to the development of progressive bone disease, osteitis fibrosa cystica and soft tissue calcifications [123].

9.4.3 Tertiary Hyperparathyroidism

Introduction

Tertiary hyperparathyroidism occurs in patients with chronic renal failure and long-standing secondary hyperparathyroidism who develop relatively autonomous parathyroid function and hypercalcaemia. They occur in patients after renal transplantation and seen in about 30 % of kidney transplant patients [123], on dialysis and occasionally with long-standing osteomalacia.

9.5 Hypoparathyroidism

It is an endocrine disorder where the parathyroid glands do not produce enough hormone. Most common cause is thyroid surgery, and autoimmune hypoparathyroidism is the next common [128]. Other causes include low magnesium levels and metabolic alkalosis. The PTH is decreased, and serum phosphate levels are increased as there is decreased urinary excretion of phosphate by the kidneys. The 1.25(OH)2-vitamin levels are decreased.

Box 9.4. Key Points. Hyperparathyroidism(HPT)

- In HPT the Ca(O)2+ is reset at a higher level and is due to increase in the parathyroid mass [113].
- The fundamental biochemical parameter is persistent hypercalcaemia.
- Patients with PHPT have an increase bone turnover and decreased BMD associated with low vitamin D states and high plasma 1,25(OH)(2)D [120].
- Secondary HPT results from chronic renal failure or occasionally malabsorption states, osteomalacia and vitamin D deficiency [123, 124].
- Secondary HPT is said to result from increase in FGF-23 concentration in chronic kidney disease [126].

Tertiary HPT occurs in chronic renal failure and long-standing secondary HPT. They occur in patients after renal transplantation, in dialysis and occasionally long-standing osteomalacia [123].

Multiple Choice Questions

1. The following are true in relation to functions of the pancreas, EXCEPT:
   A. The hormones that regulate glucose metabolism include insulin, amylin derived from the beta cells and glucagon from the alpha cells of the pancreas.
   B. With ageing, independent of obesity and sex, there is a progressive impairment of glucose tolerance in the nondiabetic individual with advancing years,

and this is more related to insulin resistance rather than to decreased insulin secretion.

C. Immune-mediated diabetes most commonly occurs in childhood and adolescents, but it can occur at any age even in the 8 and 9th decades of life.
D. Lowered glucose levels result in reduced release of insulin from the pancreas and increased conversion of glycogen to glucose.

2. The following are true in relation to thyroid disease in the elderly, EXCEPT:
   A. With normal ageing, the thyroid gland undergoes changes, and consequently T4 production declines with advancing age, but the serum T4 (total and free) concentration remains unchanged.
   B. Many elderly patients have abnormal TSH levels without changes in serum thyroid hormone levels conditions termed subclinical hyperthyroidism and subclinical hyperthyroidism.
   C. Idiopathic hypothyroidism in adults is generally thought to be the result of undiagnosed Hashimoto's disease.
   D. Large multinodular goitre (Plummer's disease) accounts for an increasing proportion of cases of hyperthyroidism in middle-aged and elder persons
3. The following are true in primary, secondary and tertiary hyperparathyroidism, EXCEPT:
   A. Primary hyperparathyroidism is characterised by increase in the parathyroid hormone secretion occurring as a result of an abnormality in one or more parathyroid glands.
   B. Decrease of PTH increases bone turnover leading to irreversible loss of cortical bone due to increased endocortical resorption even in mild and asymptomatic cases.
   C. Untreated secondary hyperparathyroidism(SHPT) due to chronic renal failure leads to the development of progressive bone disease, osteitis fibrosa cystica and soft tissue calcifications.
   D. Tertiary hyperparathyroidism occurs in patients after renal transplantation, patients on dialysis and occasionally with long-standing osteomalacia.

Answers to MCQs

1 = D; 2 = B; 3 = B

References

Anatomical and Physiological Changes with Ageing-Endocrine System

1. Glaser J, Stienecker K. Pancreas and aging: a study using ultrasonography. Gerontology. 2000;46(2):93–6 (abstract).
2. Elahi D, Muller DC. Carbohydrate metabolism in the elderly. Eur J Clin Nutr. 2000;54: S112–20.

3. DI B, Taylor R. Review: deterioration of glucose tolerance with age: the role of insulin resistance. Age Ageing. 1991;20:221–5.
4. Reaven GM, Chen N, Hollenbeck C, Chen YDI. Effect of age on glucose tolerance and glucose uptake in healthy individuals. J Am Geriatr Soc. 1989;37:735–40.
5. Gong Z, Muzumdar RH. Pancreatic function, Type 2 diabetes and metabolism and aging. Int J Endocrinol. 2012;(2012). Aricle ID:320482, 13 pages. http://dx.doi.org/10.1155/2012/320482.
6. Perry 3rd HM. The endocrinology of aging. Clin Chem. 1999;45:1369–76.
7. Davidson M. The effect of aging on carbohydrate metabolism: a review of the English literature and a practical approach to the diagnosis of diabetes mellitus in the elderly. Metabolism. 1979;28:688–705.
8. Maneatis T, Condie R, Reaven G. Effect of age on plasma glucose and insulin responses to a test mixed meal. J Am Geriatr Soc. 1982;30:178–82.
9. Barbieri M, Rizzo MR, Manzella D, Paolisso G. Age-related insulin resistance: is it obligatory finding? The lesson from healthy centenarians. Diabetes Metab Res Rev. 2001;17:19–26.
10. DeFronzo R. Glucose tolerance and aging. Diabetes Care. 1981;4:493–501.
11. Fink RI, Wallace P, Olefsky JM. Effects of aging on glucose-mediated glucose disposal and glucose transport. J Clin Invest. 1986;77:2034–41.
12. Peeters RP. Thyroid hormones and aging. Hormones. 2008;7(1):28–35.
13. Herrmann J, Heinen E, Kroll HJ, Rudorff RH, Kruskemper HL. Thyroid function and thyroid hormone metabolism in the elderly people. Low T3-syndrome in old age? Klin Wochenschr. 1981;59:315–23.
14. Mariotti S, Franceschi C, Cossarizza A, Pinchera A. The aging thyroid. Endocr Rev. 1995;16:686–715.
15. Begin ME, Langlow MF, Lorrain D, Cunnarie SC. Thyroid function and cognition during ageing. Curr Gerontol Geriatr Res. 2008 (Article ID474868). http://dx.doi.org/10.1155/2008/474868.
16. Shams N, Hamad S. Case: report: hypothyroidism in the elderly. Mid East J Age Ageing. 2007;4. website: http://www.me-jaa.com/me-jaa11June07/hypothyroidism.htm.
17. Garber J. Who is at risk for thyroid disease? website: http://www.thyroidawareness.com/assessmentresource.html.
18. Tunbridge WM, Evered DC, Hall R, Appleton D, Brewis M, Clark F, et al. The spectrum of thyroid disease in a community: the Wickham survey. Clin Endorinol (Oxf). 1977;7:481–93.
19. Hijmans W, Radl J, Bottazzo GF, Doniach D. Autoantibodies in highly aged humans. Mech Ageing Dev. 1984;26:83–9.
20. Need AG, O'Loughlin PD, Morris HA, Horowitz M, Nordin BE. The effects of age and other variables on serum parathyroid hormone in postmenopausal women attending an osteoporosis center. J Clin Endocrinol Metab. 2004;89(4):1646–9 (abstract).
21. Bilezikian JP, Silverberg ST. Parathyroid hormone: does it have a role in the pathogenesis of osteoporosis? Clin Lab Med. 2000;20:559–67.
22. Alaami O, Fang TD, Song HM, Nacamuli RP. Physiological features of aging persons. Arch Surg. 2003;138:1068–976.

Diabetes Mellitus in the Elderly

23. Khinvasara LK. Diabetes in the elderly. Diabetes Today 2004;(3):5.
24. King H, Aubert RE, Herman WH. Global burden of diabetes, 1995-2025: Prevalence, numerical estimates and projections. Diabetes Care. 1998;21:1414–31.
25. Gregg EW, Mangione CM, Cauley JA, Thompson TJ, Schawartz AV, Ensrud KE, et al. Diabetes and incidence of functional disability in older women. Diabetes Care. 2002;23:1272–7.
26. Harris MI, Hadden WC, Knowler WC, Bennett PH. Mortality among diabetics in a national sample. Am J Epidemiol. 1988;128:389–401.
27. Better Health Channel. Diabetic retinopathy. State Govt of Victoria, Melbourne; 2007.

28. Rockwood K, Awalt E, Macknight C, McDowell I. Incidence and outcomes of diabetes mellitus in elderly people: report from the Canadian Study of Health and Aging. CMAJ. 2000;162(6):769–72 (abstract).
29. Kenny SJ, Aubert RE, Geiss LS. Prevalence and incidence of non-insulin dependent diabetes. In: Harris MI, editor. Diabetes in America. 2nd ed. NIH Pubication No 95–1468. National Institute of Health, National Institue of Diabetes and Digestive Diseases, Bethesda MO,1995, p. 47–67.
30. Aronoff SL, Berkowitz K, Shreiner B, Want L. Glucose metabolism and regulation. Beyond insulin and glucagon. Diabetes Spectr. 2004;17(3):183–90.
31. Perry 3rd HM. The endocrinology of aging. Clin Chem. 1999;45:1369–76.
32. Scheen AJ. Diabetes mellitus in the elderly: insulin resistance and/or impaired insulin secretion? Diab Metab. 2005;31(spec No2):5S27–34.
33. Ryan AS. Insulin resistance with ageing: effects of diet and exercise. Sports Med. 2000;30(5):327–46.
34. American Diabetes Association. Diagnosis and classification of diabetes mellitus. Diabetes Care. 2004;27:S5–10.
35. Defranzo RB. Banting lecture. From the triumvirate to the ominous octet: a new paradigm for the treatment of type 2 diabetes mellitus. Diabetes. 2009;58:773–95.
36. Mahler RJ, Adler ML. Type 2 diabetes mellitus: update in the diagnosis, pathophysiology and treatment. J Clin Endocrinol Metab. 1999;84(4):1164–71.
37. Yarlow RS, Berson SA. Immunoassay of endogenous plasma insulin in man. J Clin Invest. 1969;39:1159–62.
38. Meneily GS. Pathophysiology of type 2 diabetes in the elderly. Clin Geriatr Med. 1999; 15:239–53.
39. Chau D, Edelman SV. Clinical management of diabetes in the elderly. Clin Diabetes. 2001; 19(4):172–5.
40. Gleichman H, Zorcher B, Grenlich B, Gries FA, Henricks HR, Betrams J, et al. Correlation of islet cell antibodies and HKA-DR phenotypes in diabetes mellitus in adults. Diabetologia. 1984;27:90–2.
41. Yared Z, Chiasson JL. Ketoacidosis and the hyperosmolar hypeglycaemic state in adult diabetic patients. Diagnosis and treatment. Minerva Med. 2003;94(6):409–18.
42. Magee MF, Bhatt BA. Management of decompensated diabetes: diabetic ketoacidosis and hyperglycaemic hyperosmolar syndrome. Crit Care Clin. 2001;17:75–106.
43. Gouni-Berthold I, Krone W. Diabetic ketoacidosis and hyperosmolar hyperglycaemic state. Med Klin (Munich). 2006;101:100–5.
44. Clayton W, Elasy TA, Tom A. A review of the pathophysiology, classification and treatment of foot ulcers in diabetic patients. Clin Diabetes. 2009;27(2):52–8.
45. Kuroki T, Isshiki K, King G. Oxidative stress: the lead or supporting actor in the pathogenesis of diabetic complications. J Am Soc Nephrol. 2003;14:S216–20.
46. Ishii H, Jirousek MR, Koya D, Takagi C, Xia P, Clermont A, et al. Amelioration of vascular dysfunctions in diabetic rats by an oral PKC an inhibitor. Science. 1996;72:728–31.
47. Koya D, Haneda M, Nakagawa H, Isshiki K, Sato H, Maeda S, et al. Amelioration of accelerated diabetic mesangial expansion by treatment with a PKC beta inhibitor in diabetic db/db mice, a rodent model for type 2 diabetes. FASEB J. 2000;13:2329–37.
48. King KD, Jones JD, Warthen J. Microvascular and macrovascular complications in diabetes mellitus. Amer J Pharm Edu. 2005;69(5):Article 87.
49. Kikkawa R. Chronic complications in diabetes mellitus. Br J Nutr. 2000;84 Suppl 2:S183–5.
50. Nishio Y, Kashiwagi A, Taki H, Shinozaki K, Maeno Y, Kojima H, et al. Altered activities of transcription factors and their related gene expression in cardiac tissues of diabetic rats. Diabetes. 2000;47:1318–25.
51. Vinik AI. Diagnosis and management of diabetic neuropathy. Clin Geriatr Med. 1999;15: 293–320.
52. Odenthal U, Haehn S, Tunggal P, Merke B, Schomburg D, Frie C, et al. Molecular analysis of laminin N-terminal mediating self-interactions. J Biol Chem. 2006;279(43):44504–12 (abstract).

53. Young MJ, Boulton AJM, Macleod AF, Williams DR, Sonksen PH. A multicentre study of the prevalence of diabetic peripheral neuropathy in United Kingdom hospital clinic population. Diabetologia. 1993;36:150–4.
54. Tesfaye S. Epidemiology and etiology of diabetic peripheral neuropathy. Adv Stud Med. 2004;4(10G):S1014–21.
55. Ziegler D, Gries FA, Spuler M, Lessmann F. The epidemiology of diabetic neuropathy. Diabetic cardiovascular autonomic neuropathy Multicentre Group. J Diabetes Complications. 1992;6(1):49–59 (abstract).
56. Vinik AL, Park TS, Stansberry KB, Pittenger GL. Diabetic neuropathies. Diabetologia. 2000;43(8):957–73 (abstract).

Thyroid Disease in the Older Patient

57. Empson M, Flood V, Ma G, Eastman CJ, Mitchell P. Prevalence of thyroid disease in older Australian population. Intern Med J. 2007;37:448–56.
58. Tunbridge WM, Evered DC, Hall R, Appleton D, Brewis M, Clark F, et al. The spectrum of thyroid disease in a community: the Wichkam survey. Clin Endocrinol (Oxf). 1977;7:481–93.
59. Canario GJ, Manowitz NR, Maypor G, Ridgway EC. The Colorado thyroid disease: prevalence study. Arch Intern Med. 2000;110:526–30.
60. Cooper DS, Biondi B. Subclinical thyroid disease. Lancet. 2012;379:1142–54.
61. Bremner AP, Feddema P, Leedman PJ, Brown SJ, Beilby JP, Lim EM, et al. Age-related changes in thyroid function: a longitudinal study of a community –based cohort. J Clin Endocrinol Metab. 2012;97:1554–62.
62. Klein I, Ojamma K. Thyroid hormone and the cardiovascular system. N Engl J Med. 2001;344:501–9.
63. Kanaya AM, Harris F, Volpato S, Perez-Stable EJ, Harris T, Bauer DC. Association between thyroid dysfunction and total cholesterol level in older bi-racial population, the health, aging and body composition study. Arch Intern Med. 2002;162:773–9.
64. Helfand M, Crapo IM. Screening for thyroid disorder. Ann Intern Med. 1990;112:840–9.
65. Brent GA, Mestman JH. Diagnosis of the major step involved in thyroid hormone synthesis and secretion. Totuwa: Humana Press; 1996.
66. Nakamura M, Ohtaki S. Molecular mechanism of thyroid hormone synthesis. Nihon Rinsho. 1994;52(4):857–63 (abstract).
67. Islam S. Thyroid gland. Norm Physiol. http://www.pathologyoutlines.com/topic/thyroidphysiology.html. Retrieved 15 Apr 2014.
68. Bonert V, Friedman TC. Chapter 65: The thyroid gland. In: Andreoli TE, editor. Cecil essentials of medicine. 5th ed. Philadelphia PA:WBaunders; 2001. pp. 543–604.
69. Roy G, Mugesh G. Thyroid hormone synthesis and anti-thyroid drugs: a bioinorganic chemistry approach. J Chem Sci. 2006;118:619–28.
70. Hennemann G, Visser TJ. Chapter 4. Thyroid hormone synthesis, plasma membrane transport and metabolism. In: Weetman AP, Grossman, editors. Pharmatherapeutics of the thyroid gland, Handbook of experimental pharmacology, vol. 128. Berlin: Springer; 1997. p. 75–7.
71. Chiovato L, Mariotti S, Pinchera A. Thyroid diseases in the elderly. Baillieres Clin Endocrinol Metab. 1997;11:251–70.
72. Hermann J, Heinen E, Kroll HJ, Rudorff KH, Kruskemper HL. Thyroid function and thyroid hormone metabolism in elderly people. Low T3 –syndrome in old age? Klin Wochenchr. 1981;59:315–23.
73. Mariotti S, Franceschi C, Cossarizza A, Pinchera A. The aging thyroid. Endocr Rev. 1995;16:686–715.
74. Wilson GR, Curry RW. Subclinical thyroid disease. Am Fam Physician. 2005;72(8):1517–24 (abstract).
75. Samuels MH. Subclinical thyroid disease in the elderly. Thyroid. 1998;8(9):803–13.

76. Faggiono A, Del Prete M, Marciello V, Marotta V, Ramundo V, Colao A. Thyroid diseases in the elderly. Minerva Endocrinol. 2011;36:211–31.
77. Rukhman N, Silverberg A. Thyroid cancer in men. Aging Male. 2011;14:91–8.
78. Hollowel JG, Staenling NW, Flanders WD, Hannon WH, Gunter EW, Spencer CA, et al. Serum TSH, T4, and thyroid antibodies in the United States Population (1988–1994) National Health and Nutrition Examination Survey (NHANES-III). J Clin Endocrinol Metab. 2002;87: 481–91.
79. Roti M, Montermini G, Robuschi G, Gardin IE, Salvo D, Gionet M, et al. Prevalence of hypothyroidism, Hashimoto's thyroiditis in two elderly populations with different dietary iodine intake. In: Pinchera A, Ongbar SH, McKenzie J, Fenzis GF, editors. Thyroid Autoimmunity New York NY: Plenum Press; 1987. pp. 555–557.
80. Diez JJ. Hypothyroidism in patients older than 55 years: an analysis of the etiology and assessment of the effectiveness of therapy. J Gerontol A Biol Sci Med Sci. 2002; 57:M315–20.
81. Almandoz JP, Gharib H. Hypothyroidism: etiology, diagnosis and management. Med Clin North Am. 2012;96:203–21.
82. Laurberg P, Andersen S, Bulow Pedersen I, Carle A. Hypothyroidism in the elderly: pathophysiology, diagnosis and treatment. Drugs Aging. 2005;22(1):23–38 (abstract).
83. Haughen BR. Drugs that suppress TSH or cause central hypothyroidism. Best Pract Res Clin Endocrinol Metab. 2009;23(6):793–800.
84. Mestman J. Disorders of the thyroid gland. Glob Libr Women's Med. (ISSN: 1756–2228) 2008. doi: 10.3843/GLOWM.10308.
85. Swain M, Swain T, Mohanty B. Autoimmune disorders-an update. Indian J Clin Biochem. 2005;20(1):9–17.
86. Marcocci C, Chiovito L. Thyroid directed antibodies. In: Braverman LE, Utiger RD, editors. The thyroid: a fundamental and clinical text. 8th ed. Philadelphia: Lipincott William and Wilkins; 2000. p. 414–31.
87. Ichikawa K, Kaneko T, Suzuki S, Komatsu M, Yamauci K, Aizawa T, et al. Aging and Hashimoto's thyroiditis. Nihon Ronen Igakkai Zasshi. 1998;35(10):771–6 (abstract).
88. Lerch M, Meier C, Staub JJ. Is there a need for treatment in subclinical hypo-hyperthyroidism? Ther Umsch. 1999;56(7):369–73 (abstract).
89. Krysiak R, Okopien B, Herman Z. Pol Merkur Lekarski. 2006;31(126):573–8. (abstract).
90. Jayme JJ, Ladenson PW. Subclinical thyroid dysfunction in the elderly. Trends Endocrinol Metab. 1994;5(2):79–82.
91. Jameson JL, Weetman AP. Disorders of the thyroid gland. In: Longo D, Fauci A, Kasper D, Haiuser S, Jameson J, Loscalzo J, editors. Harrisons principles of internal medicine. 18th ed. New York: McGraw –Hill; 2012. p. 2911–39.
92. Goldenberg LMC. Thyroid disease in late life. Thyroid Foundation of Canada. http://www.thyroid.ca/e4g.php. Retrieved 30 July 2013.
93. de Luise MA. Thyroid disease in the elderly. J Pharm Pract Res. 2003;33:228–30.
94. Diez JJ. Hyperthyroidism in patients older than 55 years: an analysis of the etiology and management. Gerontology. 2003;49:316–23. 39.
95. Parle JV, Franklyn JA, Cross KW, Jones SR, Shepperd MC. Thyroxine prescription in the community: serum thyroid stimulating hormone level assays as an indicator of under treatment or over treatment. Br J Gen Pract. 1993;43:107–9.
96. Sawin TC, Geller A, Wolf PA, Belanger AJ, Baker E, Bacharach P, et al. Low serum thyrotropin concentrations as a risk factor for atrial fibrillation in older persons. N Engl J Med. 1994;331:1249–52.
97. Muddle AA, Reijinders FJL, Nieuwenhuijzen Krusman AC. Peripheral bone density in women with untreated multinodular goiter. Clin Endocrinol. 1992;37:35–9.
98. Santos Palacios S, Pascual-Corrales E, Galofore JC. Management of subclinical hyperthyroidism. Int J Endocrinol Metab. 2012;10(2):490–6 (abstract).
99. Givelli ME, Cesara D, Rubello R, Mazzarotto R, Saladini G, Busnardo B. Differentiated thyroid cancer in the elderly, disease outcome, therapeutic approach and long-term results in a group of 314 patients. J Endocrinol Invest. 1999;22:45–6.

100. Lin JD, Chao TC, Chen ST, Weng HF, Lin KD. Characteristics of thyroid carcinomas in ageing patients. Eur J Clin Invest. 2000;30:147–53.
101. Gesing A, Lewinski A, Karbownik-Lewinska M. The thyroid gland and the process of aging: what is new? Thyroid Res. 2012;5:16. doi:10.1186/1756-6614-5-16.
102. Ito Y, Higashiyama T, Takamura Y, et al. Risk factors for recurrence to lymph node in papillary thyroid carcinoma patients without preoperatively detectable lateral node metastasis: validity of prophylactic modified radical neck dissection. World J Surg. 2007;312: 2085–91.
103. Liebner DA, Shah MH. Thyroid cancer: pathogenesis and targeted therapy. Ther Adv Endocrinol Metab. 2011;2(5):173–95.
104. Brzezianska E, Pastuzak-Lewandoska D. A minireview: the role of MAPK/ERK and P13K/Akt pathways in thyroid follicular cell-derived neoplasm. Front Biosci (Landmark Ed). 2011;16:422–39.
105. Health Encyclopedia-Diseases and Conditions. Thyroid cancer. http://www.healthscout.com/ency/68/469/main.html. Retrieved 21 July 2009.
106. Medicine.net.com http://www.medicine.net.com/ThyroidCAncer/pagC3.htm#wahat_arethe_differencetypesofthyroidcancer. Retrieved 31 July 2013.
107. University of Virginia Health System. Survival Statistics, AJCC Cancer Strategies Manual. 7th ed. http://www.cancer.orf/cancer/thyroidcancer/detailedguide/thyroid_cancer.survival. Retrieved 31 July 2013.

Hyperparathyroidism

108. Deshmukh RG, Alsagoff SA, Krishnan S, Dhillon KS, Khir ASM. Primary hyperparathyroidism presenting with pathological fractures. J R Coll Surg Edinb. 1998;43(6):424–7.
109. Yu N, Dinnan PT, Murphy J, Leese GP. Epidemiology of primary hyperparathyroidism in Europe. J Bone Miner Res. 2002;17 Suppl 2:N18–23 (abstract).
110. Bolland MJ, Grey AB, Gamble GD, Reid LR. Association between primary hyperparathyroidism and increased body weight: a meta analysis. J Clin Endocrinol Metab. 2004;90(3): 1525–30.
111. Adami S, Marcocci C, Gatt D. Epidemiology of primary hyperparathyroidism in Europe. J Bone Miner Res. 2002;17 suppl 2:N18–23 (abstract).
112. Wermier RA, Khosle S, Atkinson EG, Achenbach SJ, Oberg AL, Grant CS, et al. The rise and fall of primary hyperparathyroidism: population based study in Rochester, Minnesota. Ann Intern Med. 1997;126(6):433–40 (abstract).
113. Brown EM. The pathophysiology of primary hyperparathyroidism. J Bone Miner Res. 2002;17(Suppl 2):N24–9 (abstract).
114. Nemeth EF. Pharmacological regulation of parathyroid hormone secretion. Curr Pharm Des. 2002;8(23):2077–87 (abstract).
115. Cetani F, Picone A, Cerrai P, Vignali E, Borsans S, Pardi E, et al. Parathyroid expression of calcium sensory receptor protein and in vivo parathyroid hormone-Ca (2+) set-point in patients with primary hyperparathyroidism. J Clin Endocrinol Metab. 2000;85(2):4789–94.
116. Johnson NA, Tublin ME, Ogilivie JB. Parathyroid injury. Technique and role in the preoperative evaluation of primary hyperparathyroidism. AJR Am J Roentgenol. 2007;188:1706–15.
117. Ruda JM, Hollenbeak CS, Jr S. A systematic review of the diagnosis and treatment of primary hyperparathyroidism from 1995–2013. Otolaryngol Head Neck Surg. 2005;132:359–72.
118. Carnevale V, Romagnoli E, Pipino M, Scillitane A, D'Erasmo E, Miaisola S, et al. Primary hyperparathyroidism. Clin Ther. 2005;156(5):211–26 (abstract).
119. Hellman P, Carling T, Rask L, Akerstrom G. Pathophysiology of primary hyperparathyroidism. Histol Histopathol. 2000;15(2):619–27 (abstract).
120. Mosgaard B, Chrostensen SE, Vestergaard P, Heickendorff HL, Christiansen P, Mosekilde L, et al. Vitamin D mobility and skeletal consequences in primary hyperparathyroidism. Clin Endocrinol (Oxf). 2006;68(5):707–15 (abstract).

121. Mosekilk L. Primary hyperparathyroidism and the skeleton. Clin Endocrinol (Oxf). 2008;69(1):1–19 (abstract).
122. Marcocci C, Cianferotti L, Cetani F. Bone disease in primary hyperparathyroidism. Ther Adv Musculoskelet Dis. 2012;4(5):357–68 (abstract).
123. Pitt SC, Sippel Rebecca RS, Chen H. Secondary and tertiary hyperparathyroidism, State of the Art Surgical Management. Surg Clin North Am. 2009;89(5):1227–39.
124. Dabbagh S. Renal osteodystrophy. Curr Opin Pediatr. 1998;10(2):190–6 (abstract).
125. Pitt SC, Sippi RS, Chen H. Secondary and tertiary hyperparathyroidism: State of the Art Surgical Management. Surg Clin North Am. 2009;89(5):1227–39.
126. Cunningham J, Locatelli F, Rodriguez M. Secondary hyperparathyroidism: pathogenesis, disease progression, and therapeutic options. Clin J Am Soc Nephrol. 2011;6(4):913–21.
127. Memmos D, Williams G, Eastwood J, Gordon EM, Cochrane CL, Gower PE, et al. The role of parathyroidectomy in the management of hyperparathyroidism in patients on maintenance haemodialysis and after renal transplantation. Nephron. 1982;30:143–8.
128. Bilezkian JP, Khan I, Potts JT, Brandi ML, Clarke BL, Shoback D, et al. Hyperparathyroidism in the adult: epidemiology, diagnosis, pathophysiology. Target-organ involvement. Treatment and challenges for future research. J Bone Miner Res. 2011;26(10):2317–37.

Metabolic Bone Disorders in the Elderly

10

10.1 Bone, Bone Formation and Changes with Ageing

The mature bone consists of an outer shell called the cortex enclosed in a firmly adherent periosteal membrane. Within the cortex is a meshwork of trabeculae, the spongy or cancellous bone with its interconnecting spaces containing the marrow. Cortical and trabecular bones are composed of osteons [1], and cortical osteons are longitudinal cylindrical units called Haversian canals with branches connecting adjoining canals [2]. The trabecular osteons are called packets and are semilunar in shape [1], and the trabecular bone is made of rods and plates [3].

The bone is composed of mineral (50–70 %), organic matrix (20–40 %), water (5–10 %) and lipids (<3 %), and the mineral content is mostly hydroxyapatite [1]. There are five types of cells in the skeletal tissue, namely, osteoprogenitor cells, osteoblasts, osteocytes, osteoclasts and bone lining cells [4]. The osteoprogenitor cells give rise to the osteoblasts and they are involved in the intramembranous and endochondral bone formation. The organic matrix formed by collagen and polymucopolysaccharide is produced by the osteoblasts. The osteocytes, which are derived from the pro-osteoblasts and osteoblasts, lie in the lacunes and support bone structure and metabolism [1]. Osteoclasts originate from the haemopoietic stem cell and are related to bone resorption. They diminish in number once the erosive process is over.

The remodelling cycle is initiated by the interaction of osteoblasts and osteoclasts and involves a train of regulated events [5], and osteoclasts are activated first leading to bone resorption [6]. During each remodelling cycle, the osteoblast-mediated bone resorption takes about 2–4 weeks. Osteoclast activation and resorption is regulated by a cell surface receptor called RANK (receptor activator of NFkB) which is activated by RANK ligand (RANKL) [7]. Osteoprotegerin released by the osteoblasts [8] prevents the contact of RANK with RANKL [6]. More recently cytokines and growth factors such as interleukin-1, interleukin-6, tumour necrosis factor-a and granulocyte-macrophage colony-stimulating factor are believed to play an important role in bone formation [4, 9–11]. Successive layers of osteoblasts fill the cavity created by the resorption forming a mineralisation matrix

N. Nagaratnam et al., *Diseases in the Elderly: Age-Related Changes and Pathophysiology*, DOI 10.1007/978-3-319-25787-7_10

[12]. Bone mineralisation occurs initially as deposition of calcium and phosphorus along the length of collagen fibres surrounded by ground substance and further precipitation leads to the formation of a crystal similar to hydroxyapatite. Formation and resorption occur continuously.

Calcium homeostasis and bone metabolism are mediated through the skeleton, kidneys and intestines and regulated by hormonal factors, the more important of them being the oestrogen, parathyroid hormone, calcitonin and 1.25 OH vitamin D. Oestrogen plays a crucial role in maintaining normal bone turnover [13], and oestrogen deficiency leads to a state where resorption surpasses formation and bone mass declines [5]. The oestrogen receptor alpha (Era) a cell surface receptor binds to the hormone oestrogen forming a receptor-hormone complex assisting the entry of the hormone into the nucleus of the cell [6]. This acts to turn on the specific genes which regulate cell activity. Parathyroid hormone and 1,25 OH vitamin D play a crucial role in the metabolic functions of the skeleton. Parathyroid hormone (PTH) stimulates and controls the rate of bone remodelling and also influences the mechanisms governing control of the plasma level of calcium. The synthesis and secretion of PTH is regulated by the level of ionised calcium in the extracellular fluid. Small changes in the circulation level of Ca(2+) are detected by Ca(2+)-sensing receptor regulating the release of PTH [14]. PTH has a direct effect on mobilisation of calcium from the skeleton and on the kidney absorption of calcium and indirectly affects the intestines influencing calcium absorption through the regulation of synthesis of 1.25 OH chole calciferol metabolite in the kidney. At the cellular level it influences the osteoclasts, osteoblasts, osteocytes and the bone lining cells. A fall in the calcium level will give rise to increase parathyroid hormone which activates osteoclasts and osteocytes for bone resorption. Dihydroxy-vitamin D has a direct effect on the bone, but its greatest effects are on intestinal calcium and phosphate absorption [15].

Calcitonin secreted by the parafollicular cells of the thyroid is controlled by the serum calcium levels. Calcitonin inhibits bone resorption probably by inactivation of the osteoclasts. Other hormones regulating skeletal growth are the growth hormone, glucocorticoids and thyroid hormones [5]. Prostaglandins also stimulate both resorption and formation of the bone [16].

10.1.1 Changes with Ageing Bone and Pathophysiology

Bone changes occur with normal ageing. Although a number of mechanisms are involved, the overall result is the age-related occurrence of loss of bone mass, strength and quality. Bone mass peaks in both men and women between 25 and 30 years [17] and then plateaus for about 10 years and diminishes thereafter. The attainment of peak bone mass and subsequent rates of bone loss may be influenced by genetic factors, maternal history of vertebral fracture, a strong risk for osteoporosis in men [18], gender, exercise, diet [19, 20] and race.

Men in their fifth and sixth decade of life and women in their fourth decade develop a gradual loss of skeletal mass. Normally the loss of bone mass with ageing is about 1 % per year [21] in adults, and this loss accelerates in women postmenopause to 3–5 % for about 5–10 years [22, 23]. Thereafter, the rate of bone loss returns to the lower level seen in premenstrual women and in men [24].

Bone mass is preserved through a remarkably tight balance between resorption and formation. In ageing the osteoclastic activity is greater than osteoblastic activity and results in net bone loss. Bone mineral density decreases and the amount of the bone formed during remodelling decreases with age. Osteoblasts and adipocytes stem from the same stromal stem cell, and cells that have the capacity to form osteoblasts can be redirected to form adipocytes and become no longer available for bone formation [5]. This may be the reason why there is an increase in marrow fat with ageing and impaired osteoblast renewal [5].

Calcium homeostasis and bone metabolism are mediated through the skeleton, kidneys and intestines and the presence of hormonal factors, the more important being parathyroid hormone (PTH), calcitonin and 1.25 OH vitamin D. Several studies have shown an increase in the level of PTH with age and calcitonin, and the most active metabolites of vitamin D_3 are seen to decrease with age. Other factors include sex hormones, oestrogen deficiency following menopause and in men decrease in testosterone. Bone tissue is particularly responsive to mechanical loading, and the magnitude of the bone mass loss is a consequence of decrease physical activity [25], deconditioning or disease.

Structural changes play a significant role in the age-related alterations of bone strength and quality. Structural modifications include changes in bone architecture, changes in the protein content of the bone matrix, changes in the crystalline properties of mineral deposits, disparity in the concentration of deposited minerals, subperiosteal expansion and widening of the medullary cavity and accumulation of microfractures [25]. These factors adversely impact on the quality of bone material, its elasticity and ultimate properties [26]. It has been proposed that there are two types of structurally different forms of bone loss with different rates, a rapid and a slow [27]. With rapid bone loss, there is excessive depth of osteoclastic resorptive cavities resulting in perforation of structural elements in trabecular bone, discontinuity of bone structure and in the cortical bone to subendosteal cavitation and conversion of the inner third of the cortex to a trabecular structure [27]. Slow bone loss results from incomplete filling by the osteoblasts of resorptive cavities. These structural changes reduce the strength of the bone to a greater extent than reduction in the amount of the bone [27]. The mechanical properties of the cancellous bone tissue are largely influenced by the apparent density and trabecular architecture [28–30]. The amount of trabecular bone loss on the iliac crest and spine is alike during ageing in both genders [31].

Forces generated by muscle contractions could be an important determinant of bone quality, and there seems to be a potential interrelationship between muscle quality and skeletal health [32]. With ageing there is a decrease in muscle mass and strength. Bone mass accounts for more than 50 % of bone strength [33]. Furthermore, there is an age-related loss of collagen in the bone which parallels the loss of muscle strength [34] (Fig. 10.1).

Box 10.1. Key Points. Bone, Bone Formation and Changes with Ageing

- The bone is composed of mineral (mostly hydroxyapatite), organic matrix, water and lipids [1].
- Five types of cells in the skeletal tissue – osteoprogenitor cells, osteoblasts, osteocytes, osteoclasts and bone lining cells [4].
- Osteoprogenitor cells give rise to the osteoblasts.
- Osteocytes are derived from the pro-osteoblasts.
- Osteoclasts originate from the haemopoietic stem cells.
- The remodelling is initiated by the interaction of the osteoblasts and osteoclasts [5].
- Osteoclast activation and resorption is regulated by a cell surface receptor called RANK which is activated by RANK ligand (RANKL) [7].
- Osteoprotegerin released by the osteoblasts which prevents the contact of RANK with RANKL [8].
- Hormonal factors such as oestrogen, PTH, calcitonin and vitamin D are important [13].
- Bone mass peaks in both men and women between 25 and 30 years plateaus for about 10 years and then diminishes [17].
- The attainment of peak bone mass is influenced by genetic factors, maternal history, gender, exercise, diet and race [18, 19, 20].
- In ageing osteoclastic activity is greater than osteoblastic activity resulting in net bone loss.
- Structural changes play an important role in age-related alterations of bone strength and quality.

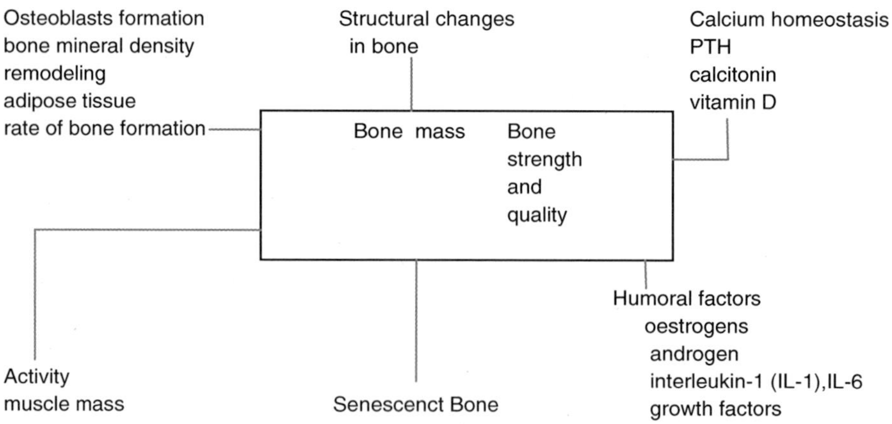

Fig. 10.1 Important factors in age-related bone changes

10.2 Osteoporosis

Osteoporosis is 'a disease characterized by low bone mass and architectural deterioration of bone tissue leading to enhanced bone fragility and a consequent increase in fracture risk' [35]. According to the World Health Organization, there is a variation in the incidence and prevalence of osteoporosis, it is estimated that 1 in 3 women and 1 in 12 men over the age of 50 years worldwide suffer from osteoporosis, and it is a major public health problem [36]. It affects people of all ethnic backgrounds [37]. In Australia it is estimated that 60 % of women and 30 % of men over the age of 60 years will suffer osteoporotic fracture in their remaining lifetime [38], that is, one in two women and one in three men will have a minimal trauma fracture (MTF) because of osteoporosis. In the United States 26 % of women aged 65 years or more and 50 % of women aged 85 years and/or more have osteoporosis [39]. With increasing age of the population the incidence of MTF will increase [40], and the financial costs for all these fractures are $1.9 billion per year [41].

Pathophysiology

The risk of osteoporosis depends on the peak bone mass attained in young adult life and the rate of bone loss in later years. The peak bone mass, excessive bone resorption and inadequate formation of new bone remodelling are the three main mechanisms by which osteoporosis develops [42]. Crucial to achieving peak bone mass are adequate nutrition, appropriate intake of calcium and vitamin D, exercise and regular menstrual cycles [37]. RANK on the cell surface nudges precursors of osteoclasts to develop into differentiated osteoclasts when RANK comes into contact with RANKL [43]. Osteoprotegerin prevents their coming together and it is believed that RANKL osteoprotegerin may play a crucial role in osteoporosis [44]. Age-related osteoporosis occurs in men and women over the age of 70 and affects cortical and trabecular bone [45]. Although there is a loss of trabecular and compact bone in older men and women after menopause, the enormity of loss of compact bone in women is greater than in men. Simultaneous reduction of trabecular bone (sponge-like bone in the ends of long bones and vertebrae) is evident, and resulting diminution of bone mass produces a decrease in strength and a proclivity to the fracture. The process of remodelling is slow normally but is a constant process and takes more than 6–8 months, from removal of mineralised bone followed by formation of bone matrix that eventually become mineralised [46]. The osteoblasts differentiated from mesenchymal cells lay down the matrix in the formation phase [47]. Parathyroid hormone, calcitriol and other hormones such as glucocorticoids, growth, thyroid and sex hormones are the major systemic regulators [46]. Furthermore, cytokines, prostaglandins and growth factors have been identified to act locally [46, 47]. The trabecular bone is more active and subject to bone turnover to remodelling. The disruption of the microarchitecture in trabecular bone, decreased density and changed bone material quality lead to bone fragility [48]. The fracture sites in osteoporosis, the wrist, the hip and the vertebra, have relatively high trabecular bone to cortical bone ratio. These areas rely on trabecular bone for strength.

The remodelling causes these areas to degenerate most when remodelling is not balanced. In Australia of all reported osteoporotic fractures, 46 % are vertebral, 16 % are hip and 16 % are wrist fractures [49].

10.2.1 Osteoporosis in Men

Osteoporosis in men although very common is less well known than osteoporosis in women. In the United States osteoporosis affects as many as 2 million men [50]. A large European study found the prevalence of vertebral deformity to be 12 % in both men and women between the ages of 59–79 years [51]. Men who develop symptoms as a result of vertebral deformity are more likely to be disabled than women [52]. In Australia 31 % of men and 50 % of women over the age of 60 years will sustain a fragility fracture due to osteoporosis throughout their remaining lifetime [38].

Pathophysiology
Both total and free testosterone levels decline with age [53]. Bone loss and reduced bone formation in men can be due to age-related decline in testosterone, adrenal androgens and growth hormone insulin-like growth factor [54]. Both adrenal and gonadal testosterone are powerful regulators of bone cell metabolism [55]. Androgen receptors suppress the release of interleukin-6 which instigates bone resorption [56]. Some degree of androgen deficiency can be found in about 50 % of older men with femoral neck fractures [57]. There may be no overt signs of hypogonadism and the diagnosis is often missed. Oestrogens play an important role in skeletal maintenance in both men and women. Mutations inactivating oestrogen receptors have been reported in men with osteoporosis [58]. In men with idiopathic osteoporosis, circulating insulin growth factor is reduced [53].

In 20–50 % of men with osteoporosis, clinical and random investigation identified no causal factors were identified [57] and could be designated as primary or idiopathic osteoporosis. Many however believe that most 'primary' osteoporosis is simply secondary osteoporosis of multiple or unknown causes or both [57]. Vertebral fractures in 30–60 % of men have other causes contributing to bone disease so that it is important that other pathological causes of osteoporosis should be excluded [53]. In man the major causes of secondary osteoporosis are hypogonadism and corticosteroid therapy. Other causes include alcoholism, cigarette smoking, malignancy, gastric surgery and recently osteoporosis related to organ transplantation. Exogenous corticosteroid therapy is now the leading cause of osteoporosis in men with multiple myeloma which induces generalised osteopenia regardless of any lytic lesions. Non-small cell lung cancer elaborates parathyroid hormone-related peptide (PTHrP) which may affect bone turnover but usually presents with hypercalcaemia [59]. There is limited evidence of usefulness of bisphosphonates in men with idiopathic osteoporosis [57]. In men with proven hypogonadism, testosterone replacement should be considered [54, 59].

Box 10.2. Key Point. Osteoporosis

- Three main mechanisms by which osteoporosis develops are peak bone mass, excessive bone resorption and inadequate formation of new bone remodelling [42].
- Age-related osteoporosis occurs in men and women over the age of 70 years and affects cortical and trabecular bone [45].
- Diminution of bone mass produces a decrease in strength and proclivity to fracture.
- PTH, calcitriol and other hormones such as glucocorticoids, growth, thyroid and sex hormones are the major systemic regulators [46].
- Osteoporosis in men [53].
- Both total and free testosterone levels decline with age [54].
- Bone loss and reduced formation in men can be attributed to age-related decline in testosterone, adrenal androgens, growth hormone and insulin-like growth factor.
- In men the major causes of secondary osteoporosis are hypogonadism and corticosteroid therapy.

10.3 Osteomalacia

Osteomalacia is a metabolic bone disorder characterised by a failure in mineralisation of the newly formed organic matrix of the bone causing an increase in unmineralised bone. The total bone mass may be normal or increased. Vitamin D deficiency is the most common cause of osteomalacia and most likely to occur in the elderly with inadequate dietary intake [60], who are housebound or institutionalised with little or no exposure to sunlight [61]. Other causes include malabsorption of calcium, phosphate and/or vitamin due to gastrointestinal disease. Poor synthesis of vitamin D can occur with liver or renal failure, i.e. failure of 1 alpha-hydroxylation of vitamin D_3 or rarely to inadequate sunlight, other causes being anticonvulsant therapy (phenytoin, phenobarbitone).

10.3.1 Pathophysiology

Vitamin D is obtained from the diet (D_2) and is absorbed in the upper small bowel. The precursor D_3 is synthesised from 7-dihydrocholesterol in the skin after exposure to sunlight and is then isomerised to D_3. The D_3 is then converted to 25 (OH) D_3 in the liver and in the kidneys to its much more metabolically active form, 1.25 $(OH)_2$ D_3 (calcitriol). Vitamin D is predominantly manufactured in the skin from absorption of UV light. Sun exposure alone would be enough for most people to maintain adequate vitamin levels. The main nutritional sources include liver, eggs, oily fish (salmon, herring) and some fortified foods such as margarine and some low-fat milk. Vitamin D increases the calcium absorption, enhances resorption by the kidney tubules, stimulates osteoblasts to produce alkaline phosphatase and inhibits parathyroid hormone secretion. Vitamin D with or without calcium contributes to muscle strength and improves balance and navigation abilities and decreases risk of falls [62].

10.4 Paget's Disease

Paget's disease is a chronic disorder of the skeletal bones characterised by localised areas which undergo excessive bone resorption with extreme osteoblastic response with formation of structurally abnormal bone. Paget's disease usually occurs past middle age [63] with increasing frequency with age [64].

Pathophysiology
There is increased resorption of the bone. This is followed by usually an intense osteoblastic response [65] to repair resulting in disordered bone formation. This process is repeated several times giving rise to a thickened, deformed and weakened bone [63] in spite of it being heavily calcified. The osteoblastic phase may occur simultaneously as the osteoclastic phase in the adjacent bone. It is slow but progressive. Any one or several bones may be affected, most often the skull, tibia, vertebrae, clavicle and humerus. The disordered bone may be exceptionally vascular [66].

Genetic [67, 68] and environmental factors are implicated [63, 64]. Deficiency in dietary calcium and repetitive mechanical loading of the skeleton are other potential triggers [68]. Examination of the enlarged muti-nucleated osteoclasts had revealed the presence of nuclear and cytoplasmic inclusions of paramyxovirus [69] suggesting a virus aetiology [70]. Genetic factors may play a role in its causation and nearly 40 % of the patients with Paget's disease have one other member of the family affected. Four genes have been identified and the most important of them is sequestosome 1 (SQSTM1) and patients with SQSTM1 mutations are severely afflicted [70].

Box 10.3. Key Points. Paget's Disease

- In Paget's disease there are localised areas which undergo excessive bone resorption with extreme osteoblastic response with formation of structurally abnormal bone [65].
- It is slow but progressive.
- Genetic and environmental factors are implicated [63–65, 68, 70].
- Four genes have been identified and the most important of them is sequestosome 1 (SQSTM1) and patients with SQSTM1 mutations are severely afflicted [65].

10.5 Related Disorders: Fractures in the Elderly

10.5.1 Hip Fracture

Hip fractures are defined as fractures occurring in the regions of the head, neck and proximal part of the femur. The incidence of hip fractures rises exponentially with increase in age irrespective of gender and ethnicity [71]. The mean age of people sustaining hip fractures is 75–80 years [72, 73]. In the United States femoral neck and intertrochanteric fractures occur with almost the same frequency in patients between the ages of 65 and 99 years [74].

Pathophysiology
There are two broad groups of hip fractures: (i) intracapsular involving the femoral head and neck and can be subcapital, transverse and basal and (ii) extracapsular involving the trochanter and can be intertrochanteric or subtrochanteric. There is very little trabecular bone in the femoral neck in contrast to large amount of trabecular bone in the intertrochanteric region. The disruption of the microarchitecture in trabecular bone, decreased density and changed in bone material quality lead to bone fragility. The common fracture sites in osteoporosis are the wrist, the hip and the vertebra, which have relatively high trabecular bone to cortical bone ratio. These areas rely on trabecular bone for strength.

In the elderly changes in stability, balance, gait disorder muscle strength and co-morbidities such as cognition concerns increase with age and are precipitating factors for falls [75]. Studies have shown that postural sway, cognition and behavioural deficits and moderate to severe disability are common to patients who fall [76]. Muscle strength decreases approximately by 50 % from age 30 to 80, and the amount of body sway increases with reduction of proprioception [75].

10.5.2 Vertebral Fractures

A 20–25 % reduction in any vertebral height (anterior, posterior or middle) is a practical method of assessing an incidence of vertebral fracture [77]. Symptomatic vertebral fractures occur in 0.2 per 1000 person years in patients under 45 years, and this increased to 1.2 per 1000 person years after 85 years [78]. The incidence of vertebral fractures increases with age in both men and women, and in both the common type of fracture was the wedge-shaped fracture [79]. In women the prevalence of vertebral fracture increases with age from 20 % in the 50-year-old menopausal women to 64.5 % in older women [80].

Pathophysiology
Vertebral fractures are the result of a combination of ageing and bone fragility [81]. In men it is associated with severe trauma; mild to moderate trauma in women [82], and there is an increased risk of further fractures in patients with vertebral fractures [77]. The majority of vertebral fractures are not connected with severe trauma, and only one in three there is a diagnosis clinically [80]. The amount of trabecular bone

in the spine with ageing is similar in both men and women [83] and in men the reduced peak bone mass and bone loss [83]. In about one-third of women and one-half of men with significant vertebral fracture, there is an underlying secondary osteoporosis [84] such as hypogonadism in men and other associated illness such as alcohol abuse, myeloma and skeletal metastasis [83]. The bone loss in the spine is mainly trabecular [85].

10.5.3 Sacral Insufficiency Fractures

Is a subtype of stress fractures [86].

Pathophysiology
It usually occurs in osteoporotic bone, metabolic bone disease and following radiotherapy [86].

Multiple Choice Questions

1. The following age-related bone changes are true, EXCEPT:
   A. Bone mass peaks in both men and women between 25 and 30 years and then plateaus for about 10 years and diminishes thereafter.
   B. Men in their fifth and sixth decade of life and women in their fourth decade develop a gradual loss of skeletal mass.
   C. Several studies have shown an increase in the level of PTH with age and calcitonin, and the most active metabolites of vitamin D_3 are seen to decrease with age.
   D. The amount of trabecular bone loss on the iliac crest and spine is different in both genders during ageing.
2. The following are true in regard to the pathogenesis of osteoporosis, EXCEPT:
   A. Age-related osteoporosis occurs in men and women over the age of 70 and affects cortical and trabecular bone.
   B. The osteoclasts differentiated from mesenchymal cells lay down the matrix in the formation phase.
   C. Parathyroid hormone, calcitriol and other hormones such as glucocorticoids, growth, thyroid and sex hormones are the major systemic regulators.
   D. The disruption of the microarchitecture in trabecular bone, decreased density and changed bone material quality lead to bone fragility.
3. The following are true of Paget's disease, EXCEPT:
   A. There is increased bone resorption.
   B. The disordered bone may be largely avascular.
   C. Genetic and environmental factors are implicated in Paget's disease.
   D. Any one of the several bones may be affected most in the skull, tibiae, vertebrae and clavicle.

4. The following in relation to fractures in the elderly with osteoporosis are true, EXCEPT:
   A. Vertebral fractures are the result of a combination of ageing and bone fragility.
   B. The fracture sites in osteoporosis are the ribs, clavicle and vertebrae.
   C. Sacral insufficiency fractures occur in osteoporotic bone, metabolic bone disease and following radiotherapy.
   D. In men vertebral fractures are associated with severe trauma.

Answers to MCQs

1 = D; 2 = B; 3 = B; 4 = B.

References

Bone, Bone Formation and Changes with Ageing

1. Clarke B. Normal bone anatomy and physiology. CJASN. 2008;3 Suppl 3:S131–9.
2. Eriksen EF, Axelrod DN, Melsen F. Bone histomorphometry. New York: Raven Press; 1994. p. 11–125.
3. Logan JG, Basett D, Cheung MS. Paediatric bone pathology and monitiring the safety and efficacy of bone drugs in children. Bone drugs paediatrics: efficacy and challenges. Klein GL, editor. US: Springer; 2014. IBSM 9978-1-4899-7435-8.
4. Munday GR. Bone remodelling and its disorders. London: Martin Dunitz; 1995.
5. Raisz LG. Physiology and pathophysiology of bone remodeling. Clin Chem. 1999;45(8): 1353–8.
6. International Osteoporosis Foundation. Pathophysiology: biological causes of osteoporosis. http://www.iofbonehealth.org/pathpphysiology-biological-causes-osteoporosis. Accessed 13 Aug 2013.
7. Yasuda H, Shima N, Nakagawa N, Yamaguchi K, Kinosaki M, Mochizuki S, et al. Osteoclast differentiation factor is a ligand for osteoprotegerin/osteoclastogenesis-inhibitory factor and is identical to TRANCE/RANKL. Proc Natl Acad Sci U S A. 1996;95:3597–602.
8. Suda Y, Takahashi N, Udagawa N, Jimi E, Gillepsi MT, Martin TJ, et al. Modulation of osteoclast differentiation and function by the new members of the tumour necrosis factor receptor and ligand families. Endocr Rev. 1999;20:345–57.
9. Bilzerkian JP, Raisz LG, Rodon GA. In: Bilezikian JP, Raisz LG, Rodan GA, editors. Principles of bone biology. San Diego: Academic; 2002. p. 979–94.
10. Boyl WJ, Simonet WS, Lacey DL. Osteoclast differentiation and activation. Nature. 2003;423:337–42.
11. Blair HC, Athanason NA. Recent advances in osteoclast biology and pathological bone resorption. Histol Histopathol. 2004;19:189–99.
12. Orwell ES. Toward an expanded understanding of the role of the periosteum in skeletal health. J Bone Miner Res. 2003;18:949–54.
13. Pacifici R. Cytokines, oestrogen and postmenopausal osteoporosis-the second decade. Endocrinology. 1998;139:2659–61.
14. Hellman P, Curling T, Rask L, Akerstrom G. Pathophysiology of primary hyperparathyroidism. Histol Histopathol. 2000;15(2):619–22.

15. Li YC, Amling M, Pirro AE, Priemel M, Mense J, Baron R, et al. Normalization of mineral ion homeostasis by dietary means prevents hyperparathyroidism, rickets and osteomalacia, but not alopecia in vitamin receptor-ablated mice. Endocrinology. 1998;139:4391–6.
16. Pilbeam CC, Harrison JR, Raisz LG. Prostaglandins and bone metabolism. In: Bilezikian JP, Raisz LG, Rodan GA, editors. Principles of biology. San Diego: Academic; 2002. p. 979–94.
17. Exton-Smith AN, Millard PH, Payne PR, Wheeler EF. Pattern of development and loss of bone with age. Lancet. 1969;2:1154–7.
18. Diaz MN, O'Neill TW, Silman T. The influence of family history of hip fracture on the risk of vertebral deformities in men and women: the European Vertebral Osteoporosis Study. Bone. 1997;20:147–9.
19. Johnston Jr CC, Slemenda CW. Pathogenesis of osteoporosis. Bone. 1995;17:195–225.
20. Handy RC, Anderson JS, Whalen KE, Harvill LM. Regional differences in bone density of young men involved in different exercises. Med Sci Sports Exerc. 1994;26:884–8.
21. Anderson FH. Osteoporosis in men. Int J Clin Pract. 1998;52:176–80.
22. Stepan T, Tesarva A, Havranek KT, Jodl J, Normankora J, Pacovsky V. Age and sex dependency of the biochemical indices of bone remodelling. Clin Chun Acta. 1985;151:273–83.
23. Nilas L, Christiansen C. Rates of bone loss in normal women. Evidence of accelerated trabecular loss after menopause. Eur J Clin Invest. 1988;18:529–34.
24. Mazess RB, Barden HS, Ettinger M, Johnston C, Dawson-Hughes B, Baran D, et al. Spine and femur density using dual photon absorptiometry in US white women. Bone Miner. 1987;2:211–9.
25. Kiebzak GM. Age-related bone changes. Experimental Gerontol. 1991;26(2):171–87 (abstract).
26. Zioupos P. Ageing human bone: factors affecting its biomechanical properties and the role of collagen. J Biomater Appl. 2001;15(1):187–229 (abstract).
27. Parfitt AM. Age-related structural changes in trabecular and cortical bone: cellular mechanisms and biomechanical consequences. Calcified Tissue Internat. 2006;36:S123–8 (abstract).
28. Carter DR, Hayes WC. Bone compressive strength: the influence of density and strain rate. Science. 1976;194:1174–6.
29. Gibson LJ. The mechanical behaviour of cancellous bone. J Biomech. 1985;18:317–28.
30. Linde F, Norgaard P, Hvid L, Odgaart A, Soballe K. Mechanical properties of trabecular bone, dependency on strain rate. J Biomech. 1991;24:803–9.
31. Seeman E. From density to structure: growing us and growing old on the surface of the bone. J Bone Min Res. 1997;12:1–12.
32. Dutta C. Significance of sarcopenia in the elderly. J Nutr. 1997;127:992S–3.
33. Pocock NA, Eisaman JA, Hopper JL, Yeates MG, Sambrook PN, Ebert S, et al. Genetic determinants of bone mass in adults: a twin study. J Clin Invest. 1987;80:706–10.
34. Bailey AJ, Sims TJ, Ebbesen JP, Mansell JP, Thomsen JS, Mosekilde L, et al. Age-related changes in the biochemical properties of human cancellous bone collagen: relationship to bone strength. Calcif Tissue Int. 1999;65:203–10.

Osteoporosis

35. Anon. Consensus development conference: diagnosis prophylaxis and treatment of osteoporosis. Sam J Med. 1993;94:646–50.
36. World Health Organisation. 5. Population nutrient intake goals for preventing diet-related chronic disease. http://www.who.int/nutrition/topics/5_population_nutrient/en/index.25html. Retrieved 10 Aug 2013.
37. Lane JM, Russell L, Kahn SN. Osteoporosis. Clin Orthop Relat Res. 2000;372:139–50 (abstract).
38. Jones G, Nguyen T, Sambrook PV, Kelly PJ, Gilbert C, Eisman JA, et al. Symptomatic fracture incidence in elderly men and women: the Dubbo Osteoporosis Epidemiological Study (DOES). Osteoporosis Int. 1994;4:277–82.

39. Gass M, Dawson-Hughes B. Preventing osteoporosis – related fractures: an overview. Am J Med. 2006;119(4):S3–11 (abstract).
40. Sanders KM, Nicholoson GC, Ugone AM, Pasco JA, Seeman E, Kotowicz MA, et al. Health burden of hip and other fractures in Australia beyond 2000. Projections made on the Geelong Osteoporosis study. Med J Aust. 1999;170:467–76.
41. Access Economics. The burden of brittle bones. Cost of osteoporosis in Australia. Canberra: Access Economics; 2001.
42. Raiz L. Pathogenesis of osteoporosis: concepts, conflicts and prospects. J Clin Invest. 2005;115(12):3318–25.
43. Yasuda H, Shima N, Nakagawa N, Yamaguchi K, Knosaki M, Mochizuki S, et al. Osteoclast differentiation factor is a ligand for osteoprotegerin/osteoclastogenesis-inhibitory factor and is identical to TRANCE/RANKL. Proc Natl Acad Sci U S A. 1998;95(7):3597–602.
44. International Osteoporosis Foundation. Pathophysiology: biological causes of osteoporosis. http://www.iofbonehealth.org/pathpphysiology-biological-causes-osteoporosis. Retrieved 13 Aug 2013.
45. Dennison E, Cooper C. The epidemiology of osteoporosis. Brit Int Clin Pract. 1996;50: 33–6.
46. Hadjidakis DJ, Androulakis II. Bone remodelling. Ann N Y Acad Sci. 2006;1092:385–96 (abstract).
47. Raisz LG. Physiology and pathophysiology of bone remodelling. Clin Chem. 1998;45(8):1353–8 (abstract).
48. Heaney RP. Pathophysiology of osteoporosis. Endocrinol Metab Clin North Am. 1998;27(2):255–65.
49. Gorman D, Poole P, Sir Scott J. Osteoporosis: it's time to 'mind the gap' Editorial. Int Med J. 2007;37:672–3.
50. Cauley JA. Osteoporosis in men: prevalence and investigation. Clin Cornerstone. 2006;8 Suppl 3:S20–5 (abstract).
51. O'Neill TW, Felsenberg D, Varlow J, Cooper C, Kanis JA, Silman AJ. The prevalence of vertebral deformity in European men and women: the European Vertebral Osteoporosis Study. J Bone Mineral Res. 1996;11:1010–8.
52. Burger H, van Dale PLA, Grashuis K, Hofman A, Grobber DE, Shutte HE, et al. Vertebral deformities and functional impairment in men and women. J Bone Mineral Res. 1997;12:152–7.
53. Ebeling PR. Osteoporosis in men. New insights into aetiology pathogenesis, prevention and management. Drugs Aging. 1998;13:421–34.
54. Seeman E. Osteoporosis in men. Baillieres Clin Rheumatol. 1997,11(3).613–29 (abstract).
55. Kasperk CH, Wakley GK, Hierl T, Ziegler R. Gonadal and adrenal androgens are potent regulators of human bone cell metabolism in vitro. J Bone Mineral Res. 1997;12:464–71.
56. Belido T, Jilka RL, Boyce BF, Girasole G, Broxmeyer N, Dalrymple SA, et al. Regulation of interleukin-6, osteoclastogenesis and bone mass by androgens the role of the androgen receptors. J Clin Invest. 1995;95:2886–95.
57. Anderson FH, Francis RM, Bishop JC, Rawlings DJ. Effect of intermittent cyclical disodium etidronate therapy on bone mineral density in men with vertebral fractures. Age Ageing. 1997;26:359–65.
58. Smith EP, Boyd J, Frank GR, Takahashi H, Cohen RM, Specker B, et al. Oestrogen resistance caused by mutation in the oestrogen-receptor gene in man. NEJM. 1994;331:1056–61.
59. Anderson FH. Osteoporosis in men. Int J ClinPract. 1998;52:176–80.

Osteomalacia

60. Binet A, Kooh SW. Persistence of vitamin D deficiency rickets in Toronto in the 1990s. Can J Pub Health. 1996;87(4):227–30.
61. Woitge HW, Scheidt Navi C, Kissling C, Leidigbruckner G, Meyer K, Grauer A, et al. Seasonal variation of biochemical of bone turnover. J Clin Endocrinol Metab. 1998;83(1):68–75.

62. Annweiler C, Montero-Odass M, Schott AM, Berrut G, Chauvire V, Le Gal D, et al. Fall prevention and vitamin D in elderly: an overview of the key role of non-bone effects. J Neuroeng Rehabil. 2010;7:50.

Paget's Disease

63. Josse RG, Hanley DA, Kendler D, Ste Marie LG, Adachi JD, Brown J. Diagnosis and treatment of Paget's disease of bone. Clin Invest Med. 2007;30(5):E210–23 (abstract).
64. Cooper C, Harvey NC, Dennison EM, van Staa TP. Update on the epidemiology of Paget's disease of bone. J Bone Miner Res. 2006;21 Suppl 2:3–8 (abstract).
65. Elgazzar AH. Diagnosis of metabolic endocrine and congenial bone disease-Paget's disease (osteitis deformans). Chapter 3 in Orthopedic Nuclear Medicine. Elgazzar AH. Heidelberg: Springer-Verlag; 2004.
66. Siris ES, Lyles KW, Singer FR, Meunoier PJ. Medical management of Paget's disease of bone: indications for treatment and review of current therapies. J Bone Miner Res. 2006;21 Suppl 2:94–8 (abstract).
67. Daroszewska A, Ralston SH. Genetics of Paget's disease of bone. Clin Sci (Lond). 2005;109(3):257–63 (abstract).
68. Ralston SH, Langston AL, Reid IR. Pathogenesis and management of Paget's disease of bone. Lancet. 2008;372(9633):155–63 (abstract).
69. Mei AP. Paramyxovirus and Paget's disease: the affirmative view. Bone. 1999;24(5 suppl): 19S–21 (abstract).
70. Abelson A. A review of Paget's disease of bone with a focus on the efficacy and safety of zoledronic acid 5 mg. Curr Med Res. 2008;24(3):695–705 (abstract).

Hip Fracture

71. Maggi S, Kelsey JL, Litvak J, Heyse SP. Incidence of hip fractures in the elderly: a cross-national analysis. Osteoporosis Int. 1991;1(4):232–41 (abstract).
72. Jensen JS, Tandevold E. Mortality after hip fractures. Acta Orthop Scand. 1979;50:161–7.
73. Cummings SR, Kelsey JL, Nevitt MC, O'Dowd KJ. Epidemiology of osteoporosis and osteoporotic fractures. Epidemiol Rev. 1985;7:178–208.
74. Karagas MR, Lu-Yao GL, Barett JA, Beach ML, Baron JA. Heterogeneity of hip fractures age, sex and geographic patterns of femoral neck and trochanteric fractures among the US elderly. Am J Epidemiol. 1996;143:617.
75. Nyberg L, Gustafosn Y. Patient falls in stroke rehabilitation. Stroke. 1995;26:838–45.
76. Sinaki M. Falls fractures and hip pads. Curr Osteoporos Rep. 2004;2(4):131–7 (abstract).

Vertebral Fractures

77. Black D, Arden NK, Palermo L, Pearson J, Cummings SR. Prevalent vertebral fractures predict hip fractures and new vertebral deformities but not wrist fractures. J Bone Miner Resl. 1999;14:521–8.
78. Cooper C, Atkinson ED, Fallon WM, Melton 3rd LT. Incidence of clinically diagnosed vertebral fractures: a population based study in Rochester Minnesota. J Bone Miner Res. 1992;7:221–7.
79. Waterloo S, Ahmed LA, Center JR, Eisman J, Morseth B, Nguyen N, et al. Prevalence of vertebral fractures in women and men in the population-based Troms Study. BMC Muscular Skeletal Disorders. 2012;14:3. doi:10.1186/1471-247-13-3.

80. Haczyski J, Jakimiuk A. Vertebral fractures: a hidden problem of osteoporosis. Med Sci Monit. 2001;7(5):1108–17 (abstract).
81. Heaney RP. Pathophysiology of osteoporosis. Endocrinol Metab Clin North Am. 1998;27(2):255–65.
82. Dennison E, Cooper C. The epidemiology of osteoporosis. BJCP. 1996;50(1):33–6.
83. Seeman E. Osteoporosis in men. Baillieres Clin Rheumatol. 1997;11(3):613–29 (abstract).
84. Francis RM, Baillie SP, Chuck AJ, Crook PR, Dunn N, Fordham JN, et al. Acute and long term management of patients with vertebral fractures. QJM. 2004;97(2):63–74 (abstract).
85. Lips P, Obrant KJ. The pathogenesis and treatment of hip fractures. Osteoporosis Int. 1991;1(4):218–31.

Sacral Insufficiency Fractures

86. Cooper KL, Beabout JW, Sweet RG. Insufficiency fractures of the sacrum. Radiology. 1985;156:15–20.

Electrolyte Disturbances and Disorders of Mineral Metabolism in the Elderly

11

11.1 Anatomical and Physiological Age-Related Changes in Mineral Metabolism

With normal ageing there are physiological alterations in water and sodium regulation which may contribute to relative frequency of water and electrolyte disorders especially hyponatraemia [1]. Because of the age-associated changes in the renal and hormonal systems involved in regulating water and sodium balance, older people are at higher risk than the young [2]. The older individuals maintain body fluid homeostasis under most circumstances [3] despite losing 20–25 % of the original kidney volume. However their ability to withstand disease-related environmental stress or iatrogenic stress becomes increasingly narrowed. With each decade the glomerular filtration falls accompanied by limitation of sodium, potassium and acid excretion and decrease in urinary concentrating ability [3]. Water homeostasis falls due to the thirst sensation decreasing with age [4], and loss of autonomy and loss of cognitive function limit the access to beverages [3]. Dehydration is a frequent cause of morbidity and mortality in the elderly. In the elderly there is a decrease in fat free mass (which is hydrated and contains 73 % of water) due to losses of muscle mass, total body water and bone mass [5].

The metabolism of calcium and vitamin D is altered in a number of ways by ageing. The intake of calcium and vitamin D, exposure to sunlight, production of vitamin D in the skin, renal production of vitamin D, intestinal absorption of calcium and the ability to adapt to a low-calcium diet may be altered in the elderly, and the elderly are prone to develop vitamin deficiency [6]. 1,25(OH)2D_3 synthesis increases in low-calcium states because of increased parathyroid hormone activity [4]. The effect of these changes is a rise in the parathyroid hormone (PTH) in the elderly [3]. As a result of the increase in the PTH, the calcium level remains normal. Independent of the parathyroid hormone, low serum phosphorus can stimulate 1,25(OH)2D_3 synthesis, and low calcium levels can directly stimulate 1,25(OH)2D_3 1 alpha-hydroxylase activity [7]. However, the balance between bone formation and bone resorption is altered in favour of resorption resulting in a decrease in bone mass with

N. Nagaratnam et al., *Diseases in the Elderly: Age-Related Changes and Pathophysiology*, DOI 10.1007/978-3-319-25787-7_11

an increased risk of osteoporosis with ageing. Vitamin D deficiency is extremely common in the older adults [6] especially those in aged care facilities, older medical inpatients and in older homebound community dwellers.

Box 11.1. Key Points. Anatomical and Physiological Age-Related Changes in Mineral Metabolism

- With normal ageing there are physiological alterations in sodium and water regulation which may contribute to relative frequency of water and electrolyte disorders [1].
- Older people are at risk because of age-associated changes in renal and hormonal systems involved in regulating water and sodium balance [1].
  - With each decade the glomerular filtration falls accompanied by limitation of sodium, potassium and acid excretion and decrease in urinary concentrating ability [3].
- Water haemostasis falls due to the thirst sensation decreasing with age [4].
- The metabolism of calcium and vitamin D is altered in many ways by ageing.
- The effect of these changes is a rise in the parathyroid hormone in the elderly [3].

11.2 Disorders of Sodium

11.2.1 Hyponatraemia

Introduction

Hyponatraemia is characterised by a fall in the sodium level below 135 mmol/l. In a study of nursing home residents, 18 % of the residents had hyponatraemia and 53 % had experienced at least one episode in the previous 12 months [8]. About 11.3 % of geriatric patents are hyponatraemic [9].

Pathophysiology

Hyponatraemia or hypernatraemia results from water loading or deprivation following the inability of the kidneys to achieve maximal urine dilution and concentration. The hormones aldosterone, antidiuretic hormone (ADH) and atrial natriuretic peptide (ANP) regulate the fluid and electrolyte balance and partly control the changes in fluid balance in the elderly [10]. The secretion of aldosterone is also altered in the elderly and ANP is increased in the elderly about fivefold [11]. ANP has the ability to suppress aldosterone [12] which stimulates sodium resorption in the distal nephron [12]. Arginine vasopressin or antidiuretic hormone (AVP/ADH) is secreted by the posterior pituitary. Plasma osmolality is the most important variable regulating AVP/

ADH secretion [10]. Increased osmolality through activation of the anterior hypothalamus and decreased blood pressure and volume through the baroreceptors stimulate the secretion of AVP. AVP acts on the collecting tubules of the kidneys to increase resorption of water. The neurons of the hypothalamus where AVP is synthesised are not affected by age-related changes; in fact its production increases with age [13].

Increase in tonicity from increase in total body sodium stimulates the thirst centre and arginine vasopressin secretion [8]. Arginine vasopressin then acts on the V2 receptors in the renal tubules causing increased water reabsorption. In diuresis the opposite occurs [14]. Serum osmolality and sodium concentration are controlled by thirst, AVP and the kidneys [15]. When the osmolality is low below the osmotic threshold, AVP secretion is suppressed and the excretion of solute free water is increased to correct the low plasma osmolality. If there is failure to suppress AVP secretion, there will be water retention and hyponatraemia if the intake of hypotonic fluids is adequate. In the syndrome of In SIADH in spite of low osmolality, AVP release is not fully suppressed [16] and AVP levels are increased. SIADH may be due to a number of causes such as infection, drugs, malignancies and central nervous system disorders [17], and the syndrome is known to occur without identifiable cause in elderly patients [17–19]. The persistence of AVP (baroreceptor-mediated) release also occurs in oedema-forming disorders (cardiac, hepatic and renal) [20] associated with hyponatraemia (hypervolaemic hyponatraemia). Non-osmotic haemodynamic stimuli may also cause a persistent release of AVP resulting in water retention and hyponatraemia with hypovolaemia.

Hyponatraemia can be classified into two groups: (i) hyponatraemia of non-osmotic hypersecretion of vasopressin (hypervolaemic hyponatraemia, euvolaemic hyponatraemia and hypovolaemic hyponatraemia) [12, 14, 21] and (ii) hyponatraemia of non-hypervasopressinaemic origin [21–23] (pseudohyponatraemia, water intoxication and cerebral salt wasting [21]) determined by measurement of plasma osmolality, glucose, lipids and proteins [21] (Box 11.3).

Box 11.2. Key Points. Disorders of Sodium

- Hyponatraemia and hypernatraemia result from water loading or deprivation following inability of the kidneys to achieve maximal urine dilution and concentration.
- The hormones aldosterone, ADH and atrial natriuretic peptide (ANP) regulate fluid and electrolyte balance and partly control the changes in fluid balance in the elderly [3].
- The secretion of aldosterone is altered in the elderly and ANP is increased fivefold [11].
- Plasma osmolality is the most important variable regulating AVP/ADH secretion [3].
- Increased tonicity from increase total body sodium stimulates the thirst centre and arginine vasopressin (AVP) secretion.

- If there is failure to suppress AVP secretion, there will be water retention and hyponatraemia if the intake of hypotonic fluids is adequate [12, 14, 21–23].
- Hyponatraemia classified as (i) hyponatraemia of non-osmotic hypersecretion of vasopressin and (ii) hyponatraemia of non-hypervasopressinaemic origin determined by measurement of plasma osmolality, glucose, lipids and proteins.

Box 11.3. Classification of Hyponatraemia and Causes

- Hypervolaemic
  - Congestive heart failure
  - Hepatic cirrhosis
  - Nephrotic syndrome
- Euvolaemic
  - SIADH due to head injury, pneumonia, small cell lung cancer, hypothyroidism and adrenal gland disorder; polydipsia due to psychogenic cause, compulsive drinking or organic cause (e.g. drugs); tuberculosis drugs; carbamazepine; amiodarone; SSRI; chlorpromazine; and theophylline
- Hypovolaemic
  - Diuretics, after severe vomiting or diarrhoea [21, 22]

11.2.2 Hypernatraemia

Introduction
Hypernatraemia is defined as serum sodium level greater than 145 mmol/l (mEq/L). In hospitalised patients the frequency ranges between 0.3 and 3.4 % [24, 25].

Pathophysiology
Like hyponatraemia, hypernatraemia results from water loading or deprivation following the inability of the kidneys to achieve maximal concentration or dilution. With increasing age the physiological responses to water deprivation may be of particular interest in understanding the pathogenesis of hypernatraemia in the elderly [26]. There is a decrease in the percentage of total body water with ageing. There is a decline in the glomerular filtration rate and an increased incidence of renal disease with advancing years. Thirst sensation decreases with ageing and this is associated with loss of water in the urine and the ability to concentrate urine declines. There is extracellular volume (ECV) expansion due to reduced capacity to respond to sodium load, and conversely there is a reduced capacity for retaining

sodium making old people sensitive to salt depletion and ECV contraction [26]. Water losses may be isolated or may occur in conjunction with sodium losses. Thus hypernatraemia may be associated with hypervolaemia, hypovolaemia or euvolaemia [27].

Box 11.4. Causes of Hypernatraemia

I. Hypervolaemic hypernatraemia
- Mineralocorticoid excess
  - Adrenal tumours secreting dexycorticosterone
  - Adrenal hyperplasia
  - Iatrogenic administration of hypertonic fluid

II. Euvolaemic hypernatraemia
- Central diabetes insipidus
- Nephrogenic diabetes insidious
- Reset osmostat
- Iatrogenic
- Primary hypodipsia (geriatric)

III. Hypovolaemic hypernatraemia
- Gastrointestinal losses
- Dermal losses – burns, excessive sweating(endurance sportsmen/women)
- Loop diuretics
- Osmotic diuresis (urea, glucose)
- Renal disease [27]

11.3 Disorders of Potassium

Potassium Metabolism

Potassium is one of the body's important ions. With normal ageing the total body potassium declines and is the reflection of the decrease in the lean muscle mass. The daily intake is between 40 and 110 mmol/l and 90 % of which is taken up by the extracellular fluid (ECF) and subsequently excreted by the kidney. The remaining 10 % is excreted by the distal colon. The amount excreted equals the amount of intake. The kidney is the major regulator of long-term potassium homeostasis [28]. Disturbances of potassium homeostasis present as low or high serum potassium and are common among hospitalised patients. Potassium is filtered in the glomerulus and is passively reabsorbed in the proximal tubule and loop of Henle. Potassium balance is regulated by alterations in excretion in the distal renal tubule [29], and the degree of potassium secretion is regulated by three factors, namely, a rise in plasma aldosterone concentration, an increase in the potassium concentration and the increased delivery of water and sodium to the distal secretory site [30]. Aldosterone by increasing the number of open sodium channels in the luminal membrane stimulates sodium reabsorption. This loss of cationic sodium makes the lumen electronegative [31] and favours the secretion of serum potassium concentration and aldosterone secretion by enhancing the electric gradient [32]. With normal ageing the ability to regulate potassium excretion is not affected.

Ninety-eight per cent of the total body potassium stores is in the intracellular fluid and only 2 % is in the extracellular fluid with a normal potassium concentration at 3.5–5.0 mmol/l [33]. This uneven distribution of potassium indicates that a 50 % change in the plasma concentration can result from a 1 % shift in its distribution [34]. The ratio of intracellular to extracellular is the major determinant of resting membrane potential and is regulated by Na-K ATPase pump in the cell membrane [30]. Insulin [29] and catecholamines among others regulate serum potassium through changes in transcellular distribution of potassium and are important regulators of internal potassium balance [28].

11.3.1 Hypokalaemia

Hypokalaemia is defined as a potassium serum level of less than 3.5 mmol/l.

Pathophysiology
There are three mechanisms associated in the pathogenesis of hypokalaemia, namely, (i) dietary deficiency, (ii) increased excretion and (iii) transcellular shift. Dietary intake in itself rarely causes hypokalaemia. Inadequate intake may occur in association with anorexia nervosa, chronic alcoholism and inappropriate intravenous therapy. Excretion of potassium is increased by aldosterone, high delivery of sodium to the collecting duct (e.g. diuretics), high urine flow (osmotic diuresis) and delivery of negatively charged ions to the collecting ducts (e.g. bicarbonate) [35]. Hypokalaemia is due to shift into the cells and may be caused by medications, normal dysregulation or raised blood pH.

11.3.2 Hyperkalaemia

Hyperkalaemia is defined as serum potassium greater than 5.0 mmol/l and serum potassium is normally regulated around a narrow range of 3.5–5.0 mmol/l. Hyperkalaemia is a frequent occurrence in hospitalised patients with a reported incidence of 1.1–10 patients per 100 hospitalised [36, 37].

A common cause is excessive potassium supplement and other causes are hypoadrenalism or renal failure [38]. Medications [39] used for cardiovascular disease in a setting of impaired glomerular filtration rate commonly cause true elevations in serum potassium [40].

Box 11.5. Key Points. Disorders of Potassium

- With normal ageing the total body potassium declines and is the reflection of the decrease in the lean muscle mass.
- Potassium balance is regulated by alterations in the excretion in the distal renal tubule [29, 30].
- The degree of potassium secretion is regulated by three factors, namely, a rise in plasma aldosterone concentration, an increase in the potassium concentration and the increased delivery of water and sodium to the distal secretory site [30].
- Three mechanisms associated in the pathogenesis of hypokalaemia are (i) dietary deficiency, (ii) increased excretion and (iii) transcellular shift.
- Hypokalaemia due to shift into the cells is caused by medications, normal dysregulation or raised blood pH.
- A common cause of hyperkalaemia is excessive potassium supplement [38].

11.4 Disorders of Calcium Metabolism

11.4.1 Calcium Metabolism

The regulation of calcium is greatly influenced by parathyroid hormone (PTH), vitamin D and ionised calcium and their corresponding receptors and calcium-sensing receptor [41]. PTH is secreted by the parathyroid glands. Any decrease in the plasma calcium concentration is sensed by the parathyroid cells which release relevant preformed PTH into the circulation. PTH increases the plasma calcium by increasing renal and intestinal absorption of calcium and mobilising calcium and phosphate from the bone. PTH converts the inactive vitamin D (25(OH) D) to active vitamin D, 1,25 (OH)2 D (1,25-dihydroxycholecalciferol) calcitriol in the kidney. In the kidneys, PTH enhances reabsorption of calcium from the distal tubules. It also decreases renal PO_4 reabsorption and increases renal PO_4 losses. The metabolism of calcium and PO_4 is closely related and interacts in several basic processes [41]. The product of the concentrations of Ca and PO_4 is normally 60, and when this exceeds 70, crystals of $CaPO_4$ form and are precipitated.

1,25 dihydroxy vitamin D is primarily responsible for regulating the amount of calcium absorbed in the small intestine, and together with the PTH it is involved in the regulation of the mineral mobilisation from the bone. Calcitonin is produced by the thyroid in response to high calcium levels. Approximately 99 % of the body calcium is in the bone where it is complexed with other ions as hydroxyapatite crystals [41]. Approximately 1 % of the bone calcium is freely exchangeable with the ECF. Homeostasis is maintained by an extracellular to intracellular gradient which is largely due to high-energy phosphate intracellularly.

Normal total plasma calcium levels range from 2.20 to 2.60 mmol/l in healthy subjects [41]. About 40 % of this is bound to plasma proteins, primarily albumin. The remaining 60 % includes ionised together with calcium complexed with citrate and phosphate. Ideally the ionised or free calcium should be determined since this the physiological active form. Alterations in the plasma concentrations affect the total calcium concentrations and also the ionised fraction. The total calcium concentration can be corrected approximately by adding 0.1 mmol/l to calcium concentration for every 4 g/l that albumin is below 4.0 g/l and a similar subtraction for raised albumin. Hypercalcaemia and hypocalcaemia are both serious diseases.

11.4.2 Hypercalcaemia

Hypercalcaemia is defined as a total serum calcium concentration of more than 2.63 mmol/l in the presence of normal plasma protein concentration or ionised calcium of 1.4 mmol/l.

Pathophysiology
Malignancy (45 %) and hyperparathyroidism (16.5 %) [42, 43] are the most common causes of hypercalcaemia [44]. In primary hyperparathyroidism, there is excess production of PTH. In cases of hypercalcaemia due to malignancy, the patient usually is known to have a tumour, in some of them the PTHrP is elevated and in others there is elevation of other systemic factors. Hypercalcaemia caused by vitamin D excess is usually due to overdosage with calcitriol characterised by elevation of calcium and PO_4 and a suppressed serum PTH. Other causes include endocrine disorders such as hyperthyroidism and hypoadrenalism and granulomatous disorders such as sarcoidosis [43], tuberculosis, histoplasmosis and coccidioidomycosis. Medically induced causes include the thiazides, vitamin A, aluminium toxicity, milk-alkali syndrome [45] and lithium among others. Immobilisation [43] and especially high-risk patients are those with Paget's disease.

11.4.3 Hypocalcaemia

Hypocalcaemia is characterised by a plasma calcium concentration <2.20 mmol/l in the presence of normal plasma concentrations or a plasma ionised calcium concentration <1.17 mmol/l.

Causes
The causes of hypocalcaemia include hypoalbuminaemia, hypomagnesaemia, medication effects, surgical effects, PTH deficiency and vitamin D deficiency [45] and resistance [46]. It is rare for hypocalcaemia to occur from poor dietary intake of

calcium. It is more likely to be due to poor intake of vitamin D. Hypocalcaemia occurs in conditions where the plasma protein level is low as in nephrotic syndrome, cirrhosis of the liver, malabsorption syndrome and malnutrition. Hypocalcaemia is associated with conditions with low PTH levels (hypoparathyroidism) and with high PTH levels (secondary hyperparathyroidism). The former occurs where there is parathyroid destruction as a result of surgery [45], radiotherapy and infiltration by metastasis. The latter occurs as a result of vitamin D deficiency, vitamin D resistance and PTH resistance (pseudohypoparathyroidism).

Multiple Choice Questions

1. The following associated with hypercalcaemia are true, EXCEPT:
   A. Malignancy and hyperparathyroidism are the most common causes of hypercalcaemia.
   B. In case of hypercalcaemia due to malignancy (to have a tumour),in some the PTHrP is elevated.
   C. Hypercalcaemia occurs with immobilisation especially high-risk patients are those associated with Paget's disease.
   D. Hypercalcaemia caused by vitamin excess is usually due to calcitriol characterised by elevation of calcium, PO_4 and serum PTH.
2. In the elderly the following which may contribute to the development of hyponatraemia are true, EXCEPT:
   A. There is increase in the percentage of body water with ageing.
   B. There is a decline in the glomerular filtration rate.
   C. There is increased incidence of renal diseases with advancing years.
   D. Thirst increases with ageing with loss of water in the urine and inability to concentrate urine.
3. The following are true in relation to hyponatraemia in the elderly, EXCEPT:
   A. The secretion of aldosterone is altered in the elderly and atrial naturetic peptide is decreased in the elderly fivefold.
   B. Serum osmolality and sodium concentration are controlled by thirst, antidiuretic hormone and the kidney.
   C. In SIADH in spite of low osmolality, antidiuretic hormone release is not fully suppressed.
   D. SIADH is known to occur without an identifiable cause in the elderly.

Answers to MCQs

1 = D; 2 = D; 3 = D

References

Anatomical and Physiological Age-Related Changes-Mineral Metabolism

1. Miller M. Hyponatraemia in the elderly: risk factors clinical consequences and management. Clin Geriatrics. 2009;17(9):34–9.
2. Miller M. Fluid and electrolyte homeostasis in the elderly: physiological changes of ageing and clinical consequences. Bailleres Clin Endocrinol Metab. 1999;7:367–87.
3. Luckey AE, Parsa CJ. Fluid and electrolytes in the aged. Arch Surg. 2003;138:1055–60.
4. Phillips PA, Rolls BJ, Ledingham JG, Forsling ML, Morton JJ, Wollner L, et al. Reduced thirst after water deprivation in healthy elderly men. N Engl J Med. 1984;311:753–9.
5. Kumar R. Metabolism of 1,25-dihydroxyvitamin D3. Physiol Rev. 1984;64(2):478–504 (abstract).
6. Janssen HCJP, Samson MM, Verhear MJJ. Vitamin deficiency, muscle function and falls in the elderly people. Am J Clin Nutr. 2002;75(4):611–5.
7. Ferry M. Strategies for ensuring good hydration in the elderly. Nutr Rev. 2005;63(6 Pt 2):S22–9 (abstract).

Disorders of Sodium

8. Miller M, Morley JE, Rubenstein LZ. Hyponatraemia in a nursing home population. J Am Geriatr Soc. 1995;43:1410–3.
9. Sunderam SG, Mankikar GD. Hyponatraemia in the elderly. Age Ageing. 1983;12:77–80.
10. Luckey AE, Parsa CJ. Fluid and electrolytes in the ages. Arch Surg. 2003;138:1055–60.
11. Ohashi M, Fujo N, Nawata H, Kato K, Ibayashi H, Kangawa K, et al. High plasma concentrations of human atrial natriuretic polypeptide in aged man. J Clin Endocrinol Metab. 1987;64:81–5.
12. Biswas M, Des JS. Hyponatraemia in clinical practice. Postgrad Med J. 2007;83(280):373–8.
13. Miller M. Hyponatraemia in the elderly. Risk factors clinical consequences and management. Clin Geriatr. 2009;17(9):34–9.
14. Goh KP. Management of hyponatraemia. Am Fam Physician. 2004;69:2387–94 (abstract).
15. Kunhle U, Lewicki S, Fuller PJ. Endocrine disorders of sodium regulation. Horm Res. 2004;61(2):68–83.
16. Bartter FC, Schwartz WB. The syndrome of inappropriate secretion of anti-diuretic hormone. Am J Med. 1967;42:790–806.
17. Ditzel J. Hyponatraemia in an elderly woman and inappropriate secretion on antidiuretic hormone. Acta Med Scand. 1966;179:407–16.
18. Crowe M. Hyponatraemia due syndrome of inappropriate antidiuretic hormone secretion in the elderly. Ir Med J. 1980;73:482–3.
19. Hirshberg B, Ben-Yehuda A. The syndrome of inappropriate antidiuretic hormone secretion in the elderly. Am J Med. 1997;103:270–3.
20. Palm C, Reiman D, Gross P. Hyponatraemia-with comments on hypernatraemia. Ther Umsch. 2000;57(6):400–7 (abstract).
21. Laczi F. Etiology, diagnostics, and therapy of hyponatraemia. Orv Hetil. 2008;149(29):1347–54 (abstract).
22. Weisberg LP. Pseudohyponatraemia: a reappraisal. Am J Med. 1989;86(3):315–8 (abstract).
23. Aw TC, Kiechie FL. Pseudohyponatraemia. Am J Emerg Med. 1985;3(3):236–9 (abstract).
24. Palevsky PM, Bhagra R, Greenberg A. Hypernatraemia in hospitalised patients. Ann Intern Med. 1996;124(2):197–203 (abstract).

25. Aiyagiri V, Deibert E, Diringer MN. Hypernatraemia in the neurologic intensive care unit: how high is too high? J Crit Care. 2000;21:163–72.
26. Andreucci V, Russo D, Cianciaruso B, Andreucci M. Some sodium potassium and water changes in the elderly and their treatment. Nephrol Dial Transplant. 1996;(11 Supp 19):9–17.
27. Rudolph EH, Pendergraft WF, Lerma EV. Hypernatraemia. Hospital Physician www.turner.white.com/pdf/brm_IM_V14P1.pdf. Retrieved 1 Mar 2015.

Disorders of Potassium

28. Rastergar A, Soleimani M. Hypokalaemia and hyperkalaemia. Postgrad Med J. 2001;77: 759–64.
29. Stockigt JR. Potassium metabolism. Anaesth Intensive Care. 1977;5(4):317–25 (abstract).
30. Rose BD, Post TW. Clinical physiology of acid-base and electrolyte disorders. 5th ed. New York: McGraw-Hill; 2001. p. 383–96.
31. Suki WN. Disposition and regulation of body potassium: an overview. Am J Med Sci. 1976;272(1):31–41 (abstract).
32. Rose BD, Sterns RH, Post TW. Causes of Hyperkalaemia. In UpToDate. Physician level topic. 2008.
33. Traeger KA, Wen S-F. Pathophysiology of potassium metabolism. http://mededconnect.com/samplechapters/9781416043911/Sample%20Chapter.pdf. Accessed 2 Mar 2015.
34. Urwin RJ, Luft FC, Shirley DG. Pathophysiology and management of hypokalaemia: a clinical perspective. Nat Rev Nephrol. 2011;7:75.
35. Lederer E, Ouseph R, Yasel L. Hypokalaemia e Medicine 2007. http://www.google.com.au/search/hl=en&q=pathophysiology+hypokalaemia&btngG=Google+Search &meta=
36. Paici B, Gray TM, McBride D, et al. Hyperkalaemia in patients in hospital. Br Med J. 1983;286:1159–92.
37. Moore ML, Bailey RR. Hyperkalaemia in patients in hospital. N Z Med J. 1989;102:557–8.
38. Willard MD. Disorders of potassium homeostasis. Vet Clin North Am Small Anim Pract. 1989;19(2):241–6 (abstract).
39. Pepin J, Shields C. Advances in diagnosis and management of hypokalaemia and hyperkalaemia in emergencies. Emerg Med Pract. 2012;14(2):1–7 (abstract).
40. Sood MM, Sood AR, Richardson R. Emergency management and commonly encountered outpatient scenarios in patients with hyperkalaemia. Mayo Clin Proc. 2007;82(12):1553–61 (abstract).

Disorders of Calcium Metabolism

41. Peacock M. Calcium metabolism in health and disease. Clin J Am Soc Nephrol. 2010; (5 Suppl 1):S23–30.
42. Frolich A. Prevalence of hypercalcaemia in normal and hospital populations. Dan Med Bull. 1998;45(4):436–9 (abstract).
43. Sexton TB, Cohen C. Hypercalcaemia and calcium metabolism in the elderly. Contem Geriatric Med. 1988;3:437–53 (abstract).
44. Koh LK. The diagnosis and management of hypercalcaemia. Ann Acad Med Singapore. 2003;32(1):129–39.
45. Cooper MS, Gittoes NJL. Diagnosis and management of hypocalcaemia. BMJ. 2008;336(7556): 1298–302.
46. Beach CB. Hypocalcaemia emedicine http://emedicine.midscape.com/activity/767260-overview. Accessed 13 Dec 2008.

Musculoskeletal Systems

12

12.1 Anatomical and Physiological Changes with Ageing

Sarcopenia is the loss of skeletal muscle mass, strength and quality [1] in unison with biological ageing [2]. Sarcopenia is common in adults over the age of 45 years and increases with age [3]. There is a reduction of muscle mass and strength in all elderly people. Muscle mass and strength reach a maximum in the second and third decade and gradually decline in middle age, and around the age of 80, the loss of muscle accelerates leading to progressive weakness [4]. By the age of 75, the muscle mass is halved and the adipose tissue doubled compared to that of a young adult. The rate and extent to which muscle changes occur are to some extent genetically determined.

The cause of sarcopenia is multifactorial [2, 5]. Several factors contribute and these include loss of neurons due to central nervous system decline, loss of muscle contractile function, humoral factors (growth hormone, testosterone and oestrogen are reduced with age), increase in catabolic mediators produced by the immune system [5] and reduced rate of skeletal muscle protein synthesis [2]. Other factors that are related to muscle loss in the elderly are reduced levels of physical activity [2, 6], increased rates of immobilisation [7] and deconditioning disease.

If sarcopenia progresses beyond a certain threshold of functional requirements, it leads to disability and frailty. It is found in 20–30 % of elderly over the age of 70 years and increases with advancing age [8]. According to Lang et al. [9], in frailty there is no single symptom crucial in its presentation, but rather it is clearly recognised by clinicians with its multiple manifestations, appearance, nutritional status, performance and health rates, among others. There is no way of knowing at what level of lean mass, sarcopenia is present. The New Mexico Health Survey measured appendicular muscle mass by dual energy X-ray absorptiometry (DEXA) in 883 Hispanic and non-Hispanic white men and women and defined sarcopenia as a muscle mass of two or more standard deviations below the mean for young healthy participants [10]. There is however a direct structure-function relationship between muscle loss and strength [6].

N. Nagaratnam et al., *Diseases in the Elderly: Age-Related Changes and Pathophysiology*, DOI 10.1007/978-3-319-25787-7_12

Muscle strength declines 20–30 % by 60 years and voluntary contractile strength of distal and proximal muscles in both men and women is decreased by 20–40 % [2]. The decline of muscle strength in old people is directly attributable to physiological and histological changes in the skeletal muscles [11, 12]. With age lipofuscin and adipose tissue are deposited in muscle tissue and the lost muscle tissue is replaced by fibrous tissue.

Ageing also affects the quality of the muscle. The muscle quality is dependent on fibre composition, contractility, fatigue characteristics and glucose metabolism and uptake [1]. Type II muscle fibres which cause forceful muscle contractions decrease to a greater extent than type I muscle fibres which maintain posture and are slow in contracting. There is an important relationship between muscle quality and muscle health. The forces generated by muscle contractions can be an important determinant of bone quality [1]; for instance, vertebral compression fractures in postmenopausal women may be due to inadequate support of the vertebral column by the surrounding back muscles [13]. The muscle may be able to attenuate the impact of forces on the bone after a fall and later the susceptibility to fracture [1]. On the other hand, it can augment the mechanical forces on the bone and thereby increase the risk of fracture [1]. Bone mass and density are lost especially in women after menopause. In both sexes bone mineral density decreases and the amount of bone formed during remodelling decreases with age. With age the joints become stiffer and less flexible. Ligaments and tendons decrease in strength. Changes are usually observed in the weight-bearing joints especially parts of the articular cartilage that are not covered by menisci. It is difficult to differentiate changes due to old age from changes of degenerative processes.

Box 12.1. Key Points. Anatomical and Physiological Changes with Ageing in the Musculoskeletal System

- Sarcopenia is the loss of skeletal muscle mass, strength and quality in unison with biological ageing [1, 2].
- Muscle mass and strength declines in middle age, and around the age of 80, the loss of muscle accelerates leading to progressive weakness [4].
- By 75 years muscle mass is halved and adipose tissue doubled.
- Several factors contribute including loss of neurons in the CNS, loss of muscle contractile function, humoral factors (growth hormone, testosterone, oestrogen are reduced with age), increase catabolic mediators and reduced rate of skeletal muscle protein synthesis [2].
- Other factors are reduced level of physical activity, increased rates of immobilisation and deconditioning disease [6, 7].
- Muscle strength declines 20–30 % by 60 years [8].
- Bone mass and density is lost.

12.2 Neck Pain (Cervical)

The most common causes of neck pain are (i) cervical spondylosis, (ii) cervical dysfunction, (iii) traumatic strain or spasm, (iv) disc prolapse and (v) fibromyalgia syndrome.

12.2.1 Cervical Spondylosis

Introduction
Cervical spondylosis is a chronic condition of the cervical spine with degenerative changes in the intervertebral discs' annulus fibrosus and calcification and formation of bony osteophytes [14] with narrowing of the spinal canal, neural foramina [15] and lateral recess, resulting in progressive spinal cord and/or nerve root compression. It is a common condition [16], and its incidence is increasing [17] and is a frequent cause of spinal cord dysfunction and nerve root compression in the elderly. It increases with age and affects both men and women. It is the most common cause of myelopathy. Ninety to ninety-five percent of the men over 50 years and 70–90 % of women over 60–65 years have radiological evidence of degenerative changes in the cervical spine [18, 19]. At the age of 60 years, half of the men and one-third of women had significant disease [20]. It had been reported that 23.6 % of patients with non-traumatic myelopathy had symptoms of cervical myelopathy [21].

Pathophysiology
Cervical spondylosis results from degenerative changes which embraces the intervertebral discs, facet joints [22], laminal arches and osteophytosis of the vertebral bodies with ligamentous and segmental instability [23]. The discs with natural processes of ageing together with other factors such as repetitive stress of occupation lose its elasticity resulting in radial fissuring of the annulus fibrosus. Herniation may occur when the inner nucleus pulposus bulges through the annulus fibrosus. Protrusions of the annulus can be posterolateral, midline posterior and far lateral. The central part of the nucleus becomes less hydrous, loses volume and degenerates. Osteophyte formation occurs in the margins of the vertebral bodies as a result of degenerative changes in the discs together with remodelling of the apophyseal joints [24]. The degeneration of the facet joints together with bony hypertrophy and thickening [25, 26] and folding [16] of the ligamentum flavum and the bulging annulus encroaches on the central canal leading to narrowing of the canal (central canal stenosis). The lateral recesses are the bony canals in which the nerve roots lie after they leave the thecal sac before they enter the nerve foramina and are associated with compression of the nerve root [27]. Further degeneration of the facet joints can cause bony outgrowths in the spine called osteophytes [24]. Thickening of the posterior longitudinal ligament decreases the cross-sectional area of the canal [28]. The ligaments, too, lose their elasticity and develop traction spurs. Facet

hypertrophy can cause stenosis of the spinal canal or where the spinal nerve roots exit [29]. The dorsal root ganglions are affected by lateral disc protrusions.

Common clinical syndromes associated with cervical spondylosis are myelopathy and radiculopathy [22, 23, 30] and both syndromes are distinct [23].

(i) Myelopathy
Cervical spondylotic myelopathy results from narrowing of the central canal resulting from degeneration of the facets with bony hypertrophy [29] and disc degeneration with bulging together with buckling of the ligament flavum [25, 26]. Although occasionally in about 5 % there is relentless progression to severe disability [31], the clinical features may improve or resolve spontaneously in about 18 % [32], and about 75 % will have a stepwise deterioration with stable periods in between [31] but complete reversal is rare once myelopathy occurs [18]. The spinal cord damage can be further aggravated by normal flexion and extension of the neck. During flexion the spinal cord lengthens stretching over the vertebral osteophytes, and extension causes buckling of the ligamentum flavum, thereby compressing the cord [33, 34].

(ii) Cervical Radiculopathy
Encroachment of the lateral recess and the neuroforamina by hypertrophy of the superior articular facet and disc fragments is the most common cause of chronic nerve root impingement. Acute herniated disc can cause cervical radiculopathy. C6 root is the most commonly affected and the next are C5 and C7 [35]. It manifests as pain in the neck radiating into either arm, forearm or hand and often accompanied by numbness. A high incidence of focal conduction block at C3–C4 and C4–C5 as compared to normal conduction at C5–C6 and C6–C7 was demonstrated characterising cervical myelopathy in the elderly [36].

Box 12.2. Key Points. Cervical Spondylosis

- Results from degenerative changes involving intervertebral discs, facet joints, laminal arches and osteophytosis of the vertebral bodies with ligamentous and segmental instability [22, 23].
- Herniation may occur.
- Clinical syndromes associated with cervical spondylosis are myelopathy and radiculopathy [23].
- Degeneration of the facet joints with bony hypertrophy and folding of the ligamentum flavum and bulging annulus encroaches on the central canal (canal stenosis) [16, 25, 26].
- In intraforaminal stenosis there is degenerative disease of the facets and hypertrophy.
- Hypertrophy of the superior anterior facet is the most common cause in lateral recess stenosis, after the nerve roots leave the thecal sac and before they enter the neuroforamen [27].

12.3 Pain in the Back

Introduction

Pain in the back, shoulders, hips and knees in the elderly are common complaints encountered by the primary care physician. The key to evaluation will require an understanding of the anatomy of the structures, a history, physical examination and knowledge of the common disorders that occur in the elderly. It is important to remember that symptomatic musculoskeletal pain may originate from many different sites. A thorough understanding of the functional anatomy of the vertebral column (the spine, intervertebral discs, spinal cord, spinal nerves, muscles and ligaments) and surrounding soft tissue is highly desirable in regard to assessment and diagnosis of musculoskeletal pain. Furthermore, a good working knowledge of the appendicular skeleton is required for thorough examination of the upper and lower limbs.

12.3.1 Low Back Pain (Lumbosacral)

In office practice prevalent estimates of the causes of low back pain [37–39] were (i) mechanical conditions (97 %) (the most common are lumbar strain and sprain followed by degenerative processes of discs and facets and herniated discs among others) and (ii) nonmechanical spinal conditions (about 1 %) such as neoplasia, infection and inflammatory arthritis and visceral disease which includes disease of the pelvic organs, renal disease, aortic aneurysm and gastrointestinal disease. As the patients get older the diagnostic probability change to malignancy/neoplasia, compression fractures, spinal stenosis and aortic aneurysms. Spinal stenosis due to hypertrophic degenerative processes and degenerative spondylolisthesis is more common in older people [37].

12.3.1.1 Muscular

(i) Lumbar strain

Lumber strain occurs in about 70 % of adults as a result of work or play and is the second most common symptom seen in the outpatients [40]. It occurs after an episode of twisting, lifting or bending with pain and tenderness in the lower lumbar area and often felt in the buttock and upper thigh. This follows the tear of muscle fibres or distal ligamentous attachments of the paraspinal muscles at the iliac crest (enthesopathy) or lower lumbar and/or upper sacral region. The terms strain and sprain have no anatomical or histological basis, and when such a diagnosis is made, it is in all probability idiopathic low back pain [37].

(ii) Piriformis syndrome

The piriformis muscle lies deep to the gluteal muscles. The sciatic nerve passes through it and is irritated by the muscle causing pain in the buttocks [41] and pain along the course of the sciatic nerve [42].

12.3.1.2 Intervertebral Discs

(i) Degenerative Disc Disease (DDD).

The discs with natural process of ageing and trauma and stress lose their elasticity, become dehydrated and become brittle. The central part of the disc becomes less hydrous and loses volume and its structure degenerates. There is fissuring of the annulus fibrosus usually radially and bulge usually diffusely. Patients with DDD complain of back pain and may complain of leg pain and numbness.

(ii) Herniated Disc

Herniation occurs when the inner nucleus pulposus bulges through the annulus fibrosus causing a protruding disc which may cause irritation of the spinal nerve. Sciatica is the hallmark of nerve root irritation and in 95 % of the cases there is disc protrusion. Depending on the nerve root involved, sciatica is characterised by pain radiating down the posterior or lateral aspect of the leg to the ankle or foot. Weakness may also occur in the areas supplied by that nerve.

(iii) Discogenic disease

This follows injury, infection and tear, and the patient usually presents with localised back pain. Infectious discitis is the primary infection of the intervertebral disc and adjoining vertebrae [14].

12.3.1.3 Spine

Spinal stenosis is the encroachment of bony or soft tissue structures in the spine on one or more of the neural elements giving rise to symptoms. It is usually associated with degenerative diseases of the discs and facets and can be classified on an anatomical basis, central canal, neuroforaminal and lateral recess [27]. (a) The most common cause of central canal stenosis is degenerative disease of the facets with bony hypertrophy, buckling of the ligament flavum and posterior longitudinal ligament and disc protrusion encroachment into the canal vertebral body (bone spurs) [43]. Severe spondylolisthesis and bony overgrowth from Paget's disease could cause central canal stenosis less commonly. (b) In neuroforaminal stenosis again there is degenerative disease of the facets and hypertrophy. Lateral disc protrusion is the most common cause of neuroforaminal stenosis with encroachment of the nerve root in the neuroforamen. (c) In lateral recess stenosis, the nerve roots after they leave the thecal sac and before they enter the neuroforamen lie in a bony canal called the lateral recess. Hypertrophy of the superior anterior facet is the most common cause, and the lateral recess is bound by the neuroforamen caudally and radially resulting in nerve root compression [27] (Fig. 12.1).

12.3.2 Osteoporotic Compression Fractures

Usually it is the middle or lower levels of the thoracic spine that are involved. Sudden back pain after a minor stress is not unusual. Patients could present with acute pain following severe flexion-compression force. Spontaneous vertebrae collapse is seen in elderly people with osteoporosis or on long-term glucocorticoids.

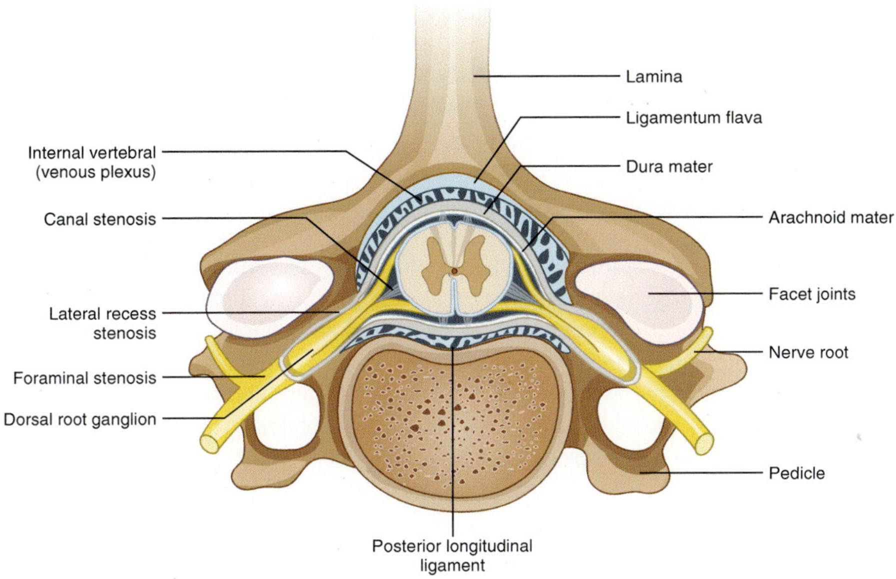

Fig. 12.1 Schematic diagram showing anatomical basis for spinal stenosis – central canal, neuroforaminal and lateral recess

(i) Neoplasia

Spinal tumours could be extradural, intradural extramedullary or intramedullary. The most common cause is metastasis and could involve the vertebral bodies and neural arches, but malignant infiltration could involve the epidural space without local bony involvement. About 80 % of the metastatic bone disease is from the breast, prostate and lung [44]. Other disseminated malignancies are multiple myeloma and lymphoma which are indistinguishable. Malignancy is often suggested by location (mid-back).

(ii) Spondylolisthesis

Spondylolisthesis is the forward subluxation of a vertebral body. In adults it results from degenerative changes and arthritis of the facet joints (degenerative) The other common type is spondylolytic [45]. Slippage usually occurs at L4 to L5 or L5 to S1.

(iii) Facet syndrome

Facet syndrome is a type of arthritis of the facet joints. There is degeneration of the facet joints with 'jamming' causing pinching of the sensitive meniscoid tabs within the joint. It may also cause pinching of the spinal nerves as they exit.

12.4 Shoulder Pain in the Elderly

Shoulder pain is usually due to injury to one of the structures comprising the joint. The exact prevalence of shoulder pain in the elderly is not known, one reason being the elderly not seeking medical attention [46, 47]. In the elderly community, the prevalence had been reported as 21 % and is more common in women than in men [47]. In cadaveric shoulders of the elderly, rupture of the tendon occurred in 20 % [48, 49]. The shoulder comprises the muscles, the glenohumeral joint, the capsules, the bones and the acromioclavicular joint. Shoulder pain is usually due to injury to one of the above-mentioned structures.

Pathophysiology
Burbank et al. [50] categorised chronic shoulder pain into six diagnostic categories, namely, rotator cuff disorders (tendinosis, tears and calcific tendinitis; adhesive capsulitis), glenohumeral osteoarthritis, acromioclavicular joint pathology and other chronic pathologies. The shoulder may be the site of referred pain – which includes heart attack, cholecystitis, Pancoast tumour, aortic aneurysm, axillary thrombosis and cervical or brachial plexus injury – and the pain is not altered by movements which are normal [51]. Basically shoulder pain in the elderly can be due to either periarthritis such as tendonitis, bursitis and capsulitis or arthritis such as osteoarthritis and rheumatoid arthritis.

12.5 Hip Pain in the Elderly

Introduction
In older adults 14.5 % of them experience significant hip pain, the women more so than man [52]. About 10 % of the population above the age of 55 years develop radiological signs of involvement during a mean follow-up of 6.6 years [53]. The incidence of symptomatic osteoarthritis has been reported as higher in women than in men, and this increased with age in both sexes until age 80 years and a slight decline thereafter [54].

Pathophysiology
Of the patients presenting with hip pain in primary care, 10–20 % can be attributed to trochanteric pain [55]. Hip pain can be categorised as anterior, lateral or posterior hip pain [56]. The common causes in the elderly are osteoarthritis, osteonecrosis, trochanteric bursitis, malignancy, osteoporosis, radiculopathy, labral tears and overuse.

12.6 Knee Pain in the Elderly

Introduction
Knee pain was twice as prevalent as hip pain in the elderly [57]. In a study comparing a random sample of 5,500 Oxfordshire residents over the age of 65 years, 19.2 % reported hip pain and 32 % reported knee pain [58]. In two other surveys the estimated annual incidence was 25 % in older adults with knee pain [59, 60]. One in six adults over the age of 55 years consults their doctor with knee pain in the course of 1 year [61].

Pathophysiology

Knee pain may be categorised as to the location of the pain. Anterior knee pain in the elderly is most commonly due to osteoarthritis of the knee which is caused by breakdown of the articular cartilage causing painful grating of the patellofemoral joint [62]. Posterior knee pain is caused by ligamentous injury, meniscal injury, bone injury, nerve injury, tendon and muscle injuries, knee cysts and bursal injury [63]. Medial knee pain results from involvement of the medial collateral ligament, medial cartilage and meniscal tear and arthritis. Lateral knee pain can be due to iliotibial band syndrome, injury to the lateral collateral ligament and lateral meniscal tear. Osteoarthritis is one of the five leading causes of disability in elderly men and women; a relatively common cause of pain in the knee in older women is osteonecrosis [64]. Knee pain in the elderly could be acute, chronic and acute or chronic.

Multiple Choice Questions

1. The following changes to the cervical spine are true, EXCEPT:
   A. Cervical spondylosis is the most common cause of myelopathy.
   B. Chronic nerve root impingement is caused by the encroachment of the lateral recess and the neuroforamina by hypertrophy of the superior articular facet and disc fragments.
   C. The dorsal root ganglions are affected by central disc protrusions.
   D. Thickening of the posterior longitudinal ligament decreases the cross-sectional area of the canal.
2. The following pathologies in relation to the spine are true, EXCEPT:
   A. The most common cause of central canal stenosis is degenerative disease of the facets with bony hypertrophy, buckling of the ligament flavum and posterior longitudinal ligament.
   B. In neuroforaminal stenosis there is degenerative disease of the facets and hypertrophy.
   C. Osteoporotic compression fractures usually occur in the upper levels of the thoracic spine.
   D. About 80 % of the metastatic bone disease in the spine is from the breast, prostate and lung.

Answers to MCQs

1 = C; 2 = C.

References

Anatomical and Physiological Changes with Aging -Musculoskeletal System

1. Dutta C. Significance of sarcopenia in the elderly. J Nutr. 1997;127:992S–3.
2. Doherty TJ. Invited review. Aging and sarcopenia. J Appl Physiol. 2003;95(4):1717–24 (abstract).

3. Iannuzzi-Sucich M, Preswood KM, Kenny AM. Prevalence of sarcopenia and prevalence of skeletal muscle mass in healthy older men and women. J Gerontol A Biol Sci Med Sci. 2002;57(12):M722–7 (abstract).
4. Spirduso WW. Physical dimensions of aging. Campaign: Human Kinetics; 1995.
5. Roubenoff R. Sarcopenia: a major modifiable cause of frailty in the elderly. J Nutr Health Aging. 2000;4(3):140–2 (abstract).
6. Roubenoff R. Sarcopenia and its implications for the elderly. Eur J Clin Nutr. 2000;54 Suppl 3:S40–S47 (b).
7. Muhiberg W, Sieber C. Sarcopenia and frailty in geriatric patients: implications for training and prevention. Z Gerontol Geriatr. 2004;37(1):2–8 (abstract).
8. Topinkova E. Aging, disability and frailty. Ann Nutr Metab. 2000;52(Suppl):1–6 (abstract).
9. Lang PO, Michel JP, Zekry D. Frailty syndrome: a transitional state in a dynamic process. Gerontology. 2009;55(5):539–49 (abstract).
10. Encyclopedia of aging. Sarcopenia 2002. website: http://www.encyclopedia.com/doc/1G2-3402200365.html.
11. Knight J, Nigam Y. Exploring the anatomy and physiology of aging. Parts-the nervous system. Nurs Times. 2008;104:3518–9.
12. Freemont AJ, Hoyland JA. Morphology mechanisms and pathology of musculo-skeletal aging. J Pathol. 2007;211(2):252–9.
13. Limburg PJ, Sinaki M, Rogers JW. A useful technique for measurement of back strength in osteoporotic and elderly patients. Mayo Clin Proc. 1991;68:39–44.

Neck Pain (Cervical)

14. Patient.co.uk. Cervical spondylosis. http://www.patient.co.uk/doctor/cervicalspondylosis-pro. Accessed 4 Mar 2015.
15. Ross J, Brant-Sawadzki M, Moore KR, Crim J, Chen MZ, Katzman GL, et al. Diagnostic neuroimaging. Spine Amursys. 2004;11(2):64–8.
16. Hirpara KM, Butler JS, Dolan RT, O'Byrne JM, Ponton AR. Nonoperative modalities to treat symptomatic cervical spondylosis. Advances Ortho. 2012;2012: Article ID 294857, 5 pages. http://dx.doi.org/10.1155/20122/294857.
17. Hid K, Yano S, Koyanagi I, Akino M, Seki T, Iwasaki Y. Surgical treatment of cervical spondylosis in the elderly. Surgical outcome, risk factors and complications. Neurol Med Chir (Tokyo). 2008;48(9):377–82 (abstract).
18. Al-Shatoury HAH, Galhom AA, Wagner FC. Cervical spondylosis. 2007. e medicine. http://www.emedicine.com/PMR/topic27.htm.
19. Gore DR, Sepic SB, Gardner GM. Roentgenographic findings of the cervical spondylotic asymptomatic people. Spine. 1986;11:521–5.
20. Holts S, Yates PO. Cervical spondylosis and nerve root lesions: incidence at routine autopsy. J Bone Joint Surg Br. 1961;48(3):407–23.
21. Moore AP, Blumhard E. A prospective survey of the causes of non traumatic spastic paraparesis and tetraparesis in 585 patient. Spinal Cord. 1997;35(6):361–7.
22. Shedid D, Benzel EC. Cervical spondylosis anatomy: pathophysiology and biomechanics. Neurosurgery. 2007;60(1 Suppl 11):S7–13 (abstract).
23. Lestini WF, Wiesel SW. The pathogenesis of cervical spondylosis. Clin Orthop Relat Res. 1989;239:69–93 (abstract).
24. Vernon-Roberts B, Pirie CJ. Degenerative changes in the intervertebral discs of the lumbar spine and their sequelae. Rheumatol Rehabil. 1977;16(1):13–21.
25. McCormack BM, Weinstein PR. Cervical spondylosis. An update. West J Med. 1996;165(1):43–51.
26. Young WT. Cervical spondylotic myelopathy: a common cause of spinal cord dysfunction in older persons. Am Fam Physician. 2000;62(5):1064–70.

27. Truumees E. Spinal stenosis: pathophysiology, clinical and radiologic classification. Instr Course Lect. 2005;54:287–302 (abstract).
28. Emery WF. Cervical spondylotic myelopathy. Diagnosis and treatment. J Am Acad Orthop Surg. 2001;9(6):376–88.
29. Cheung C. Morphopedis. http://morphopedics.wikidot.com/facet-joint-hypertrophy. Retrieved 3 Mar 2015.
30. McClure P. The degenerative spine: pathogenesis and rehabilitation concepts. J Hand Ther. 2000;13(2):165–74 (abstract).
31. Rao R. Cervical stenosis, myelopathy and radiculopathy. http://www.Knowyourback.org/pages/spinalcondition/degenerative conditions/stenosis_myelopathy_radiculopathy.
32. Kumar VG, Rea GL, Mervisl J, McGregor JM. Cervical spondylotic myelopathy: functional and radiographic long-term outcome after laminectomy and posterior fusion. Neurosurgery. 1999;44:771–8.
33. Fehlings MG, Skat G. A review of the pathophysiology of cervical spondylotic myelopathy with insights for potential novel mechanisms drawn from traumatic spinal cord injury. Spine (Phila Pa 1976). 1998;23(24):2730–7.
34. Young WF, Weaver M, Mishra B. Surgical outcome in patients with co-existing multiple sclerosis and spondylosis. Acta Neurol Scand. 1999;100(2):84–7.
35. Voorhies RM. Cervical spondylosis: recognition, differential diagnosis and management. Ochsner J. 2001;3(2):78–84.
36. Tani T, Yamamoto H, Kimora J. Cervical spondylotic myelopathy in elderly people: a high increase of conduction block C3/4 or C4/5. J Neurol Neurosurg Psychiatry. 1999;60(4):456–64 (abstract).
37. Deyo RA, Weinstein JN. Low back pain. N Engl J Med. 2001;344(5):363–6369.
38. Hart LG, Deyo RA, Cherkin DR. Physician office visits for low back pain, frequency, clinical evaluation and treatment patterns. US National Survey. Spine. 1995;20:31–9.
39. Deyo RA, Rainville J, Kent DL. What can the history and physical examination tell us about low back pain? JAMA. 1992;268:760–5.
40. Monteleone GP. Lumber strain: back to basics. http://medicine.hsc.wvh.edu/Fammed-Sports-Med//MedicalLibraries.Fammed-Sports-Med/Media/Documents/PDF/L-spine-pdf. Accessed 2 May 2014.
41. Cluett J. Piriformis syndrome. About.com.orthopedics. 2014. http://orthopedics.about.com/cs/sprainstrains/a/piriformis.htm. Retrieved 2 May 2014.
42. Boyajian-O'Neill LA, McClain RL, Coleman MK, Thomas PP. Diagnosis and management of piriformis syndrome. An osteopathic approach. J Am Osteopath Assoc. 2008;108(11):657–64.
43. Hsiang JK. Spinal stenosis. Medscape. Updated September 28, 2014. http://emedicine.medscape.com/article/1913265overview. Accessed 4 Mar 2015.
44. Maccauro G, Spineli MS, Mauro S, Perisano C, Graci C, Rosa MA. Physiopathology of spinal metastasis. Int J Surg Oncol. 2011:Article ID 107969. http://dx.doi.org/10.1155/2011/107969.
45. Orthoinfo.Acute spondylolisthesis in the low back. http://orthoinfo.aaos.org/topic.cfm?topic=A00588. Accessed 6 Mar 2015.

Shoulder Pain in the Elderly

46. Chard MD, Hazleman BL. Shoulder disorders in the elderly (a hospital study). Ann Rheum Dis. 1987;46:684–687.5.
47. Hermoso FE, Calvo E. Shoulder pain in the elderly. Aging Health. 2009;5(5):711–8 (abstract).
48. Codman EA, Akerson IB. The pathology associated with rupture of the supraspinatus tendon. Ann Surg. 1931;93:348–59.
49. Keyes EL. Anatomical observations on senile changers in the shoulder. J Bone Joint Surg Am. 1935;17:953–60.

50. Burbank KM, Stevenson JH, Czarnecki GR, Dorfman J. Chronic shoulder pain: part i. Evaluation and diagnosis. Am Fam Physician. 2008;77(4):453–60.
51. Anderson BC. Evaluation of patient with shoulder complaints. http://www.update.com/contents/evaluation-of-the-patient-with-shoulder-complaints. Accessed 4 May 2014.

Hip Pain in the Elderly

52. Christmas C, Crespo CJ, Franckowiak SC, Bathon JM, Bartlett SJ, Andersen RE. How common is hip pain among older adults? Results from the Third National and Nutrition Examination Survey. J Fam Pract. 2002;51(4):345–8.
53. Reijman M, Hazs J, Poos MJJC, Koes BW, Bierma-Zenastra SMA. X-ray findings strongly predict progression of osteoarthritis of the hip. Br Med J. 2005;380(7501):1183–5.
54. Oliveria SA, Felson DT, Reed JI, Grillo PA, Walker AM. Incidence of symptomatic hand hip and knee osteoarthritis among patients and health-maintenance organisation. Arthritis Rheum. 1995;38:1134–41.
55. Little H. Trochanteric bursitis: a common cause of pelvic girdle pain. Can Med Assoc J. 1979;120(4):456–8.
56. Roberts WN, Williams RB. Hip pain. Prim Care. 1988;15:783–93.

Knee Pain in the Elderly

57. Linsell L, Dawson J, Zondervan K, Ross P, Carr A, Randall T, et al. Population survey comparing older adults with hip versus knee pain in primary care. Br J Clin Pract. 2005;55(512):192–8 (abstract).
58. Dawson J, Linsell L, Zondervan K, Ross P, Randall T, Carr A, et al. Epidemiology of hip and knee pain and its impact on overall health status in older adults. Rheumatology (Oxford). 2004;43(4):497–504 (abstract).
59. O'Reilly SC, Muir KR, Doherty M. Screening for pain in knee osteoarthritis: which question? Ann Rheum Dis. 1996;55:931–3.
60. McAlindon TE, Cooper C, Kirwan JR, Dieppe PA. Knee pain and disability in the community. Br J Rheumatol. 1992;31:189–92.
61. Peat G, McCarney R, Croft P. Knee pain and osteoarthritis in older adults: a review of community burden and current use of primary health care. Ann Rheum Dis. 2001;60:91–7.
62. Pure Sports Medicine. http://wwwpuresportmed.com/Assets/KnowledgeFiles/001_Knowledge_Articles_Anterior Knee Pain.doc.pdf. Evaluation of acute knee pain in primary care. Ann Intern Med. 2003;139(7):575–88 (abstract).
63. English S, Perrit D. Posterior knee pain. Curr Rev Musculoskel Med. 2010;3(1–4):3–10. Retrieved 5 May 2014.
64. The Rubin Institute for Advanced Orthopedics (RIAO) Aging knee. http://www.lifebridgehealth.org/RIAO/AgingKnee.aspx. Retrieved 5 May 2014.

13 Arthritides in the Elderly

Age-Related Changes
With age, the joints become stiffer and less flexible, and ligaments and tendons decrease in strength. Changes are usually seen in the weight-bearing joints especially in parts of the articular cartilage. It is difficult to differentiate changes due to old age from changes of degenerative processes.

13.1 Rheumatoid Arthritis

Introduction
Rheumatoid arthritis (RA) is a chronic inflammatory disease characterised by uncontrolled non-suppurative proliferative synovitis and multisystem involvement. The prevalence is between 0.5 and 1 % of adult population worldwide with higher prevalence in women and the elderly [1]. It is the most common autoimmune disease in Australia and affects about 16.7 % of the population with almost 2 % disabled or handicapped with arthritis [2]. It causes severe disability, and 20–30 % become permanently work disabled within 2–3 years of diagnosis [3]. The incidence and prevalence increase with age [4], and about a third of the patients have their first symptom after the age of 60 years [5]. The peak onset is in the 3rd to 5th decades of life with an average age of onset of 42 ± 10 years [6]. There is another smaller peak in the sixth decade of life [7] 68 ± 4.6 years [6]. The prevalence increases with advancing years [7]. Elderly-onset rheumatoid arthritis (EORA) after the age of 60 [8] is distinctly different from the young-onset rheumatoid arthritis (YORA) [9, 10], genetically [7], prognostically and therapeutically [11]. In the elderly, it can take two forms: (i) continuing into old age with an 'earlier' onset and (ii) the elderly onset at the age of 60 years or over. Classical RA is twice as common in women than in men, but in EORA, there is a more balanced gender distribution [12].

N. Nagaratnam et al., *Diseases in the Elderly: Age-Related Changes and Pathophysiology*, DOI 10.1007/978-3-319-25787-7_13

Pathophysiology

RA is a systemic disease, and the pathogenesis involves autoimmunity, genetics and environmental factors [13, 14]. The pathophysiological mechanisms at the joint level involves an immune reaction leading to inflammation and associated with the formation of autoantibodies resulting through interactions of antigen-presenting cells with the adaptive immune system [15]. There is swelling and synovial proliferation with pannus formation followed by cartilage and bone destruction [15] indicating the inflammatory and autoimmune process [16]. The formation and deposition of antigen-antibody complexes within the synovium with secondary activation propagate the inflammatory response. Cytokines and chemokines are elaborated which propagate inflammation and recruit leucocytes to the synovium. Proinflammatory cytokines such as interleukin-1 (IL-1) and tissue necrosis factor-alpha (TNF-a) are central mediators in RA [16, 17]. IL-1 has been demonstrated in the synovial fluid, and disease activity correlates with IL-1 concentrations in the plasma [17, 18]. High levels of IL-1 are found in patients with erosive RA [19] and is the key indicator of synovial inflammation and pannus formation [20] and to the destruction of bone and cartilage [19, 21, 22]. Proinflammatory cytokines such as IL-1 and TNF-a play an important role in maintaining chronicity of RA mediating tissue damage [23]. EORA patients have different patterns of proinflammatory cytokines and clinical characteristics compared to YORA patients [24].

Family studies and HLA association studies have established the genetic predisposition to RA [14], and the contribution of HLA to heritability has been estimated to be 11–37 % [13]. The contribution of environmental factors has been established [14], and genetic susceptibility has also been linked with environmental factors especially smoking [13], periodontitis and viral infections [7]; Janus kinase inhibitors interfere with the signalling through type I and II cytokine receptors and has been shown to be critical in rheumatoid arthritis [25].

Box 13.1. Key Points. Rheumatoid Arthritis (RA)

- RA is a systemic disease. Pathogenesis involves autoimmunity, genetics and environmental factors [13, 14].
- Immune reaction leads to inflammation and formation of antibodies. Formation and deposition of antigen-antibody complexes within the synovium with secondary activation propagate the inflammatory response [15, 16].
- Proinflammatory cytokines such as interleukin-1 (IL-1) and tissue necrosis factor-alpha are central mediators in RA [17, 23].
- They play an important role in maintaining chronicity of RA mediating tissue damage [14].
- There is a genetic predisposition to RA [25].
- Janus kinase inhibitors interfere with the signalling through type I and II cytokine receptors and has been shown to be critical in RA.

13.2 Osteoarthritis

Introduction

Osteoarthritis is an arthropathy and is characterised by a slow and progressive degradation of the articular cartilage followed by subchondral sclerosis and formation of osteophytes on the margins of the joint. It can be monoarticular, oligoarticular or generalised. Prevalence increases to 10 % of men and 20 % of women between ages 45–60 years and to more than 50 % in women over the age of 85 year [26].

Pathophysiology

OA is characterised by an imbalance between extracellular matrix biosynthesis and extracellular matrix degradation at the molecular level, and the articular cartilage is the primary site of tissue injury response [27]. The cell/extracellular matrix (C/ECM) interactions are mediated by cell surface integrins which normally regulate growth and differentiation and maintain cartilage homeostasis [28]. In OA the integrins alter C/ECM modifying chondrocyte synthesis, and the vitality of the chondrocytes is crucial for the osteoarthritis process [29]. The ageing process is associated with declining chondrocyte function and also has an effect on cartilage extracellular matrix structure [30]. IL-1, IL-6, IL-17 and TNF-alpha and other pro-catabolic cytokines activate enzymatic degradation of cartilage matrix [28, 31]. The main enzymes involved in ECM breakdown are the collagenolytic enzymes [29] and the matrix metalloproteinases (MMPs) (MMP-1, MMP-8 and MMP-13). MMP activity is partially inhibited by the tissue inhibitors of MMPs (TIMPs) whose synthesis is low compared with MMP production in OA cartilage [28]. Growth factors such as tissue growth factor-b and insulin growth factor -1 may play a role in an attempt to repair cartilage by cartilage synthesis [32]. OA results when the cartilage breakdown exceeds cartilage synthesis.

Causes of osteoarthritis include ageing, overuse, trauma and metabolic abnormalities. Genetics may also contribute to the increased risk [33]. In certain families more recently an abnormal type of collagen gene had been recognised as a cause of OA. Chondrocalcinosis may be a factor for metabolic diseases such as haemochromatosis, hyperparathyroidism, hypothyroidism and hypomagnesaemia.

Box 13.2. Key Points. Osteoarthritis

- OA is an imbalance between extracellular matrix biosynthesis and extracellular matrix degradation at the molecular level [27].
- The articular cartilage is the primary site of tissue injury response [27].
- The cell surface intergrins alter C/ECM-modifying chondrocyte synthesis [29].
- The ageing process is associated with declining chondrocyte formation and also affects the cartilage extracellular matrix structure [30].
- The main enzymes involved in ECM breakdown are the collagenolytic enzymes [29].
- Genetics may also contribute to the increased risk [33].

13.3 Polymyalgia Rheumatica

Introduction
Polymyalgia rheumatica (PMR) is characterised by proximal myalgia of the shoulder and pelvic girdles accompanied by morning stiffness and non-specific systemic symptoms. In patients over the age of 50 years, the annual incidence was 20–50/100,000 [34].

Pathophysiology
It is of unknown aetiology. It is associated with HLA-DR4 haplotype [34] and with high levels of IL-2 and high level of IL-6 with increased disease activity. An autoimmune process may play a role. About 15 % of the patients with PMR develop giant cell arteritis (GCA), and half the patients with GCA have associated PMR. The focus for GCA appears to localise in elastin-containing arteries and can also cause myalgias [35]. About 16–20 % of patients with PMR demonstrated arteritis on histological examination requiring the diagnosis to be CGA [36]. Patients diagnosed as CGA and or PMR are found to have small vessel vasculitis and is considered a diagnostic criterion for PMR [37].

Box 13.3. Key Points. Polymyalgia Rheumatica (PMR)
- PMR is associated with HLA-DR4 haplotype and with high levels of IL-2 and IL-6 [34].
- An autoimmune process may play a role.
- Half the patients with giant cell arteritis are associated with PMR.
- PMR demonstrates arteritis on histological examination [36].
- CGA and PMR are found to have small vessel vasculitis [37].

13.4 Crystal-Induced Arthritis

13.4.1 Gout in the Elderly

Introduction
Gout is a common inflammatory arthropathy resulting from deposition of monosodium urate monohydrate crystals [38] in the tissues including the synovium and caused by overproduction and underexcretion of uric acid [39].

Gout occurs in two forms: classical gout presenting in middle age and elderly-onset gout (EOG), and because of its atypical presentation, it is often seen to be a separate entity and has been confirmed as the most common inflammatory arthropathy [40]. The former has its highest incidence in males, and men predominate in the ratio of 2:1 with females. EOG has however a more equal gender distribution [41], and women tend to develop gout at more advanced stage of life particularly after menopause. The incidence seems to be rising in the elderly, both in men and women in countries where the life expectancy is lengthening and the frequency of overuse of diuretics. The prevalence increases with age reaching 9 % in men and 6 % in women older than 81 years of age [42]. It often remains misdiagnosed, or the diagnosis is delayed despite the high prevalence [40]. In the United Kingdom, the prevalence of gout was reported as 1.4 % in 1999 and as high as 7 % in men older than 65 years in a study examining the epidemiology [43].

Pathophysiology

Gout predominately affects the middle ages and elderly people rarely occurring in young adults or children. There are two mechanisms of hyperuricaemia: (i) uric acid overproduction in 10–15 % of patients with primary gout and uric acid is a by-product of purine metabolism and (ii) impaired renal clearance of uric acid in the remainder of the patients (90 %) (Table 13.1). When the uric acid levels exceed 0.45 mmol/l with some variability depending on the pH and temperature, uric acid can crystallise. Asymptomatic hyperuricaemia is common and does not advance to clinical gout [39, 44].

Gout is caused by monosodium urate (MSU) crystal deposition in and around the joints and associated with increased blood levels of urate [45]. Urate and cation concentration levels together with changes in the extracellular matrix contribute to crystallisation, and crystal formation in the tissue fluids results in MSU deposition in the synovium and cell surface layer of cartilage [46]. Crystal-induced activation of cells appears to be the key mechanism responsible for gouty inflammation. The crystals are coated with lipoproteins apo E and apo B-100 which prevent the crystals from activating an inflammatory response [47]. According to one hypothesis, reactivation is brought about by exposure or by shedding of crystal of apo E and apo B by acute fluxes in the uric acid levels or minor trauma or can result from alcohol ingestion, trauma, haemorrhage, certain foods, starvation or medications such as diuretics. The bared areas can bind immunoglobulin M (IgM) which then stimulates neutrophils to engulf and phagocytise the crystals. This is followed by a brisk influx of neutrophils with elevated levels of interleukin -1, interleukin-6, interleukin-8, tumour necrosis factor-alpha, prostaglandin E2, leukotriene B4, kinins, C5a and other inflammatory mediators [48]. The precise roles of the individual inflammatory mediators remain unclear. Interleukin-1beta (IL-1b) and polynuclear neutrophils play an important role

Table 13.1 Causes of hyperuricaemia in gout

I. Increased uric acid production	II. Decreased uric acid clearance
Acquired causes	Acquired causes
High purine diet	Drugs (diuretics, aspirin)
Hypertriglyceridaemia	Renal disease
Myeloproliferative disorders	Hypertension
Lymphoproliferative disorders	Metabolic abnormalities
Alcohol consumption	Starvation/dehydration
Chemotherapy	Post-operative
Genetic causes	Genetic causes
Enzymatic deficiencies	Polycystic kidneys

in gout inflammation [49]. The mechanism of NLRP3 inflammasone activation remains unclear and leads to the secretion of MSU crystal-induced IL-1b although other proteases may be involved [49]. It is also envisaged that termination of attacks is brought about by recoating of the crystals by apo E and apo B [48]. Gout resolution involves several mechanisms besides protein coating on the monosodium urate crystals surface [49], but it is unclear whether the protein coating stops the inflammation or whether it cloaks the crystal surface to prevent detection by cells [50]. It is also possible that some of the mechanisms for spontaneous resolution may be brought about by clearance of apoptotic leucocytes by macrophages for triggering resolution [50]. Another mechanism is the prime mediator in active resolution of gout inflammation which is transforming growth factor –$beta_1$ [50] and may be involved in inflammation inactivity during intercritical period [51].

Box 13.4. Key Points. Gout in the Elderly

- Gout is a common inflammatory arthropathy resulting in deposition of monosodium urate monohydrate crystals in the tissues including the synovium [38, 39].
- Caused by overproduction and underexcretion of uric acid [39].
- Two mechanisms of hyperuricaemia: (i) uric acid overproduction in 10–15 % with primary gout (uric acid is a by-product of purine metabolism) and (ii) impaired clearance of uric acid in the remainder 90 %.
- Crystal-induced activation seems to be the mechanism responsible for gouty inflammation.
- The crystals are coated with lipoproteins apo E and apo B-100 which prevent the crystals from activating an inflammatory response [47].
- According to one hypothesis, activation is brought about by shedding of crystal of apo E and apo B by acute fluxes in the uric acid levels or minor trauma and by alcohol and certain food ingestion among others [48].
- Gout resolution involves several mechanisms besides protein coating on the monosodium urate crystal surface [53].

13.4.2 CPPD (Calcium Pyrophosphate Dihydrate (CPPD)) Crystal Deposition Disease:'Pseudogout'

Introduction

CPPD crystal deposition disease, a degenerative arthropathy with deposition of calcium pyrophosphate dehydrate crystals in the joints, fibrocartilage, bursae, capsules, ligaments and tendons, presents with variable manifestations, intermittent attacks of acute arthritis which may be severe or asymptomatic. The term 'pseudogout' refers to the clinical syndrome of one or more acute or subacute attacks of self-limiting inflammation caused by crystal deposition and synovitis. It is the second most common form of crystal-induced arthritis. It is common in the elderly [52], and its prevalence increases with age, 30–50 % in the 85 years and over. Both genders are equally affected.

Pathophysiology
The cause of the deposition of crystals is unclear. Majority of the patients with CPPD are over the age of 60 years where pre-existing joint damage from other metabolic conditions is common and together with the biochemical changes in ageing forms crystal nucleation. Release of CPPD crystals in the joint space is followed by phagocytosis by monocyte macrophages and neutrophils [52] resulting in the release of chemotactic and inflammatory substances. Mutation of specific genes such as ANKH and COL have been identified [53]. A minority of patients with CPPD have metabolic diseases. It is proven by the recovery of the crystals from a joint aspirate [54].

13.5 Psoriatic Arthropathy

Introduction
Psoriatic arthropathy (PsA) is a chronic inflammatory disease that develops in patients with psoriasis and involves the peripheral joints and spine and is usually seronegative for RF [55].

Pathophysiology
The arthropathy may arise before [56], with or after, and often as long as two decades after the onset of the skin disease. There is no relationship between the severity of skin changes and the severity of the arthritis. It presents as a diverse group of arthritis ranging from peripheral monoarticular and polyarticular disease to axial skeletal involvement. Despite this apparent diversity, the various presentations are bound by a continuous display of psoriasis, RF seronegativity, similar concomitance of human leucocyte antigen (HLA) and radiographic similarities. Elderly-onset PsA (EOPsA) has a more severe onset and more destructive outcome than in younger subjects [57].

Multiple Choice Questions

1. The following pathophysiological mechanisms in rheumatoid arthritis are true, EXCEPT:
   A. Swelling and synovial proliferation with pannus formation indicate inflammatory and autoimmune process in rheumatoid arthritis.
   B. Cytokines and chemokines are elevated which propagates inflammation and recruits neutrophils to the synovium.
   C. IL-1 has been demonstrated in the synovial fluid, but the disease activity does not correlate with IL-I concentrations in the plasma.
   D. Janus kinase inhibitors interfere with the signalling through type 1 and type II cytokine receptors and have been shown to be critical in rheumatoid arthritis.

2. The following pathological changes in osteoarthritis (OA) are true, EXCEPT:
   A. Ageing process is associated with declining chrondrocyte function
   B. OA is characterised by imbalance between extracellular matrix biosynthesis and extracellular matrix degradation at the molecular level.
   C. IL-1, IL-6, IL-17 and TNF-alpha inactivate enzymatic degradation of the cartilage matrix.
   D. OA results when cartilage breakdown exceeds cartilage synthesis.
3. The following statements in relation to polymyalgia rheumatica (PMR) are true, EXCEPT:
   A. PMR is associated with HLA-DR4 haplotype.
   B. Autoimmune process has no role in PMR.
   C. Patients diagnosed as giant cell arteritis (CGA) and PMR have small vessel vasculitis.
   D. Half the patients with GCA have associated PMR.
4. The following statements are true of gout, EXCEPT:
   A. Gout resolution involves several mechanisms besides protein coating on the monosodium urate crystals surface.
   B. Crystal-induced activation of cells is not the key mechanism responsible for gout inflammation.
   C. Minor trauma, alcohol, infection, haemorrhage and certain foods and medications can reactivate gout.
   D. Gout resolution involves several mechanisms besides protein coating on the monosodium urate crystals surface.

Answers to MCQs

1 = C; 2 = C; 3 = B; 4 = B.

References

Rheumatoid Arthritis

1. Kvien TK. Epidemiology and burden of illness of rheumatoid arthritis. Pharmacoeconomics. 2004;32:1–12.
2. Shanahan EM, Smith M, Roberts-Thomson L, Esterman A, Ahern M. Influence of rheumatoid arthritis on work participation in Australia. Intern Med J. 2008;38:166–73.
3. Rindfleisch JA, Muller D. Diagnosis and management of rheumatoid arthritis. Am Fam Physician. 2005;72:1036–47.
4. Negoescu A, Ostor AJ. Early recognition improves prognosis in elderly onset RA. Practitioner. 2014;258(1767):11–42 (abstract).
5. Diaz-Borjon A. Guidelines for the use of conventional and newer disease-modifying antirheumatic drugs in elderly patients with rheumatoid arthritis. Drugs Aging. 2009;26(4):273–93 (abstract).
6. Turkcapar N, Demir O, Atli T, Kopuk M, Turgay M, Kinikdi G, et al. Late onset rheumatoid arthritis: clinical and laboratory comparisons with younger onset patients. Arch Gerontol Geriatr. 2009;42(2):225–31.

7. Woodworth T, Ranganath V, Furst DE. Rheumatoid arthritis in the elderly: recent advances in understanding the pathogenesis, risk factors, comorbidities and risk-benefit of treatments. Aging Health. 2013;9(2):167–78. doi:10.2217/ahe.13.15.
8. Olivieri N, Pipitone N, D'Angelo S, Padula A, Salverani C. Late-onset rheumatoid arthritis and late-onset spondyloarthritis. Clin Exp Rheumatol. 2009;27 Suppl 55:S139–45.
9. Filipowicz-Sosnowski A, Rupinski R. Elderly onset rheumatoid arthritis. Pol Arch Med Wewn. 2008;(118 Suppl):36–42 (abstract).
10. Amador-Patarroyo MJ, Rodriguez AR, Oritz GM. How does age at onset influence the outcome of autoimmune diseases? Autoimmune Dis. 2012;2012:Article ID 251730, 7 pages. http://dx.doi.org/10.1155/2012/251730.
11. Deal CL, Meenan RF, Goldenberg DL, Anderson JJ, Sack B, Pastan RS, et al. The clinical features if elderly onset rheumatoid arthritis: a comparison with younger onset disease of similar duration. Arthritis Rheum. 1985;28(9):987–94.
12. Bajoochi G, La Corte R, Locaputo A, Goroni M, Trotta F. Elderly onset rheumatoid arthritis: clinical aspects. Clin Exp Rheumatol. 2000;18(4 Suppl 20):S49–50 (abstract).
13. Kurko J, Besenyei T, Laki J, Glant TT, Mikecz K, Szekanecz Z. Genetics of rheumatoid arthritis-a comprehensive review. Clin Rev Allergy Immunol. 2013;45(2):170–9 (abstract).
14. Kawabata K, Yamamoto K. Recent advances in the pathogenesis of rheumatoid arthritis. Clin Calcium. 2009;19(3):303–9. doi:CliCa0903303309, (abstract).
15. Agarwal SK. Biologic agents in rheumatoid arthritis: an update for managed care professionals. J Manag Care Pharm. 2011;17(9 Suppl B):S14–8 (abstract).
16. Gibofsky A. Overview of epidemiology pathophysiology and diagnosis of rheumatoid arthritis. Am J Manag Care. 2012;18:S285–302.
17. Chikanza IC, Kingsley G, Panayi S. Peripheral blood and synovial fluid monocyte expression of interleukin-1 alpha and -1 beta during active rheumatoid arthritis. J Rheumatol. 1995;22:600–8.
18. Eastgate JA, Symons JA, Wood NC, Grimlinton FM, Giovine FS, Duff GW. Correlation of plasma interleukin -1 levels with disease activity in rheumatoid arthritis. Lancet. 1988;21:706–9.
19. Fong KY, Boey ML, Koh WH, Feng PG. Cytokine concentrations in the synovial fluid and plasma of rheumatoid arthritis patients correlation with bony erosions. Clin Exp Rheumatol. 1994;12:55–8.
20. Arend WP, Dayer JM. Cytokines and cytokine inhibitors or antagonists in rheumatoid arthritis. Arthritis Rheum. 1990;33:305–15.
21. van den Beg WB. Joint inflammation and cartilage destruction may occur unrecognized. Springer Semin Immunopathol. 1998;20:149–64.
22. van den Lent PL, van De Loo FA, Holthuysen AE, van Den Berssalar LA, Vemeer H, Van Den Bergh B. Major role for IL-1 but not for TNF in early cartilage damage in immune complex in mice. J Rheumatol. 1995;22:2250–8.
23. Fantini F. New drugs and treatment strategies for rheumatoid arthritis. Recenti Prog Med. 2003;94(9):361–79 (abstract).
24. Chen DY, Hsieh TY, Chen YM, Hseih CW, Lau JL, Lin FJ, et al. Proinflammatory cytokine profiles of patients with elderly onset rheumatoid arthritis: a comparison with younger onset disease. Gerontology. 2001;55(3):250–8 (abstract).
25. O'Shea JJ, Kontzias A, Yamaoka K, Tanaka Y, Laurence A, et al. Janus kinase inhibitors in autoimmune diseases. Ann Rheum Dis. 2013;(72 Suppl 2):ii111–5.

Osteoarthritis

26. March LM, Bagga H. Epidemiology of osteoarthritis in Australia. Med J Aust. 2004;180(5 Suppl):S6–10.
27. Malemud CJ, Islam N, Haqqi TM. Pathophysiological mechanisms in osteoarthritis to novel therapeutic strategies. Cells Tissues Organs. 2003;174:34–48.

28. Iannone F, Lapadula G. The pathophysiology of osteoarthritis. Aging Clin Exp Res. 2003;15(5):364–72 (abstract).
29. Bagge E, Bjelli A, Edin S, Svanborg A. Osteoarhritis in the elderly: clinical and radiological findings in 78 and 85 years old. Ann Rheum Dis. 1991;50:535–9.
30. Hinton R, Moody RL, Davis AW, Thomas SF. Osteoarthritis: diagnosis and therapeutic considerations. Am Fam Physician. 2002;65:841–948.
31. Malemud CJ. Cytokines as therapeutic targets for osteoarthritis. BioDrugs. 2004;18(1):23–35 (abstract).
32. Manek NJ, Lane NE. Osteoarthritis: current concepts in diagnosis and management. Am Fam Physician. 2001;61:1795–804.
33. Goldring SR, Goldring MB. Clinical aspects, pathology and pathophysiology of osteoarthritis. J Musculoskelet Neuronal Interact. 2006;6:376–8.

Polymyalgia Rheumatica

34. Gardner GC. http://www.orthop.washington.edu/?q=patient-care/articles/arteries/continuing-medical–education-polmyalgia-rheumatica.html-1. Accessed 23 Aug 2013.
35. Wilske KR, Healey LA. Polymyalgia rheumatic and Giant call arteritis. The dilemma of therapy. Postgrad Med. 1985;77(8):243–8 (abstract).
36. Gonzales-Gay MA, Garcia-Porrua G, Miranda–Fillox J, Martin J. Giant cell arteritis and polymyalgia rheumatica: Pathophysiology and management. Drugs Aging. 2006;23(8):627–49.
37. Chatelain D, Duhant P, Loire R, Bosshard S, Pellet H, Piette TC, et al. Small vessel vasculitis surrounding inflamed temporal artery; a new diagnostic criterion for polymyalgia rheumatic. Arthritis Rheum. 2008;58(8):2565–73 (abstract).

Crystal-Induced Arthritis

38. Akahoshi T, Murakami Y, Kitasato H. Recent advances in crystal-induced acute inflammation. Curr Opin Rheumatol. 2007;19(2):146–50 (abstract).
39. Pitman JR, Bross MH. Diagnosis and management of gout. Am Fam Physician. 1999;59(7):1799–806 (abstract).
40. De Leonardis F, Govoni M, Colina M, Bruschi M, Trotta F. Elderly-onset gout: a review. Rheumatol Int. 2007;28:1–6.
41. Fam AG. Gout in the elderly: clinical presentation and treatment. Drugs Aging. 1998;13:229–43.
42. Arromdee E, Michel CJ, Growson CS, Fallon S, Gabriel SE. Epidemiology of gout: is the incidence rising? J Rheumatol. 2002;29:2403–6.
43. Mikuls TR, Farrar JT, Bilker WNB, Fernandes S, Schumocher Jr HC, Saag KG. Gout epidemiology: results from the United Kingdom general practice research data base 1990–1999. Ann Rheum Dis. 2005;64:267–72.
44. Eggebeen AT. Gout: an update. Am Fam Physician. 2007;76:801–8.
45. Martinin F. Mechanisms of uric acid crystal-mediated autoinflammation. Immunol Rev. 2010;233(1):218–32.
46. Choi HK, Mount DB, Reginato AM. Pathogenesis of gout. Ann Intern Med. 2005;143:499–516.
47. Terkeltaub RA, Dyer CA, Martin J, Curtiss LK. Apolipoprotein (apo)E inhibits the capacity of monosodium urate crystals to stimulate neutrophils; characterization of intra-articular apoE and demonstration of apoE binding to urate crystals in vivo. J Clin. 1991;87(1):20–6.
48. Miller AV, Ranatunge SM, Francis ML. Gout emedicine. http://emedicine.medscape.com/artile/329158-overview?src=seo_emed.

49. Ea HK. Mechanisms of gout inflammation. Presse Med. 2011;40(9 Pt 1):836–43 (abstract).
50. Martin WJ, Harper JL. Innate inflammation and resolution in acute gout. Immunol Cell Biol. 2010;88:18–9.
51. Fava R, Olsen N, Keski-Oja J, Moses H, Pincus T. Active and latent forms of for ongoing growth factor beta activity in synovial effusions. J Exp Med. 1989;169:291–6.
52. McCarty DJ. Crystal induced arthritis. Dis Mon. 1994;40(6):255–9.
53. Ea HR, Liote F. Calcium pyrophosphate dehydrate and basic calcium phosphate crystal-induced arthropathies: update on pathogenesis, clinical features and therapy. Curr Rheumatol Rep. 2004;6(3):221–7 (abstract).
54. Winzer M, Grassler J, Aringer M. Crystal-induced arthritis-old but important. Z Rheumatol. 2007;66:317–74 (abstract).

Psoriatic Arthropathy

55. Diez-Porres L, Munoz-Fernandez S, Aguado P, Alonso M, Martin-Mola E. Remitting sero-negative symmetrical synovitis with pitting oedema as he first presentation of psoriatic arthropathy. Rheumatology. 2002;41:1333–5.
56. Pitzalis C, Pipitone N. Psoriatic arthritis. J R Soc Med. 2000;93:412–5.
57. Punzi L, Pianon M, Rossini P, Schiaron FA, Gambari PF. Clinical and laboratory manifestations of elderly onset psoriatic arthritis: comparison with younger onset disease. Ann Rheum Dis. 1999;58(4):226–9 (abstract).

Organic Disorders of the Brain 14

14.1 Anatomical and Physiological Changes with Ageing: Brain

With advancing years a wide variety of changes have been described in the structure and function of the brain [1]. Different parts of the brain are affected differently and there is evidence in support of the contentions that the brain shrinks with age and the shrinkage is selective and not uniform or randomly distributed [2]. The rate of change in one region can be independent of the rate of change in another even within the brain structure [3]. The areas most susceptible to changes are the frontal and prefrontal lobe, basal ganglia, cerebellum, corpus callosum and the ventricles. Age-related brain volumes have been shown to decrease across adult age range, and after the age of 70 years, there is a stepping up of the atrophy [4]. MRI has revealed that the volume of the amygdala, hippocampus and temporal horn in healthy individuals remains relatively stable till age 60 years and then undergoes atrophy with age [5]. With age the cerebral hemispheres become atrophic. The greatest atrophy is seen in the association areas of the cortex, neostriatum and cerebellum with relative sparing of the sensory cortices and pons [2]. It is not clear whether the cortex or underlying white matter or both are accountable for the change; hence the term gyral atrophy is preferred. The ventricles and sulci become dilated with normal ageing and cerebral atrophy is variable and can vary from minimal to severe. There is a global decrease in the cortical volume with ageing and is most for superior temporal lobe, prefrontal cortex, primary visual cortex, auditory cortex and Wernicke's area [6]. In the older compared with the young, there is significant larger ventricular volume and small grey and white matter volumes in men compared to women [7]. Sulcal dilatation is typically seen with advancing age even if ventricular dilatation is not appreciable. The ventricular system increases at an average rate of 2.9 % per year compared to the total brain parenchyma; the shrinkage is only 0.18 % per annum; nevertheless, it increases with age [8].

There is a progressive loss of neural tissue with age. The ageing brain loses neurons and some of the supporting neuroglial cells. The loss of neurons is the most

N. Nagaratnam et al., *Diseases in the Elderly: Age-Related Changes and Pathophysiology*, DOI 10.1007/978-3-319-25787-7_14

significant age change in the nervous system although the traditional theories of neuronal loss with ageing have been challenged [9]. The cell loss is not confined to the cortical structures. The loss of neurons is not topographically random; the frontal poles, temporal lobes and hippocampus are more vulnerable than many brain stem structures. A significant amount of neural tissue is lost from the hippocampus [10]. The hippocampus atrophy was shown to be 29 % of the normal elderly and was strongly related to increasing age [2]. There a number of other changes as well. White matter loss also accounts for significant amount of brain shrinkage. White matter volume loss is delayed until middle adult life compared to grey matter volume loss which is constant throughout adult life [11]. White matter lesions (WML) termed *leukoaraiosis* are seen in the anterior frontal horns of the lateral ventricles in the age group 65 years and over [12]. Significant age-related differences in the white matter microstructure have been observed although the gross white matter volume remains stable across adult life [13, 14]. Two types of WML have been described, periventricular and deep white matter lesions. In the former, in early forms the lesions consist of caps around the frontal and occipital horns of the lateral ventricles. In the more advanced the changes take the form of a halo surrounding the lateral ventricles which extends into the white matter to a variable distance. They are non-vascular and are commonly seen in healthy elderly and in all dementias. The deep white matter lesions have a different pathology and are seen in many conditions such as in normal ageing and dementia The age-related differences in the regional brain volume together with the soundness of the white matter are associated with cognitive impairment [2].

The human brain can adapt itself to the ever-occurring changes by what has been termed *neuroplasticity*. It is the result of several different processes that occur throughout the lifetime. Neuroplasticity involves the reshaping of the brain not only in the developing years but throughout life and also in response to injuries or diseases. A new point of view claims that brain plasticity processes with certain constraints begin to predominate brain functioning with ageing [15, 16]. Several interrelated factors are involved in contributing to plastic changes in the brain that result in age-related functional decline [15]. Studies of adult brain plasticity have shown improvement in function and/or recovery using appropriately designed behavioural training programmes [15] from losses in cognition, memory, sensation and motor control [15]. There is increased plasticity at the nerve cell level with lengthening of the axons and sprouting of dendrites to partially compensate for the age-related loss of neurons [17]. The most plastic structures of the adult brain are the regions that present the greatest susceptibility to ageing [2]. The association areas, namely, the prefrontal, inferotemporal and posterior parietal cortices and the hippocampus are the areas where neogenesis occurs [18]. The growth-associated protein (GAP-43) is frequent in the association areas and rare in the tectum and brain stem [19, 20].

There is a deposition of a brown pigment called lipofuscin and its accumulation appears to be linear with increasing age. Other abnormal accumulations in the brain of the elderly are amyloid in the blood vessels, senile plaques and less frequently neurofibrillary tangles and Lewy bodies. There are several changes in the neurotransmitter systems throughout the life span of the individual, some related to maturation and others to senescence and which may vary from area to area as well as system to system [21]. Some of the behavioural abnormalities associated with ageing may be due to impaired transmission [22]. The four primary neurotransmitters involved in maintaining a balanced brain are acetylcholine, dopamine, gamma-aminobutyric acid (GABA) and serotonin. There is an age-related decline in the synthesis of the neurotransmitters and their receptors. At the cellular level neural death and neurochemical deficits occur in the cholinergic, serotonergic and GABAergic systems.

Acetylcholine is widely distributed in the nervous system. The central cholinergic neurons project to a widespread areas of the cortex. The cholinergic neurons of the basal forebrain complex have been described to undergo moderate degenerative changes with ageing [23]. Acetylcholine has been implicated to play a critical role in cortical activity, modulating cognitive performances, learning and memory processes [23]. In general dopamine appears to decline with age and as people age the number of dopamine receptors decrease significantly. Dopamine is a chemical transmitter and it affects function (movement), emotions, learning and behaviour. GABA is an inhibitory neurotransmitter found in multiple projections and local systems of the brain. Brain serotonergic projections are complex and embrace widespread areas of the cortex and limbic systems. Serotonin deficiency has been associated with normal ageing and neuropsychiatric disorders of late life and the occurrence of major depression [24].

Box 14.1. Key Points. Anatomical and Physiological Changes in the Ageing Brain

- The brain shrinks with age and the shrinkage is selective and not uniformly distributed [2].
- The areas most susceptible are the frontal, prefrontal, basal ganglia, cerebellum, corpus callosum and the ventricles.
- The cerebral hemispheres become atrophic.
- Sulcal dilatation is typically seen with advancing years even if ventricular dilatation is not appreciable.
- The ventricular system increases at an average rate of about 3 % per year [8].
- White matter loss also accounts for significant amount of brain damage.
- There is an age-related decline in the synthesis of neurotransmitters and their receptors.

14.2 Acute Confusional State in the Elderly

Introduction

Acute confusional state (ACS) is a disorder in which high cognitive and integrative functions become defective reflecting disturbance of global inattention and attention-directed disorders [25]. Basically it is a disorder of reduction and erratic shifting of attention [26]. Acute confusional state has also been referred to as acute delirium, acute brain syndrome, toxic psychosis and acute organic syndrome. The incidence of ACS among hospitalised patients was reported to be between 6 and 56 % [27–30]. One study found 42 % of the patients with ACS were between the ages of 70 and 75 years and 58 % in 76 years and over, with 67 % being females [31].

Pathophysiology

Elderly people are particularly vulnerable to acute confusion likely due to age-related cerebral changes and in the neurotransmitter system [32]. The presence of brain disorders associated with fewer neurons in the elderly people makes them susceptible [28]. The pathophysiology of delirium is complex and the mechanisms are poorly understood [33]. There are several observations upholding the hypothesis that multiple neurotransmitter abnormalities occur in delirium [34]. Due to abnormalities in the various neurotransmitters systems, the oxidative metabolism in the brain leads to brain dysfunction [32]. The neurotransmitters acetylcholine (ACh), dopamine, norepinephrine, glutamate, serotonin and gamma-aminobutyric acid may be involved in the development of delirium [33]. Physical stressful events giving rise to increased cortical secretion of cytokines may have a role, and some cytokines can influence the activity of the neurotransmitters and these mechanisms can interact [32]. The more important neurotransmitters are acetylcholine and dopamine. It has been demonstrated that elevated serum anticholinergic activity was independently associated with delirium and a large number of symptoms associated with delirium was associated with higher anticholinergic activity [35]. In support of ACh in the pathogenesis of delirium, anticholinergic medications or drugs with anticholinergic activity (antipsychotics, antidepressants, bladder relaxants among others) are known to cause delirium, and patients with impaired cholinergic transmission as in Alzheimer's disease are particularly susceptible to delirium. There is also increased dopaminergic activity in delirium and a reciprocal relationship exists between cholinergic and dopaminergic activity [34]. Patients with Parkinson's disease treated with L-dopa and/or dopamine agonists are frequently seen to become delirious. Delirium has been associated with disruption of the cortisol and beta-endorphin circadian rhythm. Olsson et al. [36] found that in hemispheric stroke patients with extensive limb paresis there are possible disturbances at different sites of the hypothalamic-pituitary-adrenal axis, and increased levels of dexamethasone-cortisol levels could be significantly correlated to the presence of delirium.

Those with multiple derangements are more likely to become confused, and the potential causes are innumerable with interaction of triggering factors superimposed on a susceptible patient with predisposing conditions. Some of the common risk factors that have been identified are advanced age, pre-existing underlying cognitive impairment, severe chronic illness and functional impairment [29], but the major risk factors for the development of delirium are age and dementia [37]. A number of precipitating factors have been put forward and more importantly include infections, metabolic disorders, drugs and intracerebral disease. Medications are the most common reversible cause of ACS [38, 39]. The point in question as to how inflammatory signals arising from systemic infection interact with stimuli that trigger the delirium has gained significant importance [40]. According to MacLullich et al. 2008 [41] triggers can be categorised into direct brain insults and aberrant stress responses. The inflammatory signals that arise during a systemic infection evoke a coordinated sickness behaviour response [42], and delirium is regarded as a maladaptive sickness behaviour response [40]. Severe deleterious effects on brain function can result from systemic infections; even mild infections that have minor effects in young healthy individuals can produce severe delirium in the elderly with dementia [37]. Multiple laboratory studies on aged animals too have shown that even mild acute systemic inflammation can bring about excessive sickness behaviour responses and cognitive dysfunction [40].

Box 14.2. Key Points. Acute Confusional State (ACS) in the Elderly

- ACS is a disorder of reduction and shifting of attention [25].
- Elderly people are particularly vulnerable because of age-related cerebral changes and neurotransmitter systems [32].
- The pathophysiology of ACS is complex [33].
- The more important neurotransmitters involved are acetylcholine and dopamine.
- Physical stress gives rise to increased cortical secretion of cytokines which may have a role for some cytokines can influence the activity of the neurotransmitters [32].
- Increased levels of dexamethasone-cortisol levels could be significantly correlated with delirium [36].
- Those with multiple derangements are more likely to be confused and potential causes are innumerable with interaction with precipitating factors.
- Medications are the most common reversible cause of ACS [40].
- Delirium is regarded as a maladaptive sickness behaviour response [38, 39].
- Severe deleterious effects on brain function can result from systemic infections; even mild infections that have minor effects in young healthy individuals can produce severe delirium in the elderly with dementia.

14.3 Dementia

Introduction

Dementia can be defined as a syndrome characterized by deterioration of one or more behavioural functions that leads to an incapacity for independent activity. It poses special difficulties with behavioural and psychological symptoms and debilitating psychological distress that caregivers may experience. Current demographic findings predict an increase in the elderly population more so the very elderly, and this trend is likely to continue. This means that the number of dementia patients and those with other age-related neurological disorders will increase [43]. In Europe dementia is more common than stroke in terms of both incidence and prevalence [44].

There are more than a hundred causes of dementia and classification can be a daunting task as symptoms tend to overlap. Neuropsychological examination allows the diagnosis of dementia and permits for a classification as 'cortical dementia' characterised by impairments in language (aphasia), praxis (apraxia) and visual perception (agnosia) with normal motor function and 'subcortical dementia characterised by psychomotor retardation, forgetfulness, apathy and inability to manipulate knowledge [45]. Parkinson's disease, progressive supranuclear palsy and Huntington's disease among others are associated with cognitive slowing and are examples of subcortical dementia. This concept of subcortical dementia has been challenged [46] that not all dementias can be neatly classified as either cortical or subcortical. It is not surprising that the subcortical dementias and frontal lobe syndromes are similar given their anatomical connections [47].

Drachman and Newel [48] classified the dementias on the basis of clinicopathological entities and presumed aetiological factors in two main groups, namely, 'static' occurring after a single event such as stroke, severe head trauma and encephalitis and 'progressive' which is divided into two main subtypes, 'symptomatic' and 'degenerative'. The former is caused by a known disease process, anatomical lesions such as brain tumours, normal hydrocephalus, toxic or metabolic like hypothyroidism and vitamin B_{12} deficiency and infection like Creutzfeldt-Jakob disease and human immunodeficiency virus. The latter is the degenerative dementias, namely, Alzheimer's disease, dementias associated with movement disorders, dementias associated with cortical lobar abnormalities and lastly the miscellaneous group. Although some definitions of dementia include that the cognitive impairment should be progressive, for the clinician the management problems encountered with 'static' cognitive impairment arising after an encephalitic illness or head injury are very similar to that of progressive dementias such Alzheimer's disease [49]. Most of the neuro-degenerative dementias are now identified as abnormalities of 3 proteins, the amyloid precursor protein (APP), tau and alpha-synuclein [50, 51] and classified according to their associated abnormalities [52]. In many there is an overlap of the proteins and the concomitance of tau and alpha synuclein is not rare [51]. In Alzheimer's disease A-beta peptide deposits and tau accumulate [53, 54].

14.3.1 Neurodegenerative Dementias

Introduction

The degenerative dementias include Alzheimer's disease, dementias associated with movement disorders, dementias associated with cortical lobar abnormalities and lastly a miscellaneous group. In a European study the incidence rates for possible and probable Alzheimer's disease and the most common form of dementia adjusted for age, sex and education were 1.2 per 1000 person years for 65 year old and 63.5 per 1000 person years for those above 90 years [55].

Pathophysiology
Neurofibrillary lesions made up of microtubule-associated protein tau are not only limited to Alzheimer's disease but also characterise a heterogeneous group of neurodegenerative disorders and clinically distinguished by dementia or/and motor symptoms [56] and grouped together under the general term tauopathies [56]. The degenerative dementias are now being reclassified according to the associated protein abnormalities although this classification does not necessarily help in the diagnosis but may facilitate development of strategies for the disease treatment and prevention [57]. Alzheimer's disease is a disorder of the amyloid precursor protein (APP); the frontotemporal dementia (FTD) syndromes and some of the extrapyramidal dementias (corticobasal, progressive supranuclear palsy) are associated with the microtubule-associated protein tau. Other degenerative diseases including Parkinson's disease, multiple system disease and Lewy body dementia are associated with alpha-synuclein.

14.3.1.1 Alzheimer's Disease (AD)

Introduction
Alzheimer's disease (AD) is a neurodegenerative disease characterised by progressive loss of memory and other cognitive functions and inability to perform basal activities of daily living together with behavioural and psychiatric symptoms.

Pathophysiology and genetic factors
The hallmarks of AD are the extracellular accumulation of amyloid beta (Abeta) peptides forming the core of the senile plaques and intracellular neurofibrillary tangles (NFTs) made up of the microtubule-associated protein tau in a hyperphosphorylated state [58]. This diminishes its ability to bind to tubulin resulting in destabilisation of the microtubule structure [59]. The primary function of tau is its ability to interact with alpha- and beta-globulin and stabilise the microtubules [60]. Free tau fractions are elevated when tau is hyperphosphorylated [61]. The hyperphosphorylated tau aggregates into oligomers to form paired helical filaments (PHFs) to generate NFTs [62], and several protein kinases are involved in this process [63]. Glycogen synthase kinase 3 beta (GSK-3 beta) is an important tau kinase and is overactive in AD and has been shown to hyperphosphorylate in transgenic mouse models in AD [64]. Abeta peptide arises from a large precursor, the amyloid peptide precursor (APP), and there two identified catabolic pathways for APP [65]. In the amyloidogenic pathway of APP, where the APP is cleaved by secretase enzymes, and after sequential cleavage of APP by beta and gamma secretases, neurotoxic Abeta peptides are released and amass into oligomeric aggregates [66] and induce neuronal apoptosis [65]. In the non-amyloidogenic pathway, APP is cleaved preferentially by beta-secretase [66] within the sequence of the amyloid peptide and hinders the formation of the full length Abeta found in the core of senile plaques [65].

While the mechanism in AD is unclear, several hypotheses have been postulated [67]. According to the amyloid cascade hypothesis, accumulation of senile plaques is made primarily by deposits of Abeta peptide in the initiating lesion in AD [68] and is due either to their increased production or decreased clearance of Abeta peptides [70] although the presence of tangles is essential to dementia [69]. The accumulation of Abeta is the main cause of neuronal degeneration and induces accumulation of tau in the AD brain [70]. Alternative hypothesis is the cytoskeletal changes that arise from the hyperphosphorylation of tau which leads to a cascade of events and finally causes neuronal death [66]. Neither cascade explains adequately the diversity of pathological processes underlying the disease [66, 67]. The Abeta deposits involve the neocortex while the intracellular tau accumulation mainly affects the hippocampal region [71].

Age at onset has been used to differentiate subtypes with 65 years arbitrarily used to distinguish the early from the late onset [72]. The rare autosomal dominant early-onset familial subtype occurs before the age of 65 years and is due to mutations in the genes presenilin 1 and presenilin 2 and the gene for amyloid precursor protein [73–76]. The genetic defects have been identified on chromosomes 21, 19, 14, 12 and 1. Of the early-onset cases of AD, less than 1 % of the cases are linked to chromosome 21. Presenilin 1 (PSEN1) on chromosome 14 is the most common and presenilin 2 (PSEN2) on chromosome 1 least common [75, 77]. The late onset associated with some families and the sporadic forms occurring after the age of 65 years is due to E4 variant of apolipoprotein E [73, 74].

Box 14.3. Key Points. Alzheimer's Disease (AD)

- The hallmarks of AD are the extracellular accumulation of amyloid beta (Abeta) peptides forming the core of senile plaques and intracellular neurofibrillary tangles (NFTs) made up of microtubule-associated protein tau in the hyperphosphorylated state [58].
- The hyperphosphorylated tau aggregates into oligomers to form paired helical filaments (PHFs) to generate NFTs and several protein kinases [62].
- GSK-3 beta is an important tau kinase and is overactive in AD [64].
- According to the amyloid cascade hypothesis, accumulation of senile plaques is made primarily by deposits of Abeta peptide in the initiation of AD [68].
- Alternative hypothesis is the cytoskeletal changes that give rise to hyperphosphorylation of tau which leads to a cascade of events and finally causes neuronal death [66].
- The rare autosomal dominant early-onset familial subtype is due to mutations in the genes presenilin 1 and presenilin 2 and the gene for amyloid precursor protein [73–76].

14.3.1.2 Frontotemporal Dementia and Other Focal Atrophies

Introduction

Cortical lobar atrophies are more common than realised. Localised cerebral atrophy refers to a group of degenerative disorders that present with distinctive clinical and neuropsychological features and have a high genetic element. It is debated whether some of them are part of a diffuse disease or in fact they are distinct entities.

14.3.1.3 Frontotemporal Dementia

Prominent involvement of the frontal and temporal lobes gives rise to frontotemporal dementia (FTD). FTD/Pick complex now refers to a group of diseases which include Pick's disease, frontotemporal lobar degeneration (FTLD), primary progressive aphasia (PPA), semantic dementia and corticobasal degeneration (CBD) [78]. FTD has also been described with motor neurone disease (MND). All these conditions could be considered as frontotemporal dementia, a part of Pick's complex. FTD primarily occurs between the ages of 45 and 65 years.

Pathophysiology

Aberrant mutation of tau protein is the fundamental neuropathological finding in FTD and this altered protein destabilises the microtubule structure [79]. The first mutation of the tau protein responsible for FTD and parkinsonism is linked with chromosome 17 (FTDP-17) [79]. It has been recognised that there is a clinical overlap between FTD and amyotrophic lateral sclerosis (ALS) and is characterised by neuronal inclusions that are immunoreactive to ubiquitin but not to tau and this pathogenic protein has been identified as TDP-43 [80].

14.3.1.4 Corticobasal Syndrome (CBD)

CBD is characterised by hyperphosphorylated tau forming abnormal filamentous inclusions in the neurons and glia [81].

Pathophysiology

The mean age of onset is 63 years and the youngest 45 years [82]. Both CBD and progressive supranuclear palsy (PSP) show a similar pattern of tau expression, but in CBD tau forms paired helical filaments [83]. Abnormality on chromosome may cause both diseases [84]. Corticobasal syndrome (CBS) with its constellation of features genetically, clinically and pathologically is similar to or overlaps FTD [85].

14.3.1.5 Posterior Cortical Atrophy

Posterior cortical atrophy is a progressive clinicoradiologic syndrome [86] characterised by an array of manifestations which include higher visual dysfunction and that of Balint's and Gerstmann's syndromes and transcortical sensory aphasia [87].

Pathophysiology

PCA has been attributed to the involvement of the parietal and occipital association cortices. Structural neuroimaging has demonstrated parieto-cortical atrophy, and functional imaging has revealed bilateral hypometabolism and hypoperfusion [88]. It is unclear whether the changes in white matter integrity are due to ageing process or to some other pathologies [89]. The syndrome is associated with a variety of underlying pathologies. The posterior cerebral areas show deposition of neuritic plaques and neurofibrillary tangles [90]. It is often defined as a variant or atypical form of Alzheimer's disease; however, the clinical presentation is distinctly different from Alzheimer's disease. CT and MRI demonstrate bilateral parieto-cortical atrophy but no detectable mesiotemporal atrophy as seen in Alzheimer's disease [90]. Damage to the association cortices of the occipitoparietal regions which is associated with visual-spatial integration produces disorders such as optic ataxia and simultanagnosia [91]. All the components need not be present to constitute the syndrome indicating that the syndrome does not depend upon a single brain mechanism [92].

14.3.1.6 Dementia with Lewy Bodies (DLB)

DLB also known as cortical Lewy body dementia or diffuse Lewy body dementia is a neurodegenerative disorder associated with abnormal structures (Lewy bodies) in certain parts of the brain. It is the second most common cause of dementia (15–20 %) [93, 94] after Alzheimer's disease [94, 95].

Pathophysiology

DLB is characterised in most cases with neocortical or limbic Lewy bodies and Alzheimer-type pathology below the threshold for the diagnosis of AD [96], but the cortical Lewy bodies and Lewy neuritis in DLB are the most important correlates of cognitive failure rather than the AD pathology [94]. The frequency and distribution of cortical Lewy bodies has been defined by antiubiquitin immunocytochemical staining [56]. It has been demonstrated that there is a link with 'synucleinopathies' which include Parkinson's disease and multisystem atrophy [94] and classified as a alpha-synucleinopathy [93,] and there is marked cortical reduction of acetylcholine and nigrostriatal dopamine deficiency [95].

14.3.1.7 Parkinsonism and Dementia

Parkinson's disease primarily occurs after the age of 50, carrying the 7–10 % of dementia in this age category [97, 98]. Dementia with parkinsonism poses difficulties in diagnosis. For instance, parkinsonian motor deficits encroach on the diagnostic criteria for dementia by limiting activities or increasing dependency [99]. There are three phases of dementia in Parkinson's disease, namely, (1) that of Alzheimer' disease, (2) that of cortical Lewy bodies and (3) cell loss in the nucleus basalis and remaining cells showing tangles [99]. A subgroup of PD with onset in late life demonstrates neuropathological changes of the Alzheimer's variety [100]. The prevalence rates of dementia in Parkinson's disease are said to be between 30 and 40 %, a better estimate would be 20 % [101], but this is again doubtful [102]. Depression is much more frequently seen. Clinical and neuropathological similarities to AD are seen in 10–30 % of Parkinson's disease patients.

14.3.2 Vascular Dementia (Vascular Cognitive Impairment)

Introduction

The term vascular dementia (VaD) is not only the traditional multi-infarct dementia but has a broader connotation and embraces all others due to different vascular mechanisms and changes in the brain with different causes and manifestations [103]. It has been suggested that VaD should be redefined with greater consideration to the identification of distinct vascular mechanisms in the development of dementia [104]. Currently the term vascular cognitive impairment (VCI) has been proposed. It includes a wide spectrum of cognitive declines ranging from mild deficits in one or more cognitive domains to a broad dementia-like syndrome [105]. It is a preferred term for it encompasses the complex interactions between vascular risk factors, cerebrovascular disease aetiology and cellular changes within the brain and cognition [105]. In this chapter the terms VaD and VCI are interchangeable.

The very elderly are at the highest risk for cognitive impairment and dementia and stroke is among the risk factors [106]. Vascular dementia (VaD) is probably the second most common cause of dementia after Alzheimer's disease (AD) in the Western countries but may be more common than AD after the age of 85 years [107] in countries like Japan, China and Russia [108]. Some believe that Lewy body dementia (LBD) may be more common than VaD [109, 110]. Little more than quarter of the patients with acute stroke develop dementia [111, 112]. Stroke and dementia increase exponentially with age, and hence there may be a significant overlap between VaD and AD and at very high levels may level off. It is much more common in men before the age of 75 years and the prevalence is higher in women after the age of 80 years [113, 114]. Studies have shown that 30 % of the stroke survivors over the 75 years suffer from dementia [115]. Vascular dementia and Alzheimer's disease have in common several risk factors such as hypertension, white matter lesions and lacunae among others. The prevalence of mixed vascular dementia has been underestimated more so in the elderly population [116]. Men are said to be at a higher risk of VaD than women and are a reverse of AD [117].

Pathophysiology

Its prevalence in autopsy studies has been related to cortical and/or subcortical infarcts, focal, multiple or diffuse. They often involve strategically important brain areas, thalamus, frontobasal/limbic systems [118] white matter lesions and less often large brain areas. It is now known that even a single infarction located in a strategically important area in the brain can give rise to deficits in multiple areas of cognitive function. The LADIS study demonstrated that lacunar infarcts in the putamen and globus pallidus affected memory, those in the thalamus are more likely to affect several cognitive domains and lacunar infarcts in the caudate, internal capsule and lobar white matter did not have any significant effects [119]. Several studies have shown increased white matter hyperintensities (WMH). WMH are associated with cognitive impairment even in the absence of dementia [120, 121]. In the

Rotterdam Study periventricular lesions were correlated with rapid decline [122]. The PROGRESS trail further strengthened this notion that severe leukoaraiosis portends rapid progression. The study demonstrated that those with no leukoaraiosis at study entry were associated with 4 % dementia or severe cognitive impairment after a 4-year follow-up, whereas 30 % of those with severe leukoaraiosis at study entry declined to this level [123].

MRI and autopsy studies have shown chronic hypoxia in areas of leukoaraiosis and some suggestion that hypoxia may be less pronounced in the periventricular white matter lesions and these are associated with ependymal loss [124] suggesting WMH may rise from a vascular cause [125]. Cardiovascular risk factors have an impact on vascular function and have been associated with increased WMH [118]. It appears that those factors leading to leukoaraiosis are specific to the cerebral vessels and that leukoaraiosis predicts stroke but does not predict other vascular events [126]. Endothelial dysfunction has been implicated as a mechanism underlying leukoaraiosis [125]. Leukoaraiosis on CT is seen as diffuse hypodense areas in the white matter surrounding the ventricles.

Vascular disease giving rise to relatively large infarcts enough to damage a sufficient volume of the brain causing dementia was termed multi-infarct dementia [127]. Traditionally VaD had been characterised as having a 'patchy' pattern of cognitive deficits, but this patchy pattern is associated only with one type of VaD-multiple cortical infarctions, and there are several other additional subtypes each aspecting a characteristic pattern of deficits [128]. Meyer et al. [129] proposed eight subtypes of VaD. It is now known that even a single infarction located in a strategically important area in the brain could give rise to deficits in multiple areas of cognitive function. Other recognised strategic areas in the brain are the genu of the internal capsule, thalamus, caudate, globus pallidus, basal forebrain and hippocampus. Strategic infarctions have unique features that reflect the specific brain region affected.

The penetrating arterioles and lenticulostriate arteries supplying the deeper structures of the basal ganglia and white nuclei are susceptible to arteriosclerotic injuries giving rise to lacunar infarctions, and it has been shown that multiple lacunar infarctions can give rise to full dementia [130]. Lacunar state and Binswanger's disease are two types of VaD associated with small vessel disease [131]. Binswanger's disease is the result of multiple cumulative occlusions of the deep penetrating arterioles supplying the white matter. Both produce dementia syndrome with characteristic subcortical dementia including slowing of information processing, impaired memory and poor sustained attention; parkinsonism with prominent gait disturbances in conjunction with pyramidal tract signs, dysarthria, pseudobulbar affect, and incontinence are frequent motor manifestations of VaD with small vessel disease [131]. In Binswanger's disease there is a wide spectrum of presentation, including dementia, seizures are not uncommon and there is a gait disorder. BD is characterised by hypertension, discrete strokes, acute with or without recovery, subacute deficits, plateau periods and insidious memory loss leading to dementia [132, 133].

Several genetic factors of vascular origin contributing to stroke seem to be polygenic and in particular polymorphisms in the genes encoding methylene tetrahydrofolate reductase (MTHFR), angiotensin-converting enzyme (ACE) [134, 135], Factor V Leiden, prothrombin and PAI 1 [135]. MTHFR gene regulates homocysteine metabolism [136], and elevated homocysteine levels have been suggested as risk factors for atherosclerosis and cardiovascular disease [137]. Another facet of VaD's pathophysiology is the role of inflammation, the incidence of which is influenced by the gene polymorphism of the inflammatory markers, namely, interleukin-1, interleukin-6, P-selectin, E-selectin and C-reactive protein [135].

14.3.2.1 Mixed VaD and AD

Mixed type of dementia refers to a combination of Alzheimer's disease (AD) and vascular encephalopathy and other dementia disorders [138]. The coincidence of AD and vascular disorders giving rise to a mixed dementia accounts for means of 6–12 % [138], but 25–60 % of dementia cases show both AD and vascular lesions [118]. The diagnosis of mixed dementia is based on clinical and neuroimaging criteria of possible Alzheimer's disease together with cerebrovascular disease [139]. AD and vascular dementia involve the subcortical regions or with several microinfarcts. Mixed dementia however is associated with large/hemispheric infarcts as well as microinfarcts [139]. The pathological diagnosis is based on autopsy-proven Alzheimer's disease and multiple vascular brain lesions [138].

Box 14.4. Key Points. Vascular Dementia

- Currently the term vascular cognitive impairment (VCI) has been proposed [105].
- Its prevalence has been related to cortical and/or subcortical infarcts, focal, multiple or diffuse [108].
- Several studies have shown increased white matter hyperintensities.
- Endothelial dysfunction has been implicated as a mechanism underlying leukoaraiosis [125].
- Several genetic factors of vascular origin contributing to stroke seem to be polygenic and in particular polymorphisms in the genes encoding methylene tetrahydrofolate reductase (MTHFR), angiotensin-converting enzyme (ACE), Factor V Leiden, prothrombin and PAI 1 [134, 135].
- Another facet of VaD's pathophysiology is the role of inflammation [135].

14.3.3 Symptomatic Dementias

14.3.3.1 Prion Diseases

Introduction

A prion is an infectious protein particle capable of transmitting an infectious disease in both humans and animals. The prion diseases affecting humans are Creutzfeldt-Jakob disease (CJD), Gerstmann-Straussler-Scheinker syndrome (GSS), kuru, fatal familial insomnia (FFi) and Alpers' syndrome, and these constitute 90 % of sporadic prion disease [140].

14.3.3.2 Creutzfeldt-Jakob Disease (CJD)

CJD is a rapidly progressive neurodegenerative disease with spongy degeneration of the brain and death within a year.

Pathophysiology

CJD is a neurodegenerative brain disorder which is a type of transmissible spongiform encephalopathy (TSE) [141]. The agent associated with CJD is the prion protein (PrP) encoded by the gene on chromosome 20. This is converted via a conformational change to an abnormal protein PrPsc [142], and this accumulates as an abnormal protein designated PrPres which accounts for the degenerative changes in the cerebral cortex. The age incidence ranges from 16 to 90 years with a median age of 60–65 years [143]. There are four types: sporadic, iatrogenic, inherited and variant. The sporadic form affects both men and women with symptoms appearing often between age 50 and 75 years [144]. The variant type is acquired by eating beef contaminated with bovine spongiform encephalopathy (BSE), and the prion protein is detectable outside the central nervous system [145].

14.3.3.3 Normal-Pressure Hydrocephalus (NPH)

The syndrome of normal-pressure hydrocephalus is characterised by the classical triad of gait disturbances, progressive mental deterioration and urinary difficulties. As the disease progresses, unsteadiness leads to falls, apathy, lack of spontaneity and depressive symptoms [146]. Psychiatric and behavioural symptoms characterised by agitation, paranoidal delusions, visual hallucinations and belligerence occur in association with NPH [147, 148].

Pathophysiology

There may be a precedent history of meningitis, subarachnoid haemorrhage or head injury. In most instances such a history is lacking. A number of changes have been noted as possible links with NPH. The pathophysiology of NPH has been attributed to a number of factors both mechanical [149] and ischaemic [150, 151]. Ventricular dilatation which occurs in NPH is the most noted physiological change [152]. It has been suggested that the ventricular enlargement follows the damage to the deep white matter due to vascular disease associated with ischaemia [153] resulting in tissue loss [152]. It can also be due to close down of the arterioles in the deep white matter due to ageing [152]. Currently there is general acceptance of a close association between NPH and a global reduction in cerebral blood flow (CBF) [152], and it has been interpreted that the CBF reduction in NPH is secondary to ventricular dilatation [154]. According to Bateman [152], ageing causes reduction in the craniospinal compliance, and in those with very low compliance, the venous pressure is markedly elevated making the cortical veins stiffer thereby reducing the craniospinal compliance further. When the sagittal sinus pressure increases, the pressure gradient required to reabsorb CSF is exceeded and CSF absorption through the granulations ceases [155]. Ischaemia in the deep venous territory is not a prerequisite for NPH [152]. Slow absorption of the CSF, ventricular dilatation and frontal lobe abnormalities may result from a scarring of the arachnoid villi over convexities of the frontal lobes. Severe damage to the frontal lobes gives rise to clinical features very similar to that of normal-pressure hydrocephalus which in effect a frontal lobe syndrome consequent to periodically raised intraventricular pressure [156]. Figure 14.1 shows generalised enlargement of the ventricles and rounding of the anterior horns in normal-pressure hydrocephalus.

Box 14.5. Key Points. Normal-Pressure Hydrocephalus (NPH)

- There may be precedent history of meningitis, subarachnoid haemorrhage or head injury.
- Ventricular dilatation occurs and is the most noted physiological change [152].
- There is a close association between NPH and a global reduction of cerebral blood flow (CBF) and is said to be secondary to ventricular dilatation [152].
- Ageing causes reduction in craniospinal compliance, and in those with low compliance, the venous pressure rises making the cortical veins stiffer with further reduction of craniospinal compliance. When the sagittal sinus pressure increases, the pressure gradient required to reabsorb CSF is exceeded and CSF absorption ceases [152].
- Severe damage to the frontal lobes gives rise to clinical features similar to NPH [156].

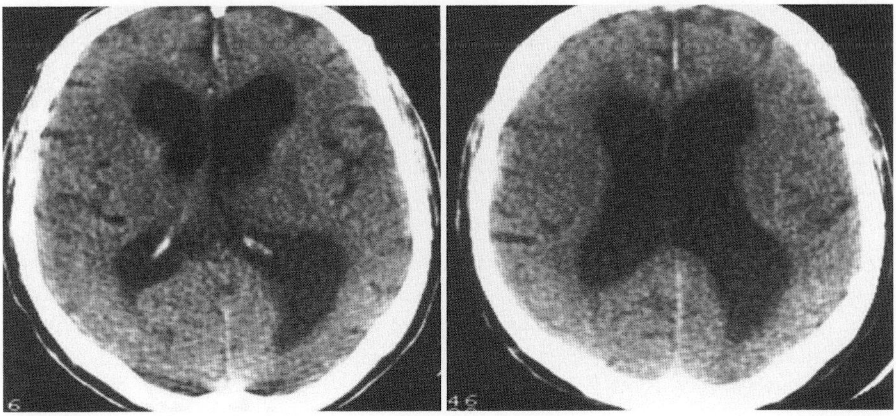

Fig. 14.1 Shows generalised enlargement of the ventricles and rounding of the anterior horns in normal-pressure hydrocephalus

14.4 Mild Cognitive Impairment (MCI)

Introduction

Although there is no common consensus in defining MCI, clinicians and researchers refer to MCI as a category with objective evidence of impairment on cognitive testing that do not meet the criteria for dementia [157]. It is believed to be an intermediate state between normal memory loss of ageing and conditions such as Alzheimer's disease [158, 159].

Pathophysiology

Several labels have been used to categorise non-disabling memory deficits in the elderly [160]. These include age-associated memory impairment (AAMI), age-associated cognitive decline (AACD), mild cognitive disorder (MCD), age-related cognitive decline (ARCD) and mild cognitive impairment (MCI) among others and are within the limits of normal ageing. In spite of the deficits, they did not exhibit the characteristics of dementia. Clinicians and researchers till recently were unable to provide firm answers concerning the significance of these categories and what they mean for the future. Unlike AAMI, MCI is assumed to have a pathological basis and is at high risk of developing dementia. The aetiology of MCI is multifactorial and includes neurodegenerative, vascular, neurological, psychiatric, traumatic and iatrogenic [161]. MCI has been classified into amnestic and nonamnestic forms [161, 162]. Memory impairment predominates in the former and is frequently a prodrome of Alzheimer's disease and in some cases autopsy studies have demonstrated an increase in proteins forming amyloid plaques and neurofibrillary tangles. The nonamnestic form is characterised by a variety of cognitive impairments involving single or multiple cognitive domains. More recently multiple subtypes of MCI had been proposed, namely, amnestic MCI with single domain, amnestic MCI with multiple domains, nonamnestic MCI with single domain and nonamnestic MCI with multiple domains [161, 163, 164] based on intention to indicate the heterogeneity in aetiology of different subtypes of dementia [165]. It is believed that each subtype is associated with an increased risk for a specific type of dementia [166]. MCI has now been expanded to include other cognitive domains and other potential causes like normal ageing, frontotemporal dementia and vascular dementia [167]. Nonamnestic forms may be due to cerebrovascular disease, Parkinson's disease, Lewy body dementia and frontotemporal dementia among others [162].

Box 14.6. Key Points. Mild Cognitive Impairment (MCI)

- It is believed to be an intermediate stage between normal memory loss of ageing and conditions such as Alzheimer's disease [158, 159].
- MCI is assumed to have a pathological basis and is at high risk of developing dementia.
- MCI is classified into amnestic and nonamnestic forms [161, 162].
- MCI has been expanded to include other cognitive domains and other potential causes like normal ageing, frontotemporal dementia and vascular dementia [167].
- Nonamnestic forms may be due to cerebrovascular disease, Parkinson's disease, Lewy body dementia and frontotemporal dementia among others [162].

Multiple Choice Questions

1. The following in relation to the pathophysiology of acute delirium in the elderly are true, EXCEPT.
   A. Elderly are particularly vulnerable to acute delirium due to age-related cerebral changes and in the neurotransmitter systems.
   B. The presence of brain disorders associated with fewer neurons makes them more susceptible.
   C. The more important neurotransmitters in the pathogenesis of acute delirium are serotonin and glutamate.
   D. Physical stressful events can influence the activity of the neurotransmitters.
2. The following age-related changes in the brain are true, EXCEPT:
   A. The loss of neurons is not topographically random.
   B. Significant white matter changes occur and gross white matter volume decreases across adult life.
   C. Neuroplasticity involves the reshaping of the brain not only in the developing years but throughout life.
   D. Age-related brain volumes decrease across adult age range, and after the age of 70 years, there is stepping up of the atrophy.
3. The following in relation to the pathophysiology of Alzheimer's disease are true, EXCEPT:
   A. Senile plaques are primarily made of microtubule-associated protein tau.
   B. Accumulation of Abeta is the main cause of neuronal degeneration and induces accumulation of tau in Alzheimer's disease brain.
   C. Abeta deposits involve the neocortex, while intracellular tau mainly affects the hippocampal region.
   D. According to the amyloid cascade hypothesis, accumulation of senile plaques is the initiating lesion in Alzheimer's disease.
4. The following are true of the neurodegenerative dementias, EXCEPT:
   A. Aberrant mutation of the tau protein is the fundamental neuropathological finding in frontotemporal dementia.
   B. Both corticobasal degeneration (CBD) and progressive supranuclear palsy (PSP) show a similar pattern of tau expression but in CBD tau forms paired helical filaments.
   C. The syndrome of posterior cortical atrophy is associated with Alzheimer's disease pathology with detectable mesiotemporal atrophy.
   D. Dementia of Lewy body is characterised in most cases with neocortical or limbic Lewy bodies.
5. The following physiological changes in normal-pressure hydrocephalus (NPH) are true, EXCEPT:
   A. Ventricular dilatation is the most obvious finding.
   B. Global reduction in cerebral blood flow is the starting point in the pathogenesis.
   C. The superficial venous pressure may be elevated.
   D. Idiopathic NPH tends to occur in the young.

6. The following are true of vascular dementia, EXCEPT:
   A. Currently the preferred term is vascular cognitive impairment.
   B. Lacunar state is one type of vascular dementia associated with small vessel disease.
   C. The coincidence of Alzheimer's disease and vascular disorders giving rise to mixed dementias accounts for more than 80 % of all dementias.
   D. Deficits in multiple areas of cognitive function could rise after a single infarction.

Answers to MCQs

1 = C; 2 = B;= 3 = A; 4 = C; 5 = D; 6 = C.

References

Anatomical and Physiological Changes with Ageing: Brain

1. Convit P, de Leon MJ, Hoptman MJ, Tarshish CM, De Santi S, Rusinek H. Age related changes in brain. i. Magnetic Resonance Imaging measures of temporal lobe volumes in normal subjects. Psychiat Quart. 1995;66(4):343–8.
2. Raz N, Rodrique KM. Differential aging of the brain: patterns cognitive correlates and modifiers. Neurosci Biobehav Rev. 2006;30:730–48.
3. Sullivan EV, Pfefferbaum A, Adalsteinsson E, Swan GE, Carmelle D. Differential rates of regional brain changes in callosal and ventricular size: a 4-year longitudinal MRI Study of Elderly Men. Cereb Cortex. 2002;12(4):438–45. doi:10.1093/circor/12.4.438.
4. Seahill RI, Frost C, Jenkins R, Whitwell JL, Ross MN, Fox NC. A longitudinal study of brain volume changes in normal aging using serial registered MRI. JAMA Neurol. 2003;60(7): 989–94.
5. Mu Q, Xie J, Wen Z, Shyun Z. A Quantitative MR study of the hippocampal formation, the amygdala and the temporal horn of the lateral ventricle in healthy subjects 40–90 years of age. AJNR Am J Neuroradiol. 1999;20:207–11.
6. Reid AT, van Norden AG, de Laat KF, van Oudheusden LT, Zwiers MP, Evans AC, et al. Patterns of cortical degeneration in elderly cohort with cerebral small vessel disease. Hum Brain Mapp. 2010;31(12):1983–92 (abstract).
7. Resnick S, Goldzal AF, Davatzikos C, Golski S, Kraut MA, Melter EJ, et al. One year age changes in MRI brain volumes in older adults. Cereb Cortex. 2000;10(5):464–72.
8. Raz N. The aging brain observed in viva: differential changers and their modifiers. In: Cabiza R, Nyberg L, Park DC, editors. Cognitive neuroscience of aging: linking cognitive and cerebral aging. New York: Oxford University Press; 2004. p. 17–55.
9. Brody H. Organisation of the cerebral cortex. III. A study of aging in the human cerebral cortex. J Comp Neurol. 1955;102:511–6.
10. Burke SN, Barnes CA. Neural plasticity in aging brain. Nat Rev. 2006;7:30–40.
11. Ge Y, Grossman RI, Babb JS, Rabin ML, Mannon LJ, Kolson DL, et al. Age-related total gray matter and white matter changes in normal adult brain, Part 1. Volumetric MR imaging analysis. AJNR. 2002;23:1327–33.
12. Hachinski VC, Potter P, Merskey H. Leuko-araiosis. Arch Neurol. 1987;44:21–3.

13. Kemper T. Neuroanatomical and neurophysiological changes during aging and dementia. In: Albert ML, Knoefil J, editors. Clinical neurology of aging. New York: Oxford University Press; 1994. p. 3–67.
14. Rees S. A quantitative electron microscopic study of aging of the cerebral cortex. Acta Neuropathol (Berlin). 1976;36(4):347–62.
15. Mahncke HW, Bronstone A, Merzenich MM. Brain plasticity and functional losses in the aged: scientific bases for a novel intervention. Prog Brain Res. 2006;157:81–109 (abstract).
16. Jones S, Nyberg L, Sandblom J, Stigsdotter Neely A, Ingvar M, Magnus Petersson K, et al. Cognitive and neural plasticity in aging: general and task-specific limitations. Neurosci Biobehav Rev. 2006;30(6):864–71 (abstract).
17. Joynt RJ. Aging and the nervous system. In: Merck manual of geriatrics. Whitehouse Staten: Merck. 2000.
18. Gould E, Reeves AJ, Graziano MS, Gross CG. Neurogenesis in the neocortex of adult primates. Science. 1999;286:548–52.
19. Neve RL, Finch EA, Bird ED, Benowitz LI. Growth associated protein GAP-43 is expressed selectively in association regions of the adult human brain. Proc Natl Acad Sci U S A. 1998;85:3638–42.
20. Benowitz LI, Perone-Bizzozero NI, Finkelstein SP, Bird ED. Localization of the growth associated phosphoprotein GAP-43 (B-50, Fi) in the human central cortex. J Neurosci. 1989;3:990–5.
21. McGeer EG. Neurotransmitter systems in aging and senile dementia. Prog Neuropsychopharmacol. 1981;5(5-6):435–45 (abstract).
22. Strong R. Neurochemical changes in the aging human brain: implications for behavioural impairment and neurodegenerative disease. Geriatrics. 1998;53 Suppl 1:S9–12.
23. Schiliebs R, Arendt T. The significance of the cholinergic system in the brain during aging and in Alzheimer's disease. J Neural Transm. 2003;113:1625–44.
24. Meltzer CC, Smith G, DeKosky ST, Mathis CA, Moore RY, et al. Serotonin in aging, late life depression and Alzheimer's disease, the emerging role of functional imaging. Neuropsychopharmacology. 1998;16(4):407–30 (abstract).

Acute Confusional State in the Elderly

25. Mesulam MM. Attention confusional state sand neglect. In: Mesulam MM, editor. Principles of behavioural neurology. Philadelphia: F.A. Davis; 1985.
26. Mesulam MM, Wayman SG, Geschwind N, Sabin T. Acute confusional states with right sided cerebral artery infarctions. J Neurol Neurosurg Psychiatry. 1976;39:84–95.
27. Francis J, Kapoor WW. Prognosis after discharge of older medical patients with delirium. J Am Geriatr Soc. 1992;40:601–6.
28. Levkoff SE, Evans PA, Liptzin B, Cleary PD, Lipsitz LA, Wetle TT, et al. Delirium: the occurrence and prevalence of symptoms among elderly hospitalized patients. Arch Int Med. 1922;152:334–40.
29. Inouye SK. The dilemma of delirium: clinical and research controversies regarding diagnosis and evaluation of delirium in hospitalized elderly medical patients. Am J Med. 1994;97:278–88.
30. Nagaratnam N, Cheuk G, O'Neile L. Acute confusional state in patients with and without dementia. Arch Geront Geriatr. 1999;29:139–47.
31. Johnson JC, Gottleib GI, Sullivan E, Wanich C, Kinosian B, Forcico MA, et al. Using DSM-3 criteria to diagnose delirium in elderly general medical patients. J Gerontol. 1990;45:113–9.
32. Van der Mast RC. Pathophysiology of delirium. J Geriatr Psychiatr Neurol. 1998;11(3):138–45 (abstract).
33. Flacker JM, Lipsitz LA. Neural mechanisms of delirium: current hypothesis and evolving concepts. J Gerontol A Biol Sci Med Sci. 1999;54(6):B239–46 (abstract).

34. Alagaikrishnan K, Blanchette P. Delirium. Delirium e Medicine Psychiatry. http://www.emedicine.mediscape.com.article/28890-overview. Accessed 16 Feb 2010.
35. Flacker JM, Cummings J, Mach Jr JR, Bettin K, Kiely DK, Wei J. The association of serum anticholinergic activity with delirium in elderly medical patients. Am J Geriatr Psychiatry. 1998;6(1):31–41 (abstract).
36. Olsson T, Marklund N, Gustafson Y, Nasman B. Abnormalities at different levels of hypothalamic-pituitary-adrenocortical axis early after stroke. Stroke. 1992;23(11): 1573–6.
37. Fong TG, Tulebav SR, Inouye SK. Delirium in elderly adults: diagnosis, prevention and treatment. Nat Rev Neurol. 2009;5:210–20.
38. Purdie FR, Honignan B, Rosen P. Acute organic syndrome. A review of 100 cases. Ann Emerg Med. 1981;10:455.
39. Moses H, Van Kaden BA. Neurologic consultations in general hospital: spectrum of iatrogenic disease. Am J Med. 1986;81:955–8.
40. Cunningham C, MacLullich AMJ. At the extreme end of the psychoneuroimmunological spectrum: delirium as a maladaptive sickness behaviour response. Brain Behav Immun. 2013;28:1–13.
41. MacLullich AM, Ferguson KJ, Miller T, de Rooij EE, Cunningham C. Unravelling the pathophysiology of delirium: a focus on the role of aberrant stress responses. J Psychosom Res. 2008;65:229–38.
42. Hart BL. Biological basis of the behaviour of sick animals. Neurosci Biobehav Rev. 1988;12:123–37.

Dementia

43. Rocca WA, Amaducci LA, Schoenberg BS. Epidemiology of clinically diagnosed Alzheimer's disease. Ann Neurol. 1986;19:415–24.
44. Lobo A, Launer LT, Fratiglioni L, Andersen K, di Carlo A, Breteler HM, et al. Prevalence of dementia and major subtypes in Europe. A collaborative study of population based cohorts. Neurology. 2000;54:34–9.
45. Cummings JL, Benson DF. Subcortical dementia: a review of an emerging concept. Arch Neurol. 1984;41:874.
46. Albert ML, Feldman RG, Willis AL. The 'subcortical dementia' of progressive supranuclear palsy. J Neurol Neurosurg Psychiatry. 1974;37:121–30.
47. Dunne FJ. Subcortical dementia. Br Med J. 1993;307:1–2.
48. Drachman DA, Newell KL. Case records of the Massachusetts General hospital. New Eng J Med. 1999;340:1269–76.
49. Rossor MN. Management of neurological disorders: dementia. J Neurol Neurosurg Psychiatry. 1994;57:1451–6.
50. Drzezga A. Basic pathologies of neurodegenerative dementias and their relevance for state-of-the-art molecular imaging studies. Eur J Nucl Med Mol Imaging 2008;35(suppl 1):S4–11.
51. Moussaud S, Jones R, Moussaud-Lamodiere EL, Delemclos M, Ross OA, McLean P. Alpha-synuclein and tau – team mates in neurodegeneration? Mol Neurodeg. 2014;9:43. Doi: 10.1186/1750-1326-9-43.
52. Rogan S, Lippa CE. Alzheimer's disease and other dementias: a review. Am J Alzheimers Dis Other Demen. 2002;17:11–7.
53. Taipa R, Pinho J, Melo-Pires M. Clinico-pathologic correlations of the most common neurodegenerative dementias. Front Neurol. 2012;3:68. Doi: 10.3389/neur-2012-00068.
54. Bloom GS. Amyloid beta- and tau, the trigger and bullet in Alzheier disease pathogenesis. JAMA Neurol. 2014;7(14):505–8.

Neurodegenerative Dementia

55. Launer LG, Anderson K, Dewey ME, Letenneur L, Ott A, Amaducci LA, et al. Rates and risk factors for dementia and Alzheimer's disease: results from EURODERM pooled analyses. EURODERM. Incidence Research Group and Work Groups. European Studies of Dementia. Neurology. 1999;52:78–84.
56. Tolnay M, Probst A. The neuropathological spectrum of neurodegenerative tauopathies. IUBMB Life. 2003;55(6):299–305 (abstract).
57. Ragon S, Lippa CF. Alzheimer's and other dementias: a review. Am J Alzheimers Dis Other Demen. 2002;17:11–7.

Alzheimer's Disease

58. Goedert M. Filamentous nerve cell inclusions in neurodegenerative diseases: tauopathies and alpha-synucleinopathies. Philos Trans R Soc Lond B Biol Sci. 1999;354(1386):1101–18 (abstract).
59. Johnson GV, Stoothoff WH. Tau phosphorylation in neuronal function and dysfunction. J Cell Sci. 2004;117(Pt2):5721–9.
60. Lindwall G, Cole RD. Phosphorylation affects the ability of tau protein to promote microtubule assembly. J Biol Chem. 1984;259:5301–5.
61. Duan Y, Dong S, Gu F, Hu Y, Zhao Z. Advances in the pathogenesis of Alzheimer's disease: focussing on tau-mediated neurodegeneration. Transl Neurodegener. 2012;15(1):24 (abstract).
62. Meraz-Rios MA, Lira-De Leon KL, Campos-Pena V, de Anda-Hernandez MA, Mena-Lopez R. Tau oligomers and aggregation in Alzheimer's disease. J Neurochem. 2010;112:1353–67.
63. Aprahamian I, Stella F, Forlenza OV. New treatment strategies for Alzheimer's disease: is there hope? Indian J Med Res. 2013;138:449–60.
64. Pei JJ, Braak E, Braak H, Grundke-Iqbal I, Iqbal K, Winbold B, et al. Distribution of active glycogen synthase kinase 3 beta (GSK-3 beta) in brains stages for Alzheimer disease neurofibrillary tangles. J Neuropathol Exp Neurol. 1999;58:1010–9.
65. Octave JN. Alzheimer disease: cellular and molecular aspects. Bull Mem Acad R Med Belg. 2005;160(10-12):445–9 (abstract).
66. de Paula VJR, Guimaraes FM, Diniz BS, Forlenza OV. Neurobiological pathways to Alzheimer's disease. Dement Neuropsychol. 2009;3(3):188–94.
67. Dong S, Duan Y, Hu Y, Zhao Z. Advances in the pathogenesis of Alzheimer's disease: a re-evaluation of amyloid cascade hypothesis. Transl Neurodegener. 2012;1:18. doi:10.1186/2047-9158-1-18.
68. Hardy JA. Alzheimer's disease: the amyloid cascade hypothesis: an update and reappraisal. J Alzheimers Dis. 2006;9:151–3.
69. Rao AT, Degnan AJ, Levy LM. Genetics of Alzheimer disease. ANJR Am J Neuroradiol. 2014;35(3):457–8.
70. Kuzuhara S. Treatment strategy of Alzheimer's disease: pause in clinical trials of Abeta vaccine and next steps. Brain Nerve. 2010;62(7):659–66.
71. Duyckaerts C, Perruchini C, Lebouvier T, Potier MC. The lesions of Alzheimer's disease: which therapeutic perspectives? Bull Acad Natl Med. 2008;192(2):303–18 (abstract).
72. Chui HC, Teng EL, Henderson VW, Moy AC. Clinical subtypes of the Alzheimer type. Neurology. 1986;35:1544–60.
73. Price DL, Sisodia SS. Mutant genes in familial Alzheimer's disease and transgenic models. Annu Rev Neurosci. 1998;21:479–505.
74. Lendon CL, Marinez A, Behrens I, Kosik KS, Madrigal L, Norton J, et al. L280A PS-1 mutation causes Alzheimer's disease but age of onset is modified by ApoE –alleles. Hum Mutat. 1997;10:186–95.

75. Williamson J, Goldman J, Marder KS. Genetic aspects of Alzheimer's disease. Neurologist. 2009;15:80–6.
76. Hoernicka J. Genes in Alzheimer's disease. Rev Neurol. 2006;42(5):302–5.
77. Bekris LM, Yu CE, Bird TD, Tsuang DW. Genetics of Alzheimer's disease. J Geriatr Psychiatr Neurol. 2010;23:213–27.

Fronto-Temporal Dementia

78. Kertesz A, Munoz DG. Primary progressive aphasia: a review of the neurobiology of a common presentation of Pick Complex. Am J Alzheimers Dis Other Demen. 2002;17:30–6.
79. Kowlaska A. The genetics of dementias. Part 1: Molecular basis of frontotemporal dementia and parkinsonism linked to chromosome 17 (FTDP-17). Postepy Hig Med Dosw (Online). 2009;63:278–86 (abstract).
80. Mackenzie IR. The neuropathology of FTD associated with ALS. Alzheimer Dis Assoc Disord. 2007;21(4):S44–9 (abstract).

Corticobasal Degeneration

81. Morris HR, Lees AJ, Wood NW. Neurofibrillary tangle parkinsonian disorders-tau pathology and tau genetics. Mov Disord. 1999;14:731–6.
82. Wenning GK, Litvan PJ, Jankovics J, Granata R, Mangone CA, McKee A, et al. Natural history and survival of 14 patients with corticobasal degeneration. J Neurol Neurosurg Psychiatry. 1998;64:184–9.
83. Dickson DW, Liu WR, Ksiezak-Reding H, Yin SH. Neuropathological and molecular considerations. Adv Neurol. 2000;82:9–27.
84. Mahapatra RK, Edwards MJ, Schott JM, Bhatia KP. Corticobasal degeneration. Lancet. 2004;3:736–43.
85. Kertsz A, Martinez-Lage P, Davidson W, Munoz DG. The corticobasal degeneration syndrome overlaps progressive aphasia and frontotemporal dementia. Neurology. 2000;55:1368–75.

Posterior Cortical Atrophy

86. Crutch SJ, Schott JM, Rabinovici GD, Boeve BF, Cappa SF, Dickerson BC, et al. Shining a light on posterior cortical atrophy. Alzheimers Dement. 2013;9(4):463–5.
87. Benson DF, Davis RJ, Synder BD. Posterior cortical atrophy. Arch Neurol. 1988;45:789–93.
88. Lehmann M, Crutch SJ, Ridgeway GR, Ridha BH, Barnes J, Warrington EK, et al. Cortical thickness and voxel–based morphometry in posterior cortical atrophy atypical Alzheimer's disease. Neurobiol Aging. 2011;32(8):1466–76. doi:10.1016/jneurobiolaging.2009.08.017.
89. Vernooij MW, de Groot M, van der Lugt A, Ikram M, Hrestin G, et al. White matter atrophy and lesion formation explain the loss of structural integrity of white matter in aging. Neuroimage. 2008;43(3):470–7 (abstract).
90. Croisile B. Benson's syndrome or posterior cortical atrophy. Orphanet Encyclopedia. 2004. http://www.orpha.net/data/patho/GB/uk-Benson.pdf. Accessed 24 Mar 2014.
91. Gerabrowski TJ, Damasio AR. Definition clinical features and neuroanatomical basis of dementia. In: Esirl MM, Lee VMY, Trojancwski JQ, editors. The neuropathology of dementia. 2nd ed. Cambridge: Cambridge University Press; 2004.
92. Vighetto A, Krolak-Salmon P. Balint syndrome. In: Vighetto A, Krolak-Salmon P, editors. The behavioral and cognitive neurology of stroke. 2nd ed. Oliver Godefroy, Cambridge: Cambridge University Press; 2013. p. 218–30.

Lewy Body Dementia

93. Barber R, Panikkar A, McKeith IG. Dementia with Lewy bodies: diagnosis and management. Int J Geriatr Psychiatry. 2001;16 Suppl 1:S12–8 (abstract).
94. McKeith IG, Burn DJ, Ballard CG, Collerton D, Joros E, Morris CM, et al. Dementia with Lewy bodies. Semin Clin Neuropsychiatry. 2003;8(1):46–57 (abstract).
95. Arsland D. Dementia with Lewy bodies. Tidsskr Nor Laegeforen. 2002;122(5):525–9 (abstract).
96. Dickson DW. Dementia with Lewy bodies: neuropathology. J Geriatr Psychiatr Neurol. 2002;15(4):210–6 (abstract).

Parkinson's Disease and Dementia

97. Wang HS. Dementia in old age. In: Wells CE, editor. Dementia. 2nd ed. Philadelphia: FA Davis Co; 1977. p. 15–26.
98. Henderson AS, Kay D. The epidemiology of mental disorders in the aged. In: Kay DWK, Burrows GD, editors. Handbook of studies on psychiatry and old age. Amsterdam: Elsevier; 1984. p. 53–88.
99. Gibbs WRG. Dementia and Parkinson's disease. J Psychiatry. 1989;154:596–614.
100. Hakim AM, Matheison G. Dementia in Parkinson's disease: a neuropathological study. Neurology. 1979;29:1219–4.
101. Brown RG, Marsden CD. How common is dementia in Parkinson's disease? Lancet. 1984;ii:1262–5.
102. Lees AJ. Parkinson's disease and dementia. Lancet. 1985;i:43–4.

Vascular Dementia

103. Scheinberg P. Dementia due to vascular disease-a multifactorial disorder. Stroke. 1988;19:1291–9.
104. Hennerici MG. What are the mechanisms for post stroke dementia? Lancet Neurol. 2009;8(11):973–5.
105. Erkinjuntti T, Gauthier S. The concept of vascular cognitive impairment. Front Neurol Neurosci. 2009;24:79–85 (abstract).
106. Zhu L, Fratiglioni L, Guo Z, Ma T, Hou R, Ma X, et al. Association of stroke with dementia, cognitive impairment and functional disability in the very old: a population based study. Stroke. 1998;29:2094–9.
107. Skoog I, Nilsson L, Palmertz B, Anfreasson L-A, Svanborg A. A population based study of dementia in 85 year olds. N Engl J Med. 1993;328:153–8.
108. Jorm AF, Korten AE, Henderson AS. The prevalence of dementia: a quantitative integration of the literature. Acta Psychiatr Scand. 1987;76:465–78.
109. Rocca WA. The prevalence of vascular dementia in Europe-facts and fragments from 1980-1990 studies. Ann Neurol. 1991;30:817–24.
110. McKeith IG, Perry RH, Fairbain AF, Iabeen S, Perry EK. Operational criteria for senile dementia of Lewy body type. Psychol Med. 1992;22:911–22.
111. Tatemichi TK, Paik M, Bagiella E, Desmond DW, Starn Y, Sano M, et al. Risk of dementia after stroke in a hospitalized cohort: results of a longitudinal study. Neurology. 1994;44:1885–92.
112. Pohjasvaara T, Erkinjunti T, Ylikoski R, Hietanen M, Vataja R, Kaste M. Clinical determinants of poststroke dementia. Stroke. 1998;29:75–81.
113. Rocca WA, Bonaiuto S, Lippi A, Luciani P, Turtu F, Cavarzeran F, et al. Prevalence of clinically diagnosed Alzheimer's disease and other dementing disorders: a door-to-door survey in Appignano Macerata Province, Italy. Neurology. 1990;40:626–31.

114. Magnusson H. Mental health of octogenarians in Iceland. An epidemiological study. Acta Psychiatr Scand Suppl. 1989;79:1–112.
115. Cherubini A, Senin U. Elderly stroke patient at risk for dementia: in search of a profile. Editorial Comment. Stroke. 2003;34:2245.
116. Rockwood K, Bowler J, Erkinjuntti T, Hachinski V, Walin A. Subtypes of vascular dementia. Alzheimer Dis Assoc Disord. 1999;13:S59–63.
117. Gorelick PB. Stroke prevention. Arch Neurol. 1995;52:347–54.
118. Jellinger KA. Pathology and pathophysiology of vascular cognitive impairment. A critical update. Panminerva Med. 2004;46(4):217–26 (abstract).
119. Benisty S, Gouw AA, Porcher R, Madureira S, Hernandez K, Poggesi A, LADIS Study Group, et al. Location of lacunar infarcts correlates with cognition: the LADIS Study. J Neurol Neurosurg Psychiatry. 2009;80:478–83.
120. Paul RH, Haque O, Gunstad J, Tate DF, Grieve SM, Hoth K, et al. Subcortical hyperintensities impact cognitive function among a select subset of healthy elderly. Arch Clin Neuropsychol. 2005;20:697–704.
121. Gunning-Dixon PM, Raz N. Neuroanatomic correlates of selected executive functions in middle-aged and older adults. Neuropsychologia. 2003;41:1929–41.
122. van Dijk EJ, Prins ND, Vrooman HA, Hofman A, Koudstaal PJ, Breteler MM. Progression of cerebral small vessel disease in relation to risk factors and cognitive consequences: Rotterdam Scan Study. Stroke. 2008;39:2712–0.
123. Dufouil C, Godin O, Chalmers J, Coskun O, Macmohon S, Tzourio-Mazayer N, Progress MRI Substudy Investigators, et al. Severe cerebral white matter hyperintensities predict severe cognitive decline in patients with cerebrovascular disease. Stroke. 2009;40:2219–21.
124. Bowler JV, Gorelick PB. Advances in vascular cognition impairment-2006. Stroke. 2007;38:241–4.
125. Hoth KF, Tate DF, Poppas A, Forman DE, Gunstad J, Moser DJ. Endothelial function and white matter hyperintensities in older adults with cardiovascular disease. Stroke. 2007;38:308–12.
126. Buyckb J-F, Dudouil C, Mazoyer B, Maillard P, Ducimetiere P, Alperovitch AH, et al. Cerebral white matter lesions are associated with risk of stroke but not with other vascular events: 3-City Dijon Study. Stroke. 2009;40:2327–31.
127. Hachinski VC, Lassen NA, Marshall J. Multi-infarct dementia- a case of mental deterioration in the elderly. Lancet. 1974;ii:207–9.
128. McPherson SE, Cummings JL. Neuropsychological aspects of vascular dementia. Brain Cogn. 1996;31:269–82.
129. Meyer J, Shirai T, Akiyama H. Neuroimaging for differentiating vascular from Alzheimer's dementia. Cerebrovasc Brain Metab Rev. 1996;8:1–10.
130. Scott TM, Folstein MF. Cognition and neuropsychology. In: Chiu E, Gustafan L, Ames D, Folstein MF, editors. Cerebrovascular disease and dementia. London: Martin Dunitz Ltd.; 2001. p. 131–44.
131. Cummings JL. Vascular subcortical dementias. clinical aspects. Dementia. 1994;5:177–80.
132. Caplan LR, Schene WC. Clinical features subcortical arteriosclerotic encephalopathy (Binswanger's Disease). Neurology. 1979;28:1206–18.
133. Nagaratnam N, Beves A, Nagaratnam S. Binswanger's disease presenting as progressive speech disorder with CT and MRI findings. Eur J Int Med. 1994;5:321–3.
134. Panza F, Solfrizzi V, D'Introno A, Capurso C, Colacicco AM, Torres F, et al. Genetics of late-onset alzheimer's disease: vascular risk and beta-amyloid metabolism. Recenti Prog Med. 2002;93:489–97 (abstract).
135. Iemolo F, Duro G, Rizzo C, Castigha L. Pathophysiology of vascular dementia. Immun Aging. 2009;6:13. doi:10.1186/1742-4933-6-13.
136. Guclu O, Yazuz C, Karahan O. Multi-genetic origins of phenotype markers of the risk of cardiovascular disease. Hellenic J Cardiol. 2013;54:331–2.
137. Varga EA, Sturm AC, Misita CP, Moll S. Homocysteine and MTHFR mutations relation to thrombosis and coronary artery disease. Circulation. 2005;111:289–93.

138. Jellinger KA. The enigma of mixed dementia. Alzheimers Dement. 2007;3(1):40–53 (abstract).
139. Jellinger KA, Attems J. Neuropathological evaluation of mixed dementia. J Neurol Sci. 2007;257(1-2):80–7 (abstract).

Symptomatic Dementias

140. Puoti G, Bizzi A, Forloni G, Safar JG, Tagliavini F, Gambeti P. Sporadic prion disease: molecular insights and diagnosis. Lancet Neurol. 2012;11:618.
141. Trevitt CR, Singh PN. Variant Creutzfeldt-Jakob disease: pathology, epidemiology, and public health implications 1'2'3'4. Am J Clin Nutr. 2003;78(3):6515–65.
142. Pan KM, Baldwin M, Nguyen I, Gasset M, Serban A, Groth D, et al. Conversion of a helices into b –sheets features in the formation of the scrapie prion proteins. Proc Natl Acad Sci U S A. 1993;90:10962–6.
143. Zerr I, Poser S. Epidemiology and risk factors of transmissible spongiform encephalopathies in man. Prions. 2001;7:93–104.
144. HelpGuide.org. Creutzfeldt-Jakob Disease (CJD). http://www.helpguide.org/articles/alzheimers-dementia/creutzfeld-jakob-disease.ht. Accessed 22 Mar 2015.
145. Pathology of variant Creutzfeldt –Jakob Disease. http://springer.com/chapter/10.1007%2F4-431-29402-3_1. Accessed 22 Mar 2015.
146. Price TR, Tucker GJ. Psychiatric and behavioural manifestations of normal pressure hydrocephalus: a case report and brief review. J Nerv Ment Dis. 1977;164:51–5.
147. Rice E, Gendelman S. Psychiatric aspects of normal pressure hydrocephalus. J Am Med Ass. 1973;223:409–12.
148. Nagaratnam N, Verma S, Nagaratnam K. Psychiatric and behavioural manifestations of normal pressure hydrocephalus. Brit J Clin Pract. 1994;48:122–4.
149. Hakim S, Vengas JG, Burton JD. The physics of the cranial cavity, hydrocephalus and normal pressure hydrocephalus: mechanical interpretation and mathematical model. Surg Neurol. 1970;5:187.
150. Graff-Radford NR, Godersky JC. Idiopathic normal hydrocephalus and systemic hypertension. Neurology. 1987;37:868–71.
151. Casmiro M, D'Alessandro R, Cacciatore FM, Daidone R, Calbuci F, Lugaresi E. Risk factors for the syndrome of ventricular enlargement with gait apraxia (idiopathic normal pressure hydrocephalus): a case-control study. J Neurol Neurosurg Psychiatry. 1989;52:847–52.
152. Bateman GA. The pathophysiology of idiopathic normal pressure hydrocephalus: cerebral ischaemia or altered venous hemodynamics. AJNR Am J Neuroradiol. 2008;29:198–203.
153. Mathew NT, Meyer JS, Hartman A, Otto EO. Abnormal cerebrospinal fluid –blood flow dynamics: implications in diagnosis, treatment, and prognosis in normal pressure hydrocephalus. Arch Neurol. 1975;32:657–64.
154. Owler BK, Pickard JD. Normal pressure hydrocephalus and cerebral blood flow: a review. Acta Neurol Scand. 2001;104:325–42.
155. Benabid AL, de Rougemont J, Barge M. Cerebral venous pressure, sinus pressure and intracranial pressure (in French). Neurochurgie. 1974;20:623–32.
156. Damasio AR, Anderson SW. The Frontal lobes. In: Heillman KM, Valenstein E, editors. Clinical neuropsychology. 3rd ed. New York: Oxford University Press; 1993. p. 439.

Mild Cognitive Impairment

157. Petersen RC, Smith GE, Waring SC, Ivaik RJ, Tangalos EG, Kokmen E. Mild cognitive impairment: clinical characteristics and outcome. Arch Neurol. 1999;56:303–8.

158. Panza F, Capurso C, D'introno A, Colacicco AM, Capurso A, Solfrizzi V. Heterogeneity of mild cognitive impairment and other predementia syndromes in progression to dementia. Neurobiol Aging. 2007;28(10):1631–4 (abstract).
159. Maioli F, Coveri M, Pagni P, Chiandetti C, Marchetti C, Ciarrocchi R, et al. Conversion of mild cognitive impairment to dementia in elderly subjects: a preliminary study in a memory and cognitive disorder unit. Arch Gerontol Geriatr. 2007;44 Suppl 1:233–41 (abstract).
160. Panza F, D'Introno A, Colaccio AM, Capurso C, Del Parigi A, Caselli RJ, et al. Current epidemiology of mild cognitive impairment and other predementia syndromes. Am J Geriatr Psychiatry. 2005;13:633–44.
161. Pavlovic DM, Pavlovic AM. Mild cognitive impairment. Srp Arh Celok Lek. 2009;137:434–9 (abstract).
162. Petersen RC. Mild cognitive impairment. N Engl J Med. 2011;364:2227–34.
163. Busse A, Bischkoff J, Riedel-Heller SG, Anger Meyer MC. Mild cognitive impairment: prevalence and incidence according to different diagnostic criteria. Results of the Leipzig Longitudinal Study of the Aged (LEILA 75+). Br J Psychiatry. 2003;182:449–54 (abstract).
164. Clark LR, Delano-Wood L, Libon DJ, McDonald CR, Nation DA, Bangen KJ, et al. Are empirically-derived subtypes of mild cognitive impairment consistent with conventional subtypes? J Int Neuropsychol Soc. 2013;19:1–11.
165. Luis CA, Lownstein DA, Acevedo A, Barker WW, Duara R. Mild cognitive impairment: directions for future research. Neurology. 2003;61:438–44.
166. Busse A, Hensel A, Guhne U, Angermeyer MC, Reidel-Heler SG. Mild cognitive impairment: long –term course of four clinical types. Neurology. 2006;67(12):2176–85 (abstract).
167. Allegri RF, Gliser FB, Taragarro FE, Buschhkel I. Mild cognitive impairment: believe it or not? Int Rev Psychiatr. 2008;20(4):357–63 (abstract).

Psychiatry of Older Adults

15

15.1 Introduction

Psychiatric illnesses can be broadly categorised as: (1) Organic disorders characterised by confusion which may be acute (acute confusional state/delirium) or chronic (dementia). Organic disorder is a disorder associated with increasing age. (2) Functional disorders such as depression, psychotic disorders such as late-onset schizophrenia (paraphrenia) anxiety disorders, alcohol and substance abuse and dependence can like many disorders continue into old age or surface for the first time when the individual is older.

The rates of both organic and functional disorders are much increased at about 30 % each type among residents in hospitals, in aged care facilities or in other institutional care [1]. Although the psychiatric disorders of the elderly have some special features, they do not differ significantly from psychiatric disorders in younger adults. The older people however have some unique features that can confound the diagnosis [2, 3]. Some of the features associated with old age psychiatry are physical illnesses, sensory deficits, disabilities, social isolation, cognitive decline, polypharmacy [4], bereavement, retirement and increased risk of institutionalisation.

15.2 Mood Disorders (Major Depression, Bipolar Disorder)

15.2.1 Depression

Introduction

Currently the accepted types of depression are (1) primary versus secondary, (2) unipolar versus bipolar, (3) depressive illness versus depressive symptoms and (4) dysthymic versus depressive illness [5]. Primary depression is not the result of any medical or psychological cause and secondary depression is caused by a medical condition. Unipolar depression is another name for major depressive disorder. Bipolar disorder is a disorder characterised by cycles of depression and highs or

N. Nagaratnam et al., *Diseases in the Elderly: Age-Related Changes and Pathophysiology*, DOI 10.1007/978-3-319-25787-7_15

mania with two subtypes: type 1 is characterised when at least one manic episode has been diagnosed and type 2 is related to recurring episodes of depression but no manic episode [6]. Dysthymic disorder is a less severe type of depression with long-term fluctuating chronic symptoms of at least 2 years of depressed mood. There is no general agreement in the classification of depression. Depression disorders have been classified variously according to the symptoms, the course and the cause of the disorder. The ICD and DSM have adopted different criteria for the classification of depression. ICD-10 divides depression into mild to moderate and severe depressive episodes.

Pathophysiology
Primary depressive disorder has been divided into 'early-onset' (EOD) and 'late-onset' (LOD) disorders. Major depression depicts a new condition arising in about half of the patients in old age (late-onset depression) and in half or less had their first experience of depression before old age (early-onset depression) [7]. The age used to cut off between EOD and LOD varies, in the United Kingdom [8] and Australia [9], it is 60 years and in the United States of America, it is 50 years [8]. Late-life depression develops as a result of complex interactions of risk factors such as age-associated neurobiological changes, stressful events [7], a higher interaction with cognitive decline and impaired effect of genes [7, 10]. A family history of depression is more likely with EOD than with LOD [11]. The LOD is closely linked to clinical and neuroimaging evidence of cerebrovascular disease [12]. The 'vascular hypothesis' is upheld by co-morbidity of depression, vascular risk factors, vascular disease and the association with ischaemic lesions to characteristic behavioural symptom [13]. In a study to compare the frequency of depression, 670 geriatric rehabilitation patients were grouped into those with no evidence of vascular disease, those with cerebrovascular risk factors but no stroke and those with stroke only [14]. The study revealed the frequency of depression in patients without stroke increased as cerebrovascular risk factors increased. Hence the term 'vascular depression' is often used to describe this syndrome [15].

Neuroanatomic correlates – Major depression is said to be significantly more frequent with left anterior lesions (frontal or basal ganglia), whereas minor depression occurs with either right or left occipital lesion [16] but has not been demonstrated in further epidemiological studies [17]. Recent studies have revealed that either left anterior cerebral or subcortical lesions may lead to development of major depression, and the pre-existing subcortical atrophy may play an important role [18]. Severe affective depression was associated with left frontal lobe lesions, whereas apathetic depression mostly involved the basal ganglia [19]. A recent study revealed lacunar infarcts within the thalamus, basal ganglia and deep white matter which may be more important than single infarcts in the prediction of post-stroke depression [20, 21]. Structural imaging changes vary considerably between LOD and EOD [22] with more severe vascular pathology associated with LOD compared to EOD [20]. LOD has been associated with white matter and periventricular hyperintensities causing frontostriatal disruption [23] and significant atrophy in the cortical and subcortical regions [24]. More lately there has been considerable move towards embodying structural brain changes and cerebrovascular pathology in the frontal, subcortical and medial temporal structures [12, 25, 26].

Neurotransmitters – PET scan findings have shown a difference in the biochemical response in the two hemispheres to stroke. The serotonin receptor binding is increased in the right hemisphere compared to the left suggesting that the lower the serotonin binding, the more severe the depression [18]. Several factors increase the likelihood of PSD – localisation and severity of the brain lesion, reduction in serotonin and dopamine and other transmitter levels, premorbid personality, patient's age and social isolation [27, 28] and possibly a family history of major depression [29]. For several years, the increase in the synaptic concentrations of serotonin, noradrenaline and/or dopamine was the basis for pathophysiological models of depression [30]. Dopamine circuits have an important role [31], and there is considerable evidence that the suboptimal therapeutic response to SSRI and SNRI is due to lack of effect on dopamine circuits [32]. There is ample evidence of reduced serotonergic activity in depression, and it had been demonstrated that there is a reduction of serotonin transporter binding sites as well as a reduction in the number and/or function of both presynaptic and postsynaptic receptor densities [33, 34]. Noradrenergic containing circuits are also involved in the aetiology of mood disorders [35], and autopsy findings support a role for norepinephrine dysfunction in depression [32]. There is evidence that increased glutamate receptor activation has an important role in major depression [36]. Muller and Schwarz [36] hypothesised incorporating current concepts of dysregulation of neurotransmission and hypothalamus-pituitary-adrenal axis with immunological and brain morphology alterations in major depression. Type 1/type 2 immune response imbalance associated with astrocyte/microglia imbalance leads to serotonergic deficiency and glutaminergic overproduction [36].

Box 15.1. Key Points. Mood Disorders (Major Depression)

- Currently the accepted types of depression are (1) primary versus secondary, (2) unipolar versus bipolar, (3) depressive illness versus depressive symptoms and (4) dysthymic versus depressive illness [5].
- Primary depressive disorder has been divided into 'early-onset' (EOD) and 'late-onset' (LOD) disorders.
- Late-life depression develops as a result of complex interactions of risk factors such as age-associated neurobiological changes, stressful events, a higher interaction with cognitive decline and impaired effect of genes [7, 10].
- A family history of depression is more likely with EOD than with LOD [11].
- The LOD is closely linked to clinical and neuroimaging evidence of cerebrovascular disease [12].
- The term 'vascular depression' is often used to describe this syndrome [15].

- More lately there has been considerable move towards embodying structural brain changes and cerebrovascular pathology in the frontal, subcortical and medial temporal structures [15, 25].
- For several years, the increase in the synaptic concentrations of serotonin, noradrenaline and/or dopamine was the basis for pathophysiological models of depression [30].
- Muller and Schwarz hypothesised incorporating current concepts of dysregulation of neurotransmission and hypothalamus-pituitary-adrenal axis with immunological and brain morphology alterations in major depression [36].

15.2.2 Mania in Old Age

Introduction
Mania is characterised by abnormally elevated mood, inappropriate elation, increased irritability often to frank hostility, severe insomnia, speech often rapid, disconnected and racing thoughts, increased sexual desire and inappropriate social behaviour. Thought disorders are expansive, inflated self-esteem and may be accompanied by grandiose delusions. Bipolar affective disorder is not uncommon in the elderly, and in the United States, the prevalence ranges from 0.1 to 0.4 % and accounts for 10 to 25 % of all elderly patients with mood disorders [37].

Pathophysiology
After many years of depression, many are converted to bipolarity and suffer from mania in late life [38]. Mania usually occurs as a phase of manic-depressive disorder, but it can occur in association with medical and pharmacological states. They are called secondary manias. There is considerable supporting clinical and neuroimaging evidence of cerebrovascular disease that link it with 'late-onset' depression [39]. There is now a growing awareness of the influence of vascular-based LOD and LOM lending support to distinct vascular subtypes. The 'vascular syndromes' are the most distinctive and can be caused by cerebral infarction, including silent infarction, transient ischaemic attack and small vessel disease. They often demonstrate small vessel ischaemic changes or white matter hyperintense lesions on magnetic resonance imaging. Late-onset mania is closely associated with other medical disorders, most commonly stroke, dementia or hypothyroidism, and also the use of medications such as antidepressants, steroids and oestrogens [40].

The concept of secondary mania in old age continues to be debated with unresolved issues such as lateralisation, localisation, age of onset disinhibition syndromes and others [41]. Several neurological conditions have been correlated with secondary mania. A study of the incidence of silent cerebral infarction (SCI) in patients with major depression found half the cases of LOM to be secondary mania related to SCI and was often associated with larger areas of brain damage as compared with late-onset depression [42]. With post-stroke mania the strongest association is with a lesion in the right hemisphere. However there are reports of secondary mania following left hemispheric stroke [41, 43–46]. The lesions in secondary mania following stroke are in the limbic or limbic-controlled areas (orbitofrontal, basotemporal cortex, head of caudate and thalamus), but secondary mania has been reported after ventral pontine infarction [47]. A manic-like syndrome was produced following a thalamic lesion causing an ipsilateral frontal dysfunction via deafferentation. This dysfunction manifested as hypoperfusion of the frontal lobe imaged by cerebral SPECT [48]. In a review of reported cases, it was noted that mania was similar to orbitofrontal syndrome and could be caused by lesions in the thalamus or orbitofrontal regions [49]. The main areas involved were the limbic or limbic-related areas, orbitofrontal, basotemporal and basal ganglia regions, all of which have frontal connections [50]. In two studies of patients with sexually related behaviours following stroke, all had two or more of the core features of mania [51]. The cerebral components of secondary mania and disinhibition syndrome are very similar. Secondary mania occurs with lesions affecting the orbitofrontal subcortical circuit [52]. Lesions of the temporobasal regions including the amygdala also produce mania.

Several transmitters and modulators are involved in the fronto-subcortical circuits. Overall the character of the symptoms is better defined by the location rather than the particular neurotransmitter. For instance, left anterior lesions (frontal, basal ganglia) give rise to major depression, whereas minor depression occurs with right or left parieto-occipital region [44], obsessive-compulsive behaviours with bilateral basal ganglia [53] and pathological crying and laughing with bi-hemispheric or other lesions [51]. In secondary mania there is a strong association with orbitofrontal [49, 50], basal ganglia [44], thalamus [48], frontotemporal and temporal regions [53]. Although nearly all lesions producing secondary mania and disinhibition syndromes involved the right cerebral hemisphere, they can also be produced by left hemispheric lesions. The cerebral components of secondary mania and disinhibition syndromes are very similar; it could be said that disinhibition syndromes, secondary hypomania and secondary mania with psychotic symptoms are simply a continuum of severity of mood disorder, and secondary mania may be the extreme form. Lesion location appears to play a critical role in the development of secondary mania and disinhibition syndromes.

The high occurrence of medical and neurological conditions in old people compared with the low incidence of late-onset mania (LOM) has made the term 'manic syndromes' in old age one of continuous debate. Manic syndrome in old age is often underdiagnosed. It has been categorised into three groups, namely, (1) middle-age-onset depression who after a latency of several years converts to bipolarity, (2) mixed-aged bipolar patients and (3) late-onset mania (LOM) in association with a heterogeneous group of neurological disorders [45]. Although bipolar disorder is uncommon in old age, it may occur in the absence of an earlier history. Late-onset bipolar disorders are more likely to have an organic pathology such as vascular lesions than the early-onset functional bipolar disorder.

In bipolar disorders full-fledged mania and major depressive episodes alternate. In the depressive phase the symptoms are that seen in unipolar depression but hypersomnia, psychomotor retardation and stupor at times which are distinctive. Mania is characterised by elevation of mood, increased activity and often with frank hostility, the speech is often rapid and in the severe form of the disorder, there is flight of ideas. Sleep is reduced, appetite is increased and so is sexual desire but in older persons there is less sexual preoccupation. Apart from this age has little influence on the symptomatology between old and young [54]. Thought activities are expansive and may be accompanied by grandiose delusions. The patient, for example, is convinced that he is all powerful, a man of wealth, a leader or one who had an aristocratic ancestry. Auditory and visual hallucinations may occur.

There are three stages in the course of the manic disorder based on the severity – mild, moderate and severe. In the mild form there is increased physical activity compared to the severe stage with uncontrolled overactivity; thinking is muddled with delusions and hallucinations [55]. There is occasionally senseless agitation known as 'delirious mania', or the patient is in a stupor and is mute and immobile – 'manic stupor'.

There is a strong resemblance of mania to disinhibition syndromes [56]. Nearly all lesions producing disinhibition syndromes and secondary mania have involved the right hemisphere [57]. In two studies of five and six patients following stroke [58, 59], all had two or more of the core features of mania, namely, elated mood, aggression, irritability and hostility, decreased sleep, impulsive behaviour, overtalkativeness, restlessness, increased activity and increased sexual activity. The mean age was 73 years. The lesions were located in the right thalamus, right posterior cerebral artery territory, left orbital-frontal, left dorsolateral, left mesencephalothalamic and left middle cerebral artery territory.

Box 15.2. Key Points. Mania in Old Age

- Mania usually occurs as a phase of manic-depressive disorder but it can occur in association with medical and pharmacological states.
- Late-onset mania is closely associated with other medical disorders, most commonly stroke, dementia or hypothyroidism, and also the use of medications such as antidepressants, steroids and oestrogens [40].
- With post-stroke mania the strongest association is with a lesion in the right hemisphere.
- Secondary mania occurs with lesions affecting the orbitofrontal subcortical circuit, and several transmitters and modulators are involved in the fronto-subcortical circuits [52].
- Mania in old age has been categorised into three groups, namely, (1) middle-age-onset depression who after a latency of several years converts to bipolarity, (2) mixed-aged bipolar patients and (3) late-onset mania (LOM) in association with a heterogeneous group of neurological disorders [45].
- There is a strong resemblance of mania to disinhibition syndromes [38].

15.3 Anxiety and Anxiety Disorders

Introduction

Anxiety disorder is characterised as anxiety or worry lasting for at least for 6 months and is a group of conditions rather than a single disorder. Pooled 1 year prevalence rate for total anxiety disorder was found to be 10.6 %; overall and lifetime prevalence was 16.6 %[60]. Less than 30 % seek treatment even though anxiety disorders are the most prevalent psychiatric disorder [61]. The current prevalence rate of panic disorder was 0.4 %, OCD 3.2 %, post-traumatic stress disorder 2.5 %, social phobia 2.8 %, specific phobias 11.5 % and generalised anxiety disorder (GAD) 6.0 % [62]. In another study the overall prevalence of anxiety disorders was estimated at 10.2 %, GAD 7.3 % and phobic disorders 3.1 %. Both OCD and panic disorder are rare [63]. Some major epidemiological studies have excluded generalised anxiety disorder (GAD) although it is the most prevalent anxiety disorder in older people [64]. 3.1 % of Australian adults experience GAD which represent 3.7 % of the female and 2.4 % of the male population [65]. There is scanty epidemiologic data on the prevalence of post-traumatic stress disorder (PTSD) and the first occurrence of GAD and PSTD in late life [66]. The first prevalence of panic disorder occurs commonly early and is uncommon after the age of 50 years when it usually associated with a physical cause [67]. The 1-year prevalence of social phobia in Australians is 2.7 % [68]. Co-morbidity of depression and anxiety disorders is highly prevalent [64]. Anxiety disorders were found in 38 % of patients with early dementia, 38 % with Parkinson's disease and 8 % with chronic obstructive airway disease, and 27 % with atypical chest pain had panic disorder [69]. There are a number of drugs associated with anxiety.

Pathophysiology

Anxiety problems are found to have physiological, behavioural and cognitive features. Everyone experiences at some time or other fear and anxiety. Some degree of anxiety is essential and is often helpful, but beyond a certain level, it is unessential and gives rise to hardship and incapacity and becomes a disorder. Pathological anxiety may occur as a component of specific anxiety disorders, other psychiatric disorders or physical illness [70, 71]. In the elderly physical and mental disorders [72] and drugs are the most common causes of anxiety and are often mistaken for an anxiety disorder. Chronic physical problems, cognitive impairment [72] and emotional losses which are nonparalleled to ageing process are the vulnerabilities that generate anxiety [73]. Thus recognising an anxiety disorder in the older adult presents difficulties [74, 75] for advancing age brings with it a higher prevalence of medical conditions, concern about physical symptoms and excessive use of prescription medications [76], and distinguishing the symptoms of anxiety from the medical condition can be arduous [72, 73, 75]. Newly onset anxiety of the elderly with the exception of phobia is routinely combined with physical disorder, depression [77], cognitive dysfunction or personality disorder [78]. Some of the medical conditions which present commonly with anxiety include cardiac arrhythmias, cardiac failure, hyperthyroidism, hypoglycaemia, recurrent pulmonary emboli and rare conditions such as phaeochromocytoma and carcinoid [70, 79].

15.4 Suicide in the Elderly

Introduction

Suicidal behaviour is characterised as a spectrum that ranges from fleeting suicidal thoughts to completed suicide. Suicide can be defined as an act of deliberately or intentionally causing one's own death [80–82]. Nock et al. [81] categorised nonfatal suicidal thoughts and behaviour into (1) suicide ideation, (2) suicide plan and (3) suicide attempt. Suicide ideation almost always used to refer to having the intent to commit suicide including planning as to how it will be done [83]. Suicidal attempts can be defined as self-injurious behaviour without fatal outcome accompanied by evidence (either explicit or implicit) that the person intended to die [84, 85]. Suicidal attempts at the lower end of the spectrum are referred to as suicide gestures. According to Havens [86], there are different degrees of suicidal intent and can be distinguished by the manifestations of different degrees of intent. Suicidal thoughts may represent the least pathological manifestation; others include suicidal threats, plans, gestures and attempts, all of which fall short of completed suicide [86]. Suicide rates increase progressively with age.

The highest suicide rates occur among persons aged 65 years and older and are about 50 % higher than in young people. The annual suicide rates in the United States in the year 2002 were 13.1 per 100,000 individuals in those aged 65–69 years. This number increases further to 17.8 for the aged 75–79 and to 21.0 among persons aged 85 and over [87]. Over 80 % of suicides in white males over the age of 65 years have had no psychiatric referral [88], and the suicide risk in this group was five times that of the general population [89]. The second highest suicide rate is for Australian males over the age of 85 years (39.8 for 100,000 men); the highest is among the younger men age 20–30 years (42.3 for 100,000) [90]. Women attempted suicide 2–3 times as often but men commit suicide three times as often as women, and suicide attempts in the elderly are much more lethal than in the young [91]. The prevalence of suicide ideation in the community-dwelling elderly ranges from 1 to 12 % depending on the definition and assessment method [91]. Incidence of suicide varies also by marital status. Single, widowed, separated, divorced and married without children are more likely to commit suicide than the married elderly [92]. Widowers are significantly more at risk than elderly widows [93].

Pathophysiology

Studies have shown that suicidal behaviour is associated with (1) 5-HT (serotonin) neurotransmitter system [94–96], (2) hyperactivity of the hypothalamic-pituitary-adrenal (HPA) axis [96] and (3) noradrenergic neurotransmission [96]. Dysregulation of the serotonergic system shown by reductions in the brain cerebrospinal fluid (CSF) 5-hydroxyindoleacetic acid (HIAA) was evident on autopsy findings in suicide victims [95]. Lower CSF 5-HIAA levels have been shown to predict future suicidal attempts and completed suicide [97] and suicide attempts after a failed attempt [95]. In suicidal elderly there has only been a single study showing significantly lower CSF 5-HIAA and homovanillic acid (HVA) compared with non-suicidal and normal controls [94].

A number of factors contribute to suicide in older people: bereavement, serious illness, isolation, retirement, organic brain disease and depression. Suicide is generally associated with major depression and is a major problem in the elderly especially elderly males [98]. Suicidal thoughts and depression are sometimes considered by physicians and family members as a natural part of ageing [99].

Box 15.3. Key Points. Suicide in the Elderly

- Studies have shown that suicidal behaviour is associated with (1) 5-HT (serotonin) neurotransmitter system, (2) hyperactivity of the hypothalamic-pituitary-adrenal (HPA) axis and (3) noradrenergic neurotransmission [94–96].
- Lower CSF 5-HIAA levels have been shown to predict future suicidal attempts and completed suicide and suicide attempts after a failed attempt [97].
- Suicide is generally associated with major depression and is a major problem in the elderly especially elderly males [98].

15.5 Substance Abuse in the Elderly

Introduction

Substance abuse in the elderly includes alcoholism, to a lesser degree illicit substances, prescription medications and over-the-counter medications. An estimated 10 % of all cases treated by geriatric mental health facilities are alcohol and substance abuse and together with mental health problems are concurrent and interactive [100]. Alcohol consumption is said to decrease with increasing age. However there is a general consensus that with ageing of the ‘baby boomers’ generation these figures will reach a high level [101]. Demographic data predicts that in the first half of the next century there will be an increase in the absolute number of elderly people with alcohol-related problems [102]. Prescription and over-the-counter drug abuse increase with advancing age, and half of all sedatives are used by people over the age of 60 years. Abuse of tranquillisers and sedatives increased with age and was consistent with prescription drug use in the elderly especially when combined or with alcohol and so did referral to treatment by health-care providers [103]. As the baby boomers age and experience physical disability, shrinking special activities and lower standards of living, substance abuse-related problems may spiral higher [104]. Furthermore it had been suggested that the baby boomers are more likely to have been exposed to drug and alcohol and consume at greater rates after the age of 65 [105].

Alcohol metabolism and ageing
In the elderly population the pattern of alcohol consumption may not change, yet age-related changes may increase the likelihood of adverse reactions [106] with alcohol consumption. There is a decrease in the gastric alcohol dehydrogenase (ADH) with ageing [107, 108] so much so the amount of alcohol metabolised in the stomach is reduced resulting in an increase in the load to the liver. The liver may not be able to metabolise the extra alcohol and the blood levels of alcohol will rise [107]. Alcohol is distributed only in the body water. There is a decrease in the lean body mass as one ages [109] with an increase in the total body fat [110, 111]. Each drink will therefore cause higher blood levels [112] as there is smaller area in which to be distributed.

Pathophysiology
The liver and to a lesser extent the gastrointestinal tract are the sites of alcohol metabolism. Alcohol dehydrogenase (ADH) and aldehyde dehydrogenase (ALDH) are two principle enzymes involved in the ethanol metabolism [113], and both exhibit genetic heterogeneity [114]. Three enzyme systems can oxidise alcohol, the cytosolic alcohol dehydrogenase (ADH) in the liver and stomach, the microsomal ethanol oxidising system and the peroxisomal catalase. Acetaldehyde is the product of all three reactions which is further metabolised to acetate by the mitochondrial enzyme aldehyde dehydrogenase (ALDH) [113, 115]. The acetaldehyde is a reactive metabolite that can produce injury in a variety of ways. The acetaldehyde may have effects on the cells producing it or in various tissues where it had been transported by blood stream [116]. The ALDH isozyme (ALDH2) is often in an immature form and is responsible for the increase in acetaldehyde levels in the body [113]. The Caucasian and Negroid population do not show this enzyme abnormality but about half of the Japanese and Chinese livers possess this abnormality [114].

Neurotransmitters dopamine, gamma-amino butyric acid and glutamate, opioid and serotonergic system are involved in the variability among individuals for susceptibility to alcohol dependence [117, 118]. Alcohol metabolism may differ among individuals and this may be due to different enzymes [118]. The susceptibility to alcohol dependence involves heredity, genetic encoding of alcohol, enzymes [117] and influence of alcohol in the different neurotransmitter systems [119]. ADH and ALDH cause a reduction of the nicotinamide adenine dinucleotide (NAD) to NADH (reduced form of NAD). The altered ratio of NAD/NADH promotes fatty liver through inhibition of gluconeogenesis and fatty acid oxidation. The hepatic macrophages are also activated by chronic alcohol exposure which in turn produces tissue necrosis factor-alpha (TNF-α) [120]. TNF-α causes increased production of reactive

O_2 species resulting in oxidative stress which fosters hepatocyte necrosis and apoptosis which worsened in alcoholics who are deficient in oxidants such as vitamin E and glutathione. Acetaldehyde incites inflammation so do free radicals causing inflammation and fibrosis.

Box 15.4. Key Points. Substance Abuse in the Elderly

- Alcohol dehydrogenase (ADH) and aldehyde dehydrogenase (ALDH) are two principle enzymes involved in the ethanol metabolism, and both exhibit genetic heterogeneity [113, 114].
- Acetaldehyde is the product of all three reactions which is further metabolised to acetate by the mitochondrial enzyme aldehyde dehydrogenase (ALDH) [113, 115].
- Neurotransmitters dopamine, gamma-amino butyric acid and glutamate, opioid and serotonergic system are involved in the variability among individuals for susceptibility to alcohol dependence [117, 118].
- The susceptibility to alcohol dependence involves heredity, genetic encoding of alcohol, enzymes and influence of alcohol in the different neurotransmitter systems [117].
- Acetaldehyde incites inflammation so do free radicals causing inflammation and fibrosis.

Multiple Choice Questions

1. The following are true with depression in the elderly, EXCEPT:
   A. Late-onset depression (LOD) is due to age-associated neurobiological changes, stressful events, a higher interaction with cognitive decline and impaired effect of genes.
   B. A family history of depression is more likely with early-onset depression (EOD) than late-onset depression.
   C. Late-onset depression is closely linked to clinical and neuroimaging evidence of cerebrovascular disease.
   D. Structural imaging changes vary considerably between LOD and EOD with more severe vascular pathology associated with EOD compared to LOD.
2. The following statements are true with mania in late life, EXCEPT:
   A. After many years of depression, many are converted to bipolarity and suffer from mania in late life.
   B. Late-onset mania is closely associated with medical disorders, most commonly stroke, dementia or hypothyroidism and also the use of medications.

C. Secondary manias are used to describe late-onset mania associated with medical and pharmacological states.
D. There is no supporting clinical and neuroimaging evidence of cerebrovascular disease that link it with 'late-onset' depression.
3. The following are true in relation to major depression, EXCEPT:
A. Serotonergic activity is reduced in depression.
B. There is overproduction of glutamate.
C. Dopamine circuits do not have any role in depression.
D. Noradrenergic containing circuits are involved in the aetiology of mood disorders.
4. The following are true in the metabolism of alcohol in the elderly, EXCEPT:
A. Age-related changes may increase the likelihood of adverse reactions with alcohol consumption.
B. Gastric ADH is decreased with ageing so much so the amount of alcohol metabolised in the stomach is reduced resulting in an increase in the load to the liver.
C. The liver however will not be able to metabolise the extra alcohol and the blood levels of alcohol will rise.
D. Alcohol is distributed only in the body fat.
5. The following that are associated with suicidal behaviour in the elderly are true, EXCEPT:
A. There is hyperactivity of the hypothalamic-pituitary-adrenal axis.
B. Suicide is generally associated with major depression and is a major problem in the elderly especially elderly females.
C. Factors such as bereavement, serious illness, isolation, retirement and organic brain disease contribute to suicide in older people.
D. There is dysregulation of the serotonergic system.

Answers to MCQs

1 = D; 2 = D; 3 = C, 4 = D; 5 = B.

References

Introduction

1. Psychiatry of old age. http://www.cchs.net/health/health-info/docs/2200/2268.asp?index+9313. Accessed 14 Sept 2007.
2. Beckman AT, Copeland JR, Prince MJ. Review of community prevalence of depression late life. Br J Psychiatry. 1999;174:307–11.
3. Callahan EJ, Bertakis KD, Azari R, Helms LJ, Robbins J, Miller J. Depression in primary care patient, factors that influence recognition. Fam Med. 1997;29:172–6.
4. Karim S, Byrne EJ. Treatment of psychosis in elderly people. Br J Psychiatry. 2005;11: 286–96.

Mood Disorders (Major Depression, Bipolar Disorder)

5. McAlister-Williams H. Classification of depression website: http://www.netdoctor.co.uk/diseases/depression/classification_000001.htm.
6. Vacheron-Trystram MN, Braitman A, Cheref S, Auffray L. Antipsychotics in bipolar disorders. Encephalae. 2004;30(5):417–24 (abstract).
7. Fiske A, Wetherell JL, Gatz M. Depression in older adults. Annu Rev Clin Psychol. 2009;5:363–98.
8. Baldwin RC, O'Brien J. Vascular basis of late-onset depressive disorder. Br J Psychiatry. 2002;180:157–60.
9. Brodaty H, Luscombe G, Parke G, Wihem K, Hickie I, Austin MP, et al. Early and late onset depression in old age: different aetiology same phenomenology. J Affect Disord. 2001;66:225–56.
10. Devanandan DP, Adorno E, Cheng J, Burt T, Pelton GH, Roose SP, et al. Late onset dysthymic disorder and major depression differ from early onset dysthymic disorder and major depression in elderly outpatients. J Affect Disord. 2004;78:259–67.
11. Huen R, Papassotiropoulos A, Jessen F, Maier W, Breitner JC, et al. A family study of Alzheimer disease and early- and late-onset depression in elderly patients. Arch Gen Psychiatry. 2001;58:190–6.
12. Hickie I, Naismuth S, Ward PB, Turner K, Scott E, Mitchell P, et al. Reduced hippocampal volumes and memory loss in patients with early – and late-onset depression. Br J Psychiatry. 2005;186:197–202.
13. Alexopolous GS, Meyers BS, Young RC, Kakuma T, Silbersweig D, Charlson M. Clinically defined vascular depression. Am J Psychiatry. 1997;154:497–501.
14. Mast BT, MacNeill SE, Litchenberg PA. Post-stroke and clinically defined vascular depression in geriatric rehabilitation. Am J Geriatr Psychiatry. 2004;12(1):84–92.
15. Hickie IB. Reducing the burdens of depression: are we making progress in Australia? Med J Aust. 2004;181:S4–5.
16. Starkstein SE, Robinson ER. Affective disorders in cerebrovascular disease. Br J Psychiatry. 1989;154:170–82.
17. Carod-Artel F. Post-stroke depression (ii): its differential diagnosis, complications and treatment. Rev Neurol. 2006;42(4):238–44.
18. Robinson RG, Starkstein SE. Mood disorders following stroke: new findings and future directions. J Geriatr Psychiatry. 1989;22(1):1–15.
19. Hama S, Yamashita H, Shigenobu M, Watanabe A, Hiramoto K, Taimoto Y, et al. Post-stroke affective or apathetic depression and lesion location: left frontal lobe and bilateral basal ganglia. Eur Arch Psychiatry Clin Neurosci. 2007;257:149–52.
20. House A, Dennis M, Warlow C, Hanton K, Molyneux A. Mood disorders after stroke and their relation to lesion location. Brain. 1990;113:1113–29.
21. Sharpe M, Hawton K, House A. Mood disorders in long-term survivors of stroke associations with brain lesion location and volume. Psychol Med. 1990;20:815–28.
22. Takahashi K, Oshima A, Ida I, Kumano H, Yuuki N, Fukuda M, et al. Relationship between age at onset and magnetic resonance image-defined hyperintensities in mood disorders. J Psychiatr Res. 2008;42:443–50.
23. Lin HF, Kuo YT, Chiang IC, Chen HM, Chen CS. Structural abnormality on brain magnetic resonance imaging in late-onset major depressive disorder. Kaohsiung J Med Sci. 2006;21:405–11.
24. Papazacharias A, Logroscino G, Barulli MR, Nardini M. Late life depression and late onset depression: are the same clinical and pathological picture? Psychiatr Danub. 2010;22 Suppl 1:108–10.
25. Naismuth SL, Hickie IB, Ward PB, Scott EM, Little CL. Impaired implicit sequence learning in depression: a probe for frontostriatal dysfunction? Psychol Med. 2006;36:313–23.
26. Hickie B, Naismuth SL, Ward PB, Little CL, Pearson M, Scott EM, et al. Psychomotor slowing in older patients with major depression: relationships with blood flow in the caudate nucleus and white matter lesions. Psychiatry Res. 2007;155:211–20.

27. Gottfries CG, Blennon K, Karisson I, Wallin A. The neurochemistry of vascular dementia. Dementia. 1994;5:163–7.
28. Allard P, Englund E, Marcusson J. Reduced number of caudate nucleus dopamine uptake sites in vascular dementia. Dement Geriatr Cogn Disord. 1999;10:77–80.
29. Huffman JC, Stern TA. Poststroke neuropsychiatric symptoms and pseudoseizures: a discussion. J Clin Psychiatry. 2003;5(2):85–8.
30. Hickie IB, Naismuth SL, Norrie LM, Scott EM. Managing depression across the life cycle: new strategies for clinicians and their patients. Intern Med J. 2009;39:720–3.
31. Dunlop BW, Nemeroff CB. The role of dopamine in the pathophysiology of depression. Arch Gen Psychiatry. 2007;64:327–37.
32. Nemeroff CB. Recent findings in the pathophysiology of depression. FOCUS. 2008;6:3–14.
33. Mann JJ, Malone KM, Psych MR, Sweeney JA, Brown RP, Linnolin M, et al. Attempted suicide characteristics and cerebrospinal fluid amine metabolites in depressed patients. Neuropsychopharmacology. 1996;15:576–86.
34. Drevets WC, Frank E, Price JC, Kupler DJ, Holt D, Greer PJ, et al. PET imaging of serotonin 1A receptor binding in depression. Biol Psychiatry. 1999;46:1375–87.
35. Ressler KJ, Nemeroff CB. Role of norepinephrine in the pathophysiology of neuropsychiatric disorders. CNS Spectr. 2001;6:663–6.
36. Muller N, Schwarz MJ. The immune-mediated alteration of serotonin and glutamate: towards an integrated view of depression. Mol Psychiatry. 2007;12:988–1000.

Mania in Old Age

37. Aziz R, Lorberg B, Tampi RR. Treatments for late life bipolar disorder. Am J Geriatr Pharmacother. 2006;4(4):347–64 (abstract).
38. Shulman KL, Hermann N. The nature and management of mania in old age. Psychiatr Clin North Am. 1999;22:649–63.
39. Hickie I, Scott E, Wilhelm K, Brodaty H. Subcortical hyperintensities on magnetic resonance imaging in patients with severe depression-a longitudinal evaluation. Biol Psychiatry. 1997;42:367–74.
40. Kennedy GJ. Bipolar disorder in late life: mania. Primary Psychiatry. website: http://www.primarypsychiatry.com/aspx/atrticledetail.aspx?artiicleid+=1404.
41. Nagaratnam N, Wong K-K, Patel I. Secondary mania of vascular origin in elderly patients: a report of two clinical cases. Arch Gerontol Geriatr. 2006;43:223–32.
42. Fujikawa T, Yamasaki S, Touhouda Y. Silent cerebral infarctions in patients with late-onset mania. Stroke. 1995;26:946–9.
43. Herlihy Jr CE, Herlihy CE. Lithium and organic brain syndrome. J Clin Psychiatry. 1979;40:455 (Letter to editor).
44. Fenn D, George R. Post-stroke mania late in life involving the left hemisphere. Aust N Z J Psychiatry. 1999;33:598–608.
45. Turecki G, De Mari J, Porto JAD. Bipolar disorder following a left basal ganglia stroke. Br J Psychiatry. 1993;163:690.
46. Liu CY, Wang SJ, Fuh JL, Yang YY, Lin HC. Bipolar disorder following a stroke involving the left hemisphere. Aust N Z J Psychiatry. 1996;30:688–91.
47. Drake Jr ME, Pakalnis A, Phillips B. Secondary mania after ventral pontine infarction. J Neuropsychiatry Clin Neurosci. 1990;2:322–5.
48. Bogousslavasky J, Ferrazzani M, Regli F, Assal G, Tanabe H, Delaloyebischof A. Manic delirium and frontal-lobe syndrome with paramedian infarction of the right thalamus. J Neurol Neurosurg Psychiatry. 1988;51:116–9.
49. Cummings JL. Organic delusions, phenomenology, anatomical evaluation and review. Br J Psychiatry. 1985;146:184–97.
50. Starksein SE, Fedoroff P, Berthier ML, Robinson RG. Manic depressive and pure manic states after brain lesions. Biol Psychiatry. 1991;29:149–58.

51. Nagaratnam N, Lim R, Chowdhury M. Aberrant sexual behaviour following stroke. Eur J Int Med. 1998;9:207–9.
52. Cummings JL, Mendez MF. Secondary mania with focal cerebrovascular lesions. Am J Psychiatry. 1984;141:1084–7.
53. Laplane D, Levasseur M, Pillon B, Dubois B, Baulac M, Mazoyer B, et al. Obsessive-compulsive and other behavioural changes with bilateral basal ganglia lesions. A neuropsychological, magnetic resonance imaging and positron tomography study. Brain. 1989;6:237–55.
54. Young RC, Kiosses D, Heo M, Schulberg HC, Murphy C, Klimstra S, et al. Age and ratings of manic psychopathology. Bipolar Disord. 2007;9(3):301–4.
55. Carlson GA, Goodwin FK. The stages of mania. Arch Gen Psychaitry. 1973;23:221–2.
56. Shulman KI. Mania in old age: a neuropsychiatric syndrome. Geriatrics Aging. 2004;7:34–7.
57. Steffens DC, Krishnan KRR. Structural neuroimaging and mood disorders. Recent findings, implications for classification, and future directions. Biol Psychiatry. 1991;43:705–12.
58. Nagaratnam N, Wong V, Jeyaratnam D. Left anterior choroidal artery infarction and uncontrollable crying. J Stroke Cerebrovasc Dis. 1998;7:263–4.
59. Nagaratnam N, Gayagay G. Hypersexuality in nursing care facilities- a descriptive study. Arch Gerontol Geriatr. 2002;35:195–203.

Anxiety and Anxiety Disorders

60. Somers JM, Goldner EM, Waraich P, Hsu L. Prevalence and incidence studies of anxiety disorders: a systematic review of the literature. Can J Psychiatry. 2006;51(2):100–13.
61. Lepine JP. The epidemiology of anxiety disorders: prevalence and social codes. J Clin Psychiatry. 2002;63 Suppl 14:1–4 (abstract).
62. Kimiziogh Y, Dogar O, Kugn N, Akyuz G. Prevention of anxiety disorders among the elderly. Int J Geriatr Psychiatry. 2009;24(9):1026–33.
63. Beckman AT, Bremmer MA, Deig DJ, van Balkom AM, Smit JH, De Beurs E, et al. Anxiety disorders in later life: a report from the Longitudinal Aging Study Amsterdam. Int J Geriatr Psychiatry. 1998;13(10):717–26 (abstract).
64. Beckman AT, de Beurs S, van Balkom AJL, Deeg DJ, van Dyck R, Tilburg W. Anxiety and depression in later life. Co-occurrence and commonality of risk factors. Am J Psychiatry. 2000;157:89–95.
65. Mental Health Council Inc and ORYGEN, Australian Government Department of Employment and Work Place Relations. Research Centre; 2000.
66. Flint AJ. Epidemiology and comorbidity of anxiety disorders in the elderly. Am J Psychiatry. 1994;15(15):640–9 (abstract).
67. Satcher D. Mental Health: a report of the Surgeon General US Government. Washington, DC: Department of Health and Human Services; 1999.
68. Wills JC, Tien AY, Garrisa R, Eaton W. Risk factors with incidence of social phobia as determined by Diagnostic Intervention Schedule in a Population-based study. Acta Psychiatr Scand. 1994;90:84–90.
69. Sadavoy J, Lellar JK. Treatment of anxiety disorders in late life. Can J Psychiatry. 1997;42 Suppl 1:28S–34.
70. Jefferson JW, Marshall JR, editors. Neuropsychiatric features of mental disorders. New York: Plenum; 1981. p. 6–7.
71. Hentz P. Separating anxiety from physical illness. The Clinical Advisor. 2008. www.clinicaladvisor.com.
72. Friedman MB, Furst L, Gellis Zvi D, Williams K. Social Work Today. 2013;13(4):10.
73. Anxiety in the elderly. www.healthyplace.com/anxety-panic/articles/anxiety-in-the-elderly.
74. Sable JA, Jeste DV. Anxiety disorders in older adults. Curr Psychiatry Rep. 2001;3(4):302–7.
75. Gilles Zvi D, Kim EG, McCracken SG. Master's Advanced Curriculum (MAC) Project. Mental health and aging resource review, 2014. Revision. Chap 2. Anxiety disorders in older adults. Literature review. www.CSWE.org/File.aspx?id=23485.

76. Nobili A, Garattini S, Mannuci PM. Multiple diseases and polypharmacy in the elderly: challenges for the internist of the third millennium. J Comorbidity. 2011;7:28–44.
77. Hek K, Tiemeier H, Newman RS, Luijendijk H, Hofman A, Mudder CL. Anxiety disorders and comorbid depression in community dwelling older adults. Int J Methods Rev. 2011;20(3):157–68.
78. Nakra B, Grossberg G. Management of anxiety in the elderly. Compr Ther. 1986;12:53–80.
79. Hall RCW, Hall RCW. Anxiety and endocrine disease. www.drrichardhall.com/Article/anxiety.pdf. Accessed 7 Jan 2016.

Suicide in the Elderly

80. WHO. http://www.who.int/topics/suicide/en/. Retrieved 22 Sept 2103.
81. Nock MK, Borges G, Bromet EJ, Cha CB, Kessler RC, Lee S. Cross-rational prevalence and risk factors for suicidal ideation, plans and attempts. Br J Psychiatry. 2008;192:98–115.
82. Shneidman ES. The definition of suicide. New York/London: Wiley; 1985.
83. Read K, Purse M. Suicidal ideation. About.com.Bipolar Disorder. http://bipolar.about.con/od/suicide/g/suicidalideatio.htm. Retrieved 3 July 2006.
84. American Psychiatric Association. Practice guidelines for the assessment and treatment of patients with suicide behaviours. Am J Psychiatry. 2003;160 suppl 11:1–30.
85. Jacobs D, Baldessarini R, Conwell Y, Fawcett JA, Horton L, Meltzer H, et al. Practice guidelines for the assessment and treatment of patients with suicidal behaviours. Psychiatric Online http://psycho.silverchair.com/contentsaspx?De57699. Retrieved 23 Sept 2013.
86. Havens LL. Diagnosis of suicidal intent. 2009 Annual Review website: annualreview.org/aroutine.
87. National Strategy for Suicide Prevention. Suicide in the elderly. http://mentalhealth.samhsa.gov/suicideprevention/elderly.asp. Accessed 3 Oct 2009.
88. Duckworth G, Mcbride H. Suicide in old age: a tragedy of neglect. Can J Psychiatry. 1996;41(4):217–22 (abstract).
89. Anderson RN, Smith BL. Deaths: leading causes for 2001. Natl Vital Stat Rep. 2003;52(9):1–47.
90. National Advisory Council in Suicide prevention Draft 6. It's all about living. A National partnership for the prevention of suicide and self harm 1999. Phillip ACT: Department of Health and Ageing; 1999.
91. Dombroyski AY, Szanto K. Prevention of suicide in the elderly. Ann Long term Care. website: http://www.annalsolongtermcare.com/article/5082. Accessed 3.10.09.
92. McIntosh JL. Suicide among the elderly; levels and trends. J Orthopsychiatry. 1985;55:75–82.
93. Suicide DE. A study in sociology. New York: The Free Press; 1997. Translated by John A Spaulding and George Simpson ed George Simpson, 1997.
94. Jones JS, Stanley B, Mann JJ, Francis AJ, Guido JR, Traskinan-Bendz L, et al. CSF-5-HIAA and HVA concentrations in elderly depressed patients who attempted suicide. Am J Psychiatry. 1990;147:1225–7.
95. Cattell H. Suicide in the elderly. Adv Psychiatr Treat. 2000;6:102–8. doi:10.1192/apt.6.2.102.
96. Van Heiringen K. Neurobiology of suicide and suicidality. Can J Psychiatry. 2003;48:292–300.
97. Nordstrom P, Samuelsson M, Asberg M, Traskinan-Bendz L, Alberg-Wistedt A, Nordin C, et al. CSF 5-HIAA predicts suicide risk after attempted suicide. Suicide Life Threat Behav. 1994;24:1–9.
98. Barraclough B. Suicide in the elderly. In: Kay DWK, Walk A, editors. Recent developments in psychogeriatrics. Ashford: Headley Bros; 1971. p. 87–9.
99. Institute of Medicine. Reducing scale. A national imperative. Washington DC: The National Academic Press; 2002. website: http://darwin.nap.edu. Accessed 24 July 2006.

Substance Abuse in the Elderly

100. King CJ, Ven Hasselt VB, Segal DL, Hersen M. Diagnosis and treatment of substance abuse in older adults. Correct strategies and issues. Addict Behav. 1994;19:41–55.
101. Blow FC, Walton MA, Chermacvk ST, Mudd SA, Brower KJ. Older adult treatment outcome following elder-specific in patient alcoholism treatment. J Subst Abuse Treat. 2000;19(1):67–75.
102. Johnson I. Alcohol problems in old age: a review of recent epidemiological research. Int J Geriatr Psychiatry. 2000;15(7):575–81.
103. Henderson LA. Age differences in multiple drug use. National Admissions to Publicly Funded Substance Abuse Treatment. Chap 4 http://www.ors.sanihsn.gov/aging/chap4.htm.
104. Koenig HG, George LK, Schneider R. Mental health care for older adults in the year 2020. A dangerous and topic. Gerontologist. 1994;34:674–9.
105. Levin SM, Kruger J. editors. Substance abuse among older adults: a guide for social service providers. Rockville: Substance abuse and Mental Health Services Administration; 2000.
106. Smith JW. Medical manifestations of alcoholism in the elderly. Int J Addit. 1995;309(13-14):174–1798.
107. Seitz HK, Egerer G, Simanowski VA, Waldherr R, Eckey R, Agarwal DP, et al. Human gastric alcohol dehydrogenase activity: effect of age, sex and alcoholism. Gut. 1993;34(10): 1433–7.
108. Pozzato G, Moretti M, Franzin F, Groce LS, Lacchin T, Benedetti G, et al. Ethanol metabolism and aging. The role of 'first pass metabolism' and gastric acohol dehydrogenase activity. J Gerontol A Biol Sci Med Sci. 1995. doi:10.1093/gerona/50A.3.8135.
109. Newman AB, Lee JS, Visser M, Goodpaster BH, Kritchevsky SB, Tylavsky FA, et al. Weight change and conservation of lean mass in old age: the Health Aging and Body Composition Study. 1'2'3. Am Soc Clin Nutr. 2005;82(4):872–8.
110. Skovenborg E. Alcohol consumption and the elderly, do adult responsible drinking guidelines apply? www.aim-digest.com/digest/members%20over%20yr/skovraged.pdf. Accessed 6 Jan 2016.
111. Dufour M, Archer L, Gordis E. Alcohol and the elderly. Clin Geriatr Med. 1992;8(1):127–41.
112. NIH Senior Health. Alcohol use and older adults. http://nihseniorhealth.gov/alcoholuse/alcoholandaging/0.1html. Accessed 5 Jan 2016.
113. Suddendorf RF. Research on alcohol metabolism among Asians and its implications for understanding causes of alcoholism. Public Health Rep. 1989;104(6):615–20 (abstract).
114. Agarwal DP, Goedde HVV. Pharmacogenetics of alcohol metabolism and alcoholism. Pharmacogenetics. 1992;3(2):48–62 (abstract).
115. Stewart S, Jones D, Day CP. Alcoholic liver disease: new insights into mechanisms and preventive strategies. Trends Mol Med. 2001;7:408–13.
116. Crabb DW, Matsumoto M, Chang D, You M. Overview of the role of alcohol dehydrogenase and aldehyde dehydrogenase and their variants in the genesis of alcohol-related pathology. Proc Nutr Soc. 2004;63(1):49–63 (abstract).
117. Ginter E, Simko V. Alcoholism: recent advances in epidemiology, biochemistry and genetics. Bratisl Lek Listy. 2009;110(5):307–11 (abstract).
118. Li TK. Pharmacogenetics of responses to alcohol and genes that influence alcohol drinking. J Stud Alcohol. 2000;61(1):5–12 (abstract).
119. Moussas G, Christodoulou C, Donzenia A. A short review on the aetiology and pathophysiology of alcoholism. Ann Gen Psychiatry. 2009;8:10. doi:10.1186/1744-850-8-10 (abstract).
120. Zhon Z, Wang L, Song Z, Lambert JC, McClain CJ, Kong YJ. A critical involvement of oxidative stress in acute alcohol induced hepatic tumour-necrosis factor-alpha production. Am J Path. 2003;163:1137–46.

Low and Loss of Vision in the Elderly

16

16.1 Anatomical and Physiological Changes with Ageing

Age-related changes occur in all structures of the eye causing varied effects [1]. It causes laxity of the eyelid tissues due to involutional changes of the skin; the muscles – levator and orbicularis; the tarsus and the tendons [2]. There is atrophy of the orbital fat. The horizontal eyelid fissure shortens with ageing. The most striking age-related changes occur in the lens. The major areas in the lens are the nucleus which is in the centre, surrounded by the cortex, and the capsule is the outer layer. As age advances, there is hardening of the lens (nuclear sclerosis) [1], and lens becomes thick and less pliable due to continued growth of the lens fibres. With ageing, there is increase opacity of the lens nucleus, thickness of the cortex and anterior lens capsule [3]. Eventually, there is inability to change its shape resulting in reduced accommodation which in part may also be due to atrophy of the ciliary muscles. These changes are continuous with age.

With ageing, lens opacities and changes in the vitreous often increase the scattering of light passing through the lens, and it is not unusual for the older person to complain of a glare while driving at night from the headlights of the oncoming vehicles [4]. The visual acuity is usually normal. Daytime glare often with bright light occurs where there are opacities beneath the posterior lens capsule. These opacities may subsequently increase in size and interfere with visual acuity. With ageing, the less clear lens scatter more light and thus reduce the contrast of the retinal image. The lens optical density increases with age, the lens becomes coloured due to accumulation of yellow pigments [1] and the intrinsic fluorescence increases [5]. There is a decreased ability to discriminate colours especially blue colours because of the loss of sensitivity to short wavelengths. The lens selectively absorbs more blue light causing a relative 'blue blindness' [1]. In the older person, the thickened lens responds slowly to change in tension of the elastic capsule. As a result, there is difficulty to focus on near objects (presbyopia).

The vitreous gel undergoes liquefaction and its opacities are visible as floaters, and separation of the vitreous gel from the retina with ageing may also manifest as floaters [2]. Posterior vitreous detachment (PVD) occurs when about 50 % of the

N. Nagaratnam et al., *Diseases in the Elderly: Age-Related Changes and Pathophysiology*, DOI 10.1007/978-3-319-25787-7_16

liquefaction is reached [1]. PVD by itself is innocuous, and the patients often note a spiderlike floater in front of the eye which moves in the direction of the gaze [1]. With ageing, a number of changes occur in the retina including the accumulation of melanin granules, accumulation of basal deposits on or within the Bruch's membrane, accumulation of lipofuscin and thickening of Bruch's membrane [6]. There is narrowing of the choroidal vessels, reduction in the number of photoreceptors and slow fall out of the retinal pigmentary epithelium (RPE). In the seventh decade, there appears a layer of membranous debris from the basal surface of the RPE and focal accumulation of the material forming soft drusen, and these changes have no counterpart in earlier life [7]. Bruch's membrane also becomes laden with debris from the RPE. This results in loss of elasticity and increased fragility of the Bruch's membrane. The vision deteriorates with age and is due to a combination of factors associated with ageing, changes in the ocular media, smaller pupil [1] and reduced retinal illuminance because of the smaller pupil and thicker lens occurring with age.

Box 16.1. Key Points. Age-Related Eye Changes

- Age-related changes occur in all structures of the eye causing varied effects [1].
- With ageing, there is increase opacity of the lens nucleus, thickness of the cortex and anterior lens capsule, and they are continuous with age [3].
- With ageing, lens opacities and changes in the vitreous often increase the scattering of light passing through the lens [4].
- There is decreased ability to discriminate colours especially blue colours because of the loss of sensitivity to short wavelengths ('blue blindness') [1].
- Vitreous gel undergoes liquefaction and its opacities are visible as floaters [2].
- Lipofuscin accumulates and there is thickening of Bruch's membrane [6].
- Bruch's membrane also becomes laden with debris from the RPE.
- The vision deteriorates with age and is due to a combination of factors associated with ageing [1].

16.2 Low and Loss of Vision in the Elderly

The four common causes of low vision in the elderly patients are:

1. Age-related macular degeneration
2. Glaucoma
3. Cataract
4. Diabetic retinopathy

In 2002, the number of people with visual impairment worldwide was in excess of 161 million of whom about 37 million were blind [8]. Major causes of visual impairment in the order of importance were glaucoma, age-related macular degeneration, diabetic retinopathy and trachoma [8]. According to the National Eye Institute [9] in the United States, the prevalence of cataract, age-associated macular degeneration (AMD) and glaucoma increased with age. The prevalence of blindness and low vision in the United States increased from 0.3 % in the 60–69 age group to 7.0 % in the 80 years and over and in low vision 0.9–16.7 %, respectively [9].

16.2.1 Age-Related Macular Degeneration (AMD, ARMD)

Introduction
Age-related macular degeneration (AMD, ARMD) is characterised by degenerative changes in the macula resulting in loss of central vision in the elderly. AMD occurs in older people, one in seven over the age of 50 which increases to one in three for people over the age of 75 years [10]. In the United States, it is the leading cause of loss of central vision in the 50 years and older [11]. The prevalence of AMD increases with increasing age, about 10 % in the 66–74 year group to 30 % in the 75–85 year group [12].

Pathophysiology
The pathophysiology of AMD is complex and unclear and the pathological processes implicated are accumulation of lipofuscin (with its linkage to oxidative stress), formation of drusen, neovascularisation and local inflammation [13]. Dysfunction of the retinal pigmentary epithelium (RPE) occurs early and is brought about by an inherited susceptibility and/or environmental exposure [14]. Extracellular matrix (ECM) material is produced by the RPE and plays an important role in some of the functions of this tissue. In both early and advanced AMD, there is continuous rebuilding of ECM, and the degradation and accumulation of ECM structural components result from impairment or hyperactivity of specific matrix metalloproteinases MMPs/tissue inhibitor of metalloproteinases (TIMPs) complexes [15]. Besides the RPE, other functionally interrelated tissues are the Bruch's membrane, photoreceptors and choriocapillaris [13]. There is thickening of Bruch's membrane with accumulation of membranous debris on either side of the RPE which hinders the exchange of waste products between the outer retina and the choroid [7]. The membranous debris that accumulates on either side of the RPE and the RPE correlate with the AMD, and the membranous debris is now believed to be lipoprotein-derived, and the lipoproteins are not dietary nor systemic but are waste products of retinal metabolism.

Drusen are small yellowish-white excrescences which lie under the RPE and protrude into the cells and separate the retina from the choroid capillary. They may be soft (distinct or indistinct) or hard. The soft drusen are larger and tend to be confluent (Fig. 16.1) and precede the development RPE detachment and choroidal neovascularisations (CNVs) [16] and specific for AMD. Progression to exudative maculopathy correlates with drusen characteristics such as size, number and confluence [16]. The hard drusen are small and occur in clusters and are globular in shape (Fig. 16.2) and pose a low rate of choroidal neovascularisation (CNV). The RPE cells die and an area of atrophy and choriocapillaris develops and the membranous

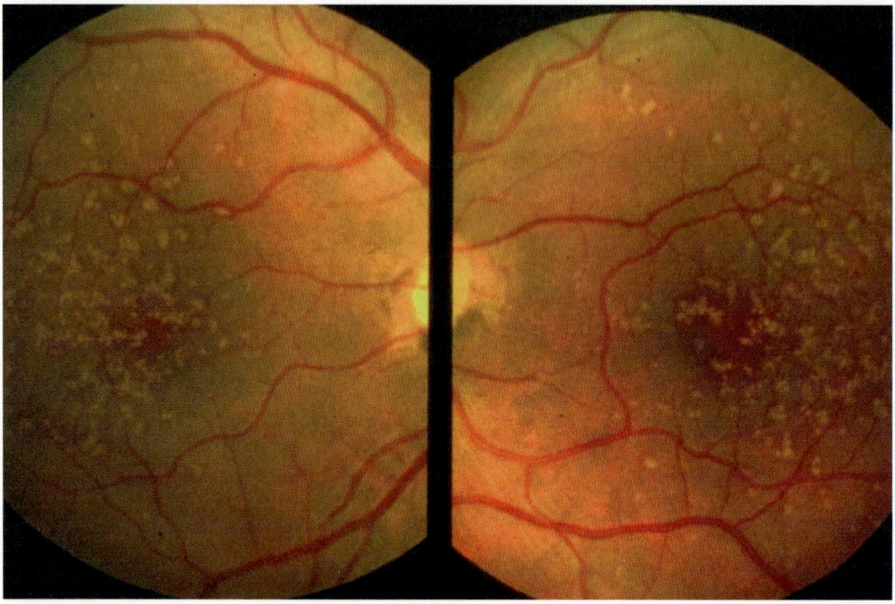

Fig. 16.1 (**a**) Soft drusen and (**b**) in clusters (Reproduced with permission from Dr. John Sarks)

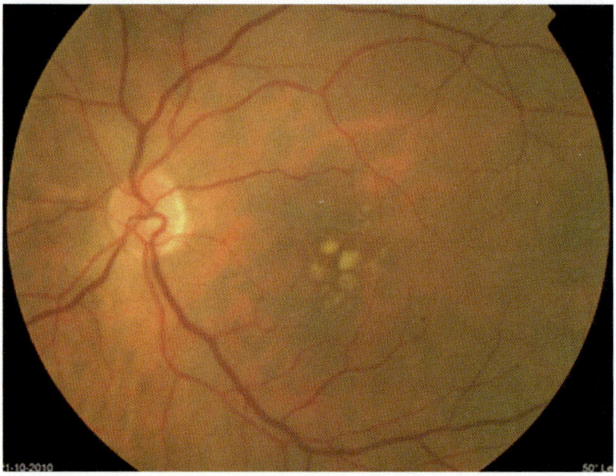

Fig. 16.2 Hard drusen (Reproduced with permission from Dr. John Sarks)

debris then disappears and drusen regresses (Fig. 16.3), but the drusen can regress without evidence of atrophy [16]. All drusen undergo a cycle of formation and regression. The loss of RPE is accompanied by loss of photoreceptors and the atrophic areas become non-functioning. In early AMD, besides the presence of soft drusen, there may be a disturbance of pigmentation. AMD can be classified as early (marked by drusen and pigmentary change and associated with normal vision) and late [17]. Focal pigmentation and systemic hypertension are associated with

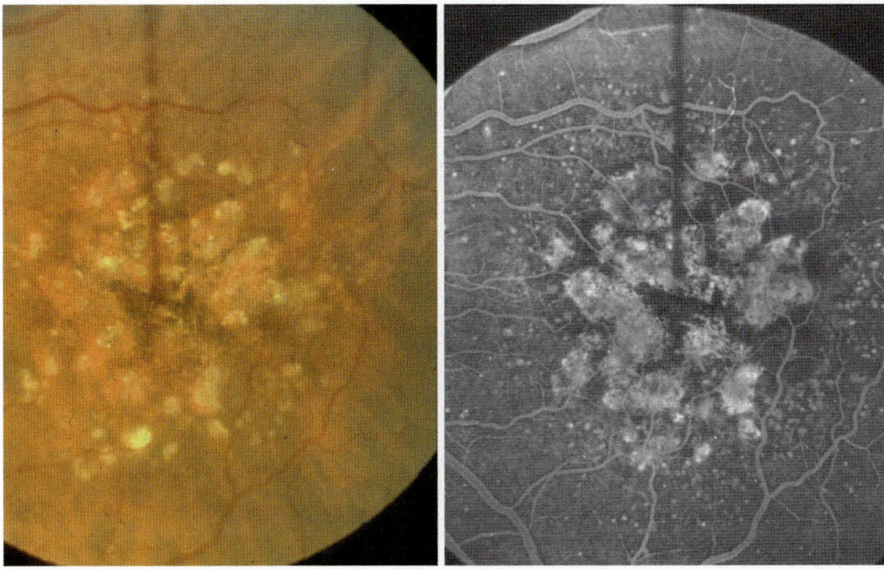

Fig. 16.3 Drusen in regression (Reproduced with permission from Dr. John Sarks)

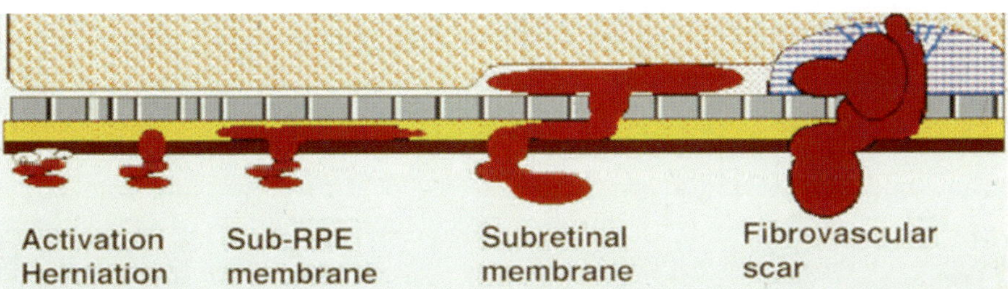

Fig. 16.4 Stages of CNV. Intrachoroidal phase. Choroidal capillaries activated vessels bulge through prepared gaps of Bruch's membrane spread beneath RPE (Gass type1) of cleavage phase; CNV breaks through RPE and forms sensory retina (Gass type2). Exudation, bleeding, fibrosclerosis, arterialisation (Reproduced with permission from the authors J Sarks and S. Sarks. Original photographs published in *How to Treat, Australian Doctor*, 2001)

increased risk of developing CNVs [16]. Individually, a significant symmetry of drusen characteristics is seen although clinical appearances may vary from one individual to another [18].

The deposition of neutral lipids in Bruch's membrane is associated with RPE detachments [18]. RPE and the choriocapillaris are on opposite sides of the Bruch's membrane and control the transfer in and out of the retina [19] and with subsequent atrophy of the choriocapillaris, calcification and fragmentation of Bruch's membrane [20]. The late stage has two forms, atrophic (or dry) characterised by geographical atrophy and exudative (wet) characterised by development of choroidal neovascularisation (CNV) (Fig. 16.4). This results in a break in the Bruch's membrane through

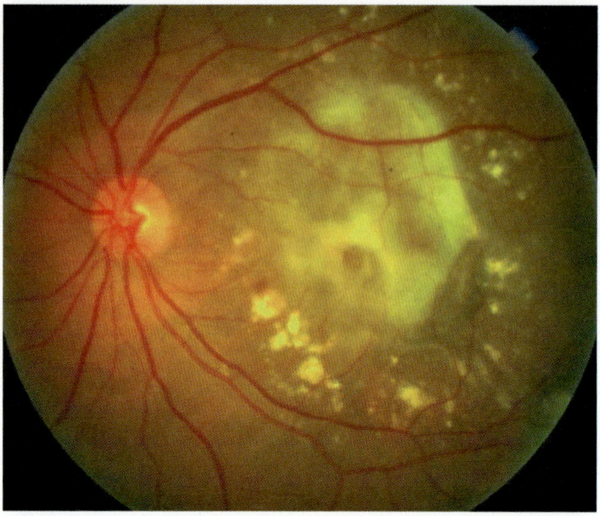

Fig. 16.5 Forming of disciform scar (Reproduced with permission from Dr. John Sarks)

which the neovascular vessels from the choroids encroach into the space below the RPE. This is followed by white hard exudates, intra-retinal haemorrhages, subretinal haemorrhages and eventually forming a disciform scar (Fig. 16.5) [21, 22]. Progression to CNVs results from angiogenic factors such as vascular endothelial group factor (VEGF) [13]. A critical balance exists between VEGF and a pigment epithelium-derived factor (PEDF – antiangiogenic factor), and a decrease in PEDF may disturb the balance and allow the formation of CNV [23].

The last few years have led to a better understanding of the molecular mechanisms underlying AMD [24] and the role of genetic factors in the aetiology of AMD [24, 25]. There has always been much speculation of the role of inflammation because chronic inflammatory cells can be found, but many have regarded this as appearing secondary to the debris produced. However, some drusen contain components of the complement system so that the current understanding is that some trigger event in genetically predisposed individuals [25], together with impaired regulation of the complement pathways [24] leads to complement activation, drusen and AMD. There is convincing evidence that the complement system especially the alternative pathway plays a vital role in the patho-aetiology of AMD [24]. The search is on to find ways of modifying these pathways.

Box 16.2. Key Points. Age-Related Macular Degeneration (AMD)

- The pathophysiology of AMD is complex and unclear [13].
- The pathological processes implicated are accumulation of lipofuscin, formation of drusen, neovascularisation and local inflammation [13].
- Dysfunction of the retinal pigmentary epithelium (RPE) occurs early [14].
- Extracellular matrix produced by the RPE plays an important role.

- Other functionally interrelated tissues are the Bruch's membrane, photoreceptors and choriocapillaris [13].
- Soft drusen precede the development of RPE detachment and choroidal neovascularisations and specific for AMD [16].
- The late stage has two forms: atrophic (or dry) characterised by geographical atrophy and exudative (wet) characterised by development of choroidal neovascularisation (CNV).
- Progression to CNVs results from angiogenic factors such as vascular endothelial group factor (VEGF) [13].
- At the molecular level, there is convincing evidence that the complement system especially the alternative pathway plays a vital role in the pathoaetiology of AMD [24].

16.2.2 Glaucoma

Introduction
Glaucoma is a group of disorders characterised largely by increased intraocular pressure causing a progressive damage to the optic nerve. It is the second most common cause of irreversible blindness next to age-related macular degeneration. The Melbourne Visual Impairment Project found the prevalence of 1.7 % in the over 40s increasing with age to 6.7 % in those in the 80s [26].

Pathophysiology
The aqueous humour which circulates in the anterior chamber is produced by the ciliary body which is located behind the iris. It flows (inward flow) between the iris and the lens and flows out (outward flow) through the sponge-like tissue called the trabecular meshwork and the canal of Schlemm and which is situated at the angle where the iris and cornea meet.

Glaucoma is caused by a group of disorders and is classified according to the mechanism of outflow obstruction as either open (wide)-angle glaucoma or closed (narrow)-angle glaucoma. A decrease of the outward flow of the aqueous humour as a result of clogging of the trabecular meshwork will result in increased pressure within the eye. With the rise in pressure in the eye, the nerve cells of the optic nerve become compressed and eventually lead to death of the nerve cells giving rise to permanent visual loss. This is the *open- or wide-angle glaucoma.* Sometimes, the lens is more forwardly placed, and in certain situations of the pupillary dilatation, the flow of the aqueous is obstructed. This is the *acute angle close glaucoma.* A subgroup is the *normal tension glaucoma* which is also an open-angle type of glaucoma and causes visual field loss due to nerve damage even though the intraocular pressure remains normal [27].

Several studies have revealed that multiple factors are involved in the development of retinal ganglion cell death (RGC), and it is unclear whether the site of primary damage is the ganglion cell body or the axons [28]. Elevated intraocular pressure (IOP) and vascular dysregulation have been put forth contributing to the initial insult by way of obstruction to axoplasmic flow within the RGC axons, changes in the laminar glial tissue and altered optic nerve microcirculation [28]. Apart from neuronal and axonal loss, glaucoma results in activation of glial cells, tissue remodelling and changes in the outer blood flow [29]. Elevation of IOP as a primary risk factor has been excluded from the definition of glaucoma for glaucoma can exist and progress despite normal or reduced levels of IOP [29]. There are several possible secondary factors which include excitotoxic damage caused by glutamate released from damaged neurons and overproduction of nitric oxide (NO) [28], immune-induced neurodestruction and disruption of neurotrophic factor transport [27]. The ultimate result is death of RGCs causing irreversible visual loss brought about by a collective interplay of multiple factors [30].

16.2.3 Cataract

Introduction
Cataract is characterised by opacity of the lens either developmental or degenerative. Age is the major risk factor for developing cataract. About 40 % of the primary cause of visual impairment in older Australians is cataract [31]. It is common in the elderly and more than two-thirds of those afflicted are over the age of 70 years and are often thought to be a normal part of ageing. Age-related cataracts usually affect both eyes with each cataract progressing at different rate.

Pathophysiology
Cataract formation begins in the third decade of life and progresses at different rates, and cataract of old age is a multifactorial disease with genetic, environmental, socioeconomic and biochemical factors which may act synergistically [32]. Ageing by reducing the metabolic efficiency of the lens makes it more vulnerable to noxious factors leading to the formation of a variety of cataracts [33]. In metabolic cataracts as in diabetes, the glucose accumulates in the aqueous humour in the lens where reduction of glucose to sorbitol takes place resulting in the accumulation of sorbitol which causes osmotic swelling of the lens fibres [34].

16.2.4 Diabetic Retinopathy

Introduction
Diabetic retinopathy (DR) is the most common chronic microvascular complication of diabetes and is due to progressive damage to the vessels in the retina caused by sustained hyperglycaemia. One in 12 persons in the United States 40 years and older have advanced vision-threatening retinopathy [35]. The overall prevalence of DR however varies across different populations [36]. It occurs in both type 1 and type 2 diabetes. DR is basically a manifestation of small vessel disease and is a function of the metabolic defect rather than the type of diabetes [37].

Pathophysiology

Diabetic retinopathy is classically defined by its vascular lesions and classified as non-proliferative diabetic retinopathy (NPDR) and proliferative diabetic retinopathy (PDR) [38]. NDPR is further subdivided into mild, moderate and severe [38]. NDPR is manifested by focal closure of retinal capillaries, microaneurysms and associated punctuate haemorrhages, serous exudates and, occasionally, cotton-wool spots secondary to acute ischaemia. These changes rarely cause serious visual problems [37]. On the other hand, PDR is more threatening and involves the growth of new blood vessels in front of the retina where they tend to bleed and through concomitant fibroblastic activity, tear and retinal detachment [37]. It is also related to the blood pressure and glycaemic control, and there is ample evidence that the effects of diabetes on the retina can be delayed or even curtailed by rigorous control of the blood sugar level, blood pressure and possibly lipids [38].

A number of biochemical pathways have been proposed as possible links between hyperglycaemia and DR [38]. There is a close association between chronic hyperglycaemia and development and progression of DR, but the underlying mechanism that leads to development of microvascular damage remains unclear [39]. Several studies in the pathophysiology of DR now reveal it is the result of a complex interplay of multiple interconnecting biochemical pathways [38] rather than any one of them acting individually. The instrumental pathways include increased polyol pathway, activation of protein kinase C, increased expression of growth factors such as vascular endothelial growth factor (VEGF) [38, 40, 41] and insulin-like growth factor-1 [38], oxidative stress [38, 41] activation of the renin-angiotensin-aldosterone system [38, 42, 43], ischaemia inducible erythropoietin (Epo) [44, 45] subclinical inflammation and haemodynamic changes [38]. VEGF plays an important role in inducing ischaemic retinal vascularisation [45] and elevated levels act as pathological angiogenic stimulus [40]. Oxidative stress-induced intracellular signalling is suppressed by Angiopoietin 1 (Ang 1) secreted by the pericytes [44] implying that Ang 1 in the pericytes is needed to maintain normal retinal vasculature [45]. A train of events are initiated which include basement membrane thickening, loss of pericytes [44] and endothelial cells, endothelial dysfunction and retinal capillary non-perfusion. The exact mechanisms by which hyperglycaemia brings about vascular disruption remain poorly defined. The two main pathological processes responsible for the development of DR are microvascular leakage and microvascular occlusion. Increased vascular permeability gives rise to mild non-proliferative abnormalities, followed by vascular closure giving rise to moderate to severe non-proliferative diabetic retinopathy (NPDR) to proliferative diabetic retinopathy (PDR) by abnormal growth of retinal vessels due to ischaemia on the retina and posterior surfaces of the vitreous [46]. Macular oedema characterised by retinal thickening from leaky blood vessels due to breakdown of the blood retinal barrier and can develop at all stages of retinopathy [47]. A better understanding of the pathophysiological mechanisms involved is crucial so that new pharmacological therapies based on any one of the underlying mechanisms can be recognised.

Box 16.3. Key Points. Diabetic Retinopathy (DR)

- DR is classified as non-proliferative diabetic retinopathy (NPDR) and proliferative diabetic retinopathy (PDR) [38].
- PDR is more threatening and involves the growth of new blood vessels in front of the retina where they tend to bleed and through concomitant fibroblastic activity, tear and retinal detachment [37].
- A number of biochemical pathways have been proposed as possible links between hyperglycaemia and DR [38].
- There is a close association between chronic hyperglycaemia and development and progression of DR, but the underlying mechanism that leads to development of microvascular damage remains unclear [39].
- The instrumental pathways include increased polyol pathway, activation of protein kinase C, increased expression of growth factors such as vascular endothelial growth factor (VEGF) and insulin-like growth factor-1, oxidative stress, activation of the renin-angiotensin-aldosterone system, ischaemia-inducible erythropoietin (Epo) subclinical inflammation and haemodynamic changes [38, 41, 43, 44].
- VEGF plays an important role in inducing ischaemic retinal vascularisation [46].

Multiple Choice Questions

1. In aged-related macular degeneration (AMD), the following pathological changes that occur are true, EXCEPT:
   A. Dysfunction of retinal pigment epithelium (RPE) occurs early.
   B. Membranous debris accumulates on either side of the RPE.
   C. Membranous debris is believed to be lipoprotein derived and the lipoproteins are dietary and systemic.
   D. Soft drusen are larger and tend to be confluent.
2. The following are true in aged-related macular degeneration (AMD), EXCEPT:
   A. Focal pigmentation and systemic hypertension increase risk of developing choroidal neovascularisation (CNV).
   B. Hard drusen pose a low rate of CNV.
   C. Progression to CNV results from angiogenic factors such as vascular endothelial growth factor (VEGF).
   D. Complement system plays an important role in the pathogenesis of AMD.
3. The following are true of diabetic retinopathy (DR), EXCEPT:
   A. There is a close association between chronic hyperglycaemia and development and progression of DR.
   B. Macular oedema always occur early in DR.
   C. Vascular endothelial growth factor (VEGF) plays an important role in ischaemic retinal vascularisation.
   D. Microvascular leakage and microvascular occlusion are responsible for the development of DR.

4. The following statements are true in glaucoma, EXCEPT:
   A. In acute angle close glaucoma in certain situations of pupillary dilatation, the flow of aqueous is obstructed.
   B. Normal tension glaucoma causes visual field loss due to nerve damage.
   C. Elevation of the intraocular pressure (IOP) is a primary risk factor for the development of glaucoma.
   D. The ultimate result of glaucoma is irreversible visual loss.

Answers to MCQs

1 = C; 2 = B; 3 = B; 4 = C

References

1. Salvi SM, Akhtar S, Currie Z. Ageing changes in the eye. Postgrad Med J. 2006;82:581–7.
2. Cassim R. The ageing eye. CME. 2007;25(10):484–9.
3. Niesel P. Visible changes of the lens with age. Trans Ophthalmol Soc UK. 1982;102:327–30 (abstract).
4. van den Berg TJTP, van Rijn LJ (Rene), Kasper-Bongers R, et al. Disability glare in the aging eye. Assessments and impact on driving. J Optom. 2009;02(03):112–8.
5. Ducan G, Weale RA. Physical changes due to aged cataracts. In: Ducan G, editor. Mechanisms of cataract formation in the human lens. London: Academic Press; 1981. p. 47–70.
6. Boniha VL. Age and disease-related structural changes in the retinal pigment epithelium. Clin Ophthalmol. 2008;2(2):413–24.
7. Sarks J, Sarks S. Age related macular degeneration. Australian doctor. 28 Sept 2001.
8. Resnikoff S, Pascolini D, Etya'ale D, Kocur I, Pararajasegaram R, Pokharel GP, et al. Global data on visual impairment in the year 2002. Bull WHO. 2004;82:844–85.
9. National Eye Institute. Facts about Age-related macular degeneration [NEI Health Information]. http://www.nei.nih.gov/health/maculardegen/armd_facts.asp.
10. Macular Degeneration Foundation 2007. Is anything more precious than your sight? Macular Degeneration Foundation. http://www.mdfoundation.com.au.
11. de Jong PT. Age-related macular degeneration. N Engl J Med. 2006;355:4474–785.
12. Wikipedia Macular degeneration. http://en.wikipedia.org/wiki/Macular_degeneration.
13. Nowak JZ. Age-related macular degeneration (AMD): pathogenesis and therapy. Pharmacol Rep. 2006;58:353–63.
14. Zarbin MA. Age-related macular degeneration: review of pathogenesis. Eur J Ophthalmol. 1998;8(4):199–206 (abstract).
15. Nita M, Strzalka-Mrozik B, Grzybowski A, Mazurek U, Romaniuk W. Age-related macular degeneration and changes in the extracellular matrix. Med Sci Monit. 2014;20:1003–16 (abstract).
16. Abdelsalam A, Del Priore L, Zarbin MA. Drusen in age-related macular degeneration: pathogenesis, natural course and laser photocoagulation-induced regression. Surv Ophthalmol. 1999;44(1):1–29 (abstract).
17. Arnold JJ, Sarks SH. Age related macular degeneration. BMJ. 2000;321:7263–741.
18. Pauleikhoff D. Drusen in Bruch's membrane. Their significance for the pathogenesis and therapy of age-associated macular degeneration. Ophthalmologe. 1992;89(5):363–86 (abstract).
19. Lutty G, Grunwalde J, Majji AB, Uyama M, Yoneya S. Changes in choriocapillaris and retinal pigment epithelium in age-related macular degeneration. Mol Vis. 1999;5:35 (abstract).

20. Spraul CW, Lang GE, Grossniklaus HE, Lang GK. Histologic and morphometric analysis of the choroid, Bruch's membrane and retinal pigment epithelium in postmortem eyes with age –related macular degeneration and histologic examination of surgically excised choroidal neovascular membranes. Surv Ophthalmol. 1999;44 Suppl 1:S10–32 (abstract).
21. Bird AC, Bressler NM, Bressler SB, Chisholm IH, Coscas G, Davis MD, de Jong PT, Klaver CC, Klein BE, Klein R, et al. International Age-Related Maculopathy. Epidemiological Study Group. An International classification and Age-Related Maculopathy and Age-Related Macular Degeneration. Surg Ophthalmol. 1995;39:367–74.
22. Macular Photocoagulation Study Group. Subfoveal neovascular lesion image-related ADM. Guidelines for evaluation and treatment in macular photocoagulation study. Arch Ophthalmol. 1991;109:1242–51.
23. Bhutto IA, McLead DS, Hasegawa T, Kim SY, Merges C, Tong P, et al. Pigment epithelium – derived factor (PEDF) and vascular endothelial growth factor (VEGF) in aged human choroid eyes with age related macular degeneration. Exp Eye Res. 2006;82(1):99–110.
24. Troutbeck R, Al-Qureshi S, Guymer RH. Therapeutic targeting of the complement system in age-related macular degeneration: a review. Clin Experiment Ophthalmol. 2012;40(1):18–26.
25. Broadhead GK, Chang A, McCluster P. Genetics in age-related macular degeneration: current research and implications for future treatment? Asia Pac J Ophthamol. 2012;5:312–8.
26. Wensor MD, McCarty CA, Stanislavsky YL, Livingston PM, Taylor HR. The prevalence of glaucoma in the Melborne Visual Impairment Project. Ophthalmology 1998;105(4):733–9.
27. Kumarasamy NA, Lam FS, Wong AL, Theoharides TC. Glaucoma: current and developmental concepts for inflammation, pathways and treatment. Eur J Inflammation. 2006;41(3):129–37.
28. Agarwal R, Gupta SK, Agarwal P, Saxena R, Agrawal SS, et al. Current concepts in the pathogenesis of glaucoma. Ind J Ophthalmol. 2001;57(4):257–66.
29. Dimitriou D, Broadway DC. Pathophysiology of glaucoma. In Glaucoma: basic and Clinical perspectives. 2013. p. 32–57. http://www.futuremedicine.com/doi/abs/10,2217/ebo.12420.
30. Kanshik S, Pandau SS, Ram J. Neuroprotection in glaucoma. J Postgrad Med. 2003;49:90–5.
31. Australian Institute and Health Welfare (AIHW). http://www.aihw.gov.au/workArea/Download.Assit.aspx?id+6442453390. Accessed 10 Jan 2015.
32. Chitkara DK, Hall AB, Rosenthal AR. Pathology and epidemiology of cataract. Section 2-Cataract. Ophthamology; 2010:269–72. Chap 35.
33. Wegener A. Pathophysiology of cataract. 98th annual meeting DOG 2000. http://www.dog.org/2000/e_abstract_2000/214html.
34. Schmitt C, Hockwin O. The mechanisms of cataract formation. J Inher Metab Dis. 1990; 13:501–8.
35. Kempen JH, O'Colman BJ, Leske MC, Haffner SM, Klein R, Moss SE, et al. The prevalence of diabetic retinopathy among adults in US. Arch Ophthamol. 2004;122(4):552–63 (abstract).
36. Access my library. Pathophysiology of diabetic retinopathy. Optician.http://www.accessmylibrary.com/coms2/summary_0286-18736025_ITM. Accessed 29 June 2008.
37. Garner A. Developments in the pathology of diabetic retinopathy: a review. J Roy Soc Med. 1981;74:427–31.
38. Tarr JM, Kaul K, Chopra M, Kohner EM, Chibber R. Pathophysiology of diabetic retinopathy. Ophthalmology; 2013. doi:http://dx.dorg/10.1155.2013/343560.
39. Mathews DR, Stratton IM, Aldington SJ, Holman RR, Kohner EM. Risks of progression of retinopathy and vision loss related to tight blood control in type 2 diabetes mellitus. cUKPDS 69. Arch Ophthalmol. 2004;122(1):1631–40.
40. Wirostko B, Wong TY, Simo R. Vascular endothelial growth factor and diabetic complications. Prog Retin Eye Res. 2008;27(6):608–21 (abstract).
41. Caldwell RB, Bartoli M, Behzadian MA, El-Remessy AE, Al-Shabrawey M, Platt DH, et al. Vascular endothelial growth factor and diabetic retinopathy: role of oxidative stress. Curr Drug Targets. 2005;6(4):511–24 (abstract).
42. Giese MJ, Speth RC. The ocular renin-angiotensin system: a therapeutic target for the treatment of ocular disease. Pharmacol Thera. 2014;142(1):11–32.

43. Simo R, Hernandez C. Advances in the medical treatment of diabetic retinopathy. Diabetes Care. 2009;32(8):1556–62.
44. Takagi H, Watanabe D, Suzuma K, Kurimoto M, Suzuma I, Ohashi H, et al. Novel role of erythropoietin in proliferative diabetic retinopathy. Diabetes Res Clin Pract. 2007;77 Suppl 1: S62–4 (abstract).
45. Takagi H. Aging and retinal vascular diseases. Nihon Ganka Gakkai Zasshi. 2007;111(3):207–30 (abstract).
46. Fong DS, Aiello L, Gardner TW, King GI, Blankenship G, Cavallerano JD, et al. Diabetic retinopathy. Diabetes Care. 2003;26:S99–102.
47. Sino R, Carrasco E, Garcia-Ramirez M, Hernandez C. Angiogenic and antiangiogenic factors in proliferative diabetic retinopathy. Curr Diabet Rev. 2006;2:71–98.

Ear-Related Problems in the Elderly 17

17.1 Anatomical and Physiological Changes with Ageing: EAR

It is often difficult to distinguish changes of normal ageing from those of other contributing factors [1]. Hearing depends on the integration of three processes – the peripheral comprising the external ear, middle ear and inner ear, auditory nerve and the central auditory processing (the brain stem and cortex). With ageing, there are a number of structural and pathophysiological processes associated with changes to functional components of the ear. Alterations include thickening of the ear drum, sclerotic changes of the muscles and joints in the middle ear, decreasing number of hair cells in the inner ear and degeneration of the eighth nerve and of the neurons of the medullary centre [2]. There is stiffening of the ossicular chain [3] and thinning and stiffening of the tympanic membrane [4, 5]. Age- related changes occur in the cochlea [6, 7] resulting in sensorineural hearing loss affecting high-frequency behaviours [6]. The vestibular system is also affected by ageing. Degenerative changes occur in the semicircular canals, utricle and saccule with advancing age. By the age of 70 years, there is a 40 % loss of vestibular hair and nerve cells which gives rise to a reduction in the function of the vestibular system [8]. In the saccule, degenerative changes occur in the otoconia and loss of hair cells and neurons together with innervating fibres of the hair cells in the vestibular ganglion. The changes are summarised in Table 17.1.

17.2 Common Ear Problems in the Elderly

Introduction

Some of the common problems related to the ear in the elderly:

1. Hearing impairment/loss
2. Imbalance and vertigo
3. Tinnitus

N. Nagaratnam et al., *Diseases in the Elderly: Age-Related Changes and Pathophysiology*, DOI 10.1007/978-3-319-25787-7_17

Table 17.1 Changes with ageing

Anatomical	Pathophysiology	Effects
External ear		
Decrease in the activity and number of cerumen glands	Cerumen becomes drier	Cerumen impaction
Middle ear		
Joints between the ossicles – cartilage becomes thin, frayed, loss of joint space, calcification	Arthritic changes	Does not interfere with conductive hearing
Inner ear		
(i) Vestibular Loss of sensory epithelium with decrease in the number of hair in utricle (cristae) and saccule (maculae), and nerves innervating	Decrease balance monitoring function – disequilibrium	Macular disequilibrium ampullary disequilibrium vestibular ataxia BPPV[a] the hair cells and rods of Scarpa's ganglion; degenerative changes in the otoconia
(ii) Cochlear Stiffening of basilar membrane, deterioration of hair cells, ganglion cells cochlear nuclei, striae vascularis	See Table 17.2	Presbycusis

Information sources: see text

[a]*BPPV*: benign paroxysmal positional vertigo

17.2.1 Hearing Loss in the Elderly

Hearing loss can be broadly defined as impairment of varying degree in the ability to recognise sound. About 25–60 % of people over the age of 65 years have sufficient hearing loss to impair communication [9]. Approximately 50 % of Australians over the age of 65 years have hearing impairment [10]. Hearing impairment may be categorised according to the anatomy and physiology involved or by cause. Any lesion in the external auditory canal or middle ear affecting the transmission of sound will give rise to conductive hearing loss. Some of the common causes of conductive deafness include cerumen, tympanosclerosis, otosclerosis and Paget's disease. Dysfunction in the sensory elements and neural structures in the inner ear, cochlea and auditory centres will give rise to sensorineural hearing loss and is the most common hearing impairment in adults [11]. Sensorineural hearing loss can be further subdivided into sensory (cochlear) or neural (retrocochlear) hearing loss. It is important to make the distinction because neural hearing loss is often caused by tumours which are potentially curable.

17.2.1.1 Presbycusis

Presbycusis is a slowly progressive bilateral and symmetrical sensorineural hearing loss that is most predominant at high frequencies. Presbycusis is the most common type of hearing impairment in the elderly and is age related.

Pathophysiology

It may arise from loss of internal ear hair cells and to degeneration of the central auditory pathways. Four different types of presbycusis have been identified based on the pathological findings in the cochlea. They are sensory presbycusis, neural

Table 17.2 Presbycusis

Type	Pathology	Functional deficit
Sensory presbycusis	Loss of hair cells at the basal end of cochlea	Decrease in the threshold of high-frequency sounds
Neural presbycusis	Loss of cochlear neurons	Severe loss of speech discrimination
Strial presbycusis	Atrophy of stria atrophy	Hearing loss – flat or slightly descending audiometric curve
Cochlear conductive presbycusis	Stiffening of the basilar membrane	Speech discrimination average linear descending audiogram

Source of information: Balasubramaniam [12]

presbycusis, strial presbycusis and cochlear conductive presbycusis [12] (Table 17.2). Besides the decline in the high frequencies (due to sensory cell loss), there is reduction in speech discrimination (due to loss of cochlear neurons) particularly in the presence of background noise resulting in significant communication difficulties [13].

17.2.1.2 Noise-Induced Sensorineural Hearing Loss (NIHL)

Noise-induced hearing loss is hearing loss due to exposure to loud and repeated sounds over an extended period resulting in damage to the inner ear.

Pathophysiology

Most common cause of NIHL is an excessively high-noise industry, but any form of sound exposure can lead to NIHL. There are three general classes of noise hazards: (1) impact noise, for instance, from a gun shot or explosion; (2) continuous noise such as from machinery working continuously or prolonged exposure to amplified music and (3) intermittent noise such as from a passing heavy vehicle [14]. Repeated and sustained sound exposure above the level of approximately 85 dBA may cause the hair cells and associated nerve fibres to degenerate and may become permanent [15]. NIHL generally affects both ears. Other causes of hearing loss are Meniere's disease and acoustic neuroma among others.

Box 17.1. Key Points. Hearing Loss in the Elderly

- Hearing loss is defined as impairment of varying degree in the ability to recognise sound.
- Presbycusis is a slowly progressive bilateral and symmetrical sensorineural hearing loss that is most predominant at high frequencies and is age related.
- Hearing loss may arise from loss of internal ear hair cells and to degeneration of the central auditory pathways.
- Noise-induced hearing loss is hearing loss due to exposure to loud and repeated sounds over an extended period resulting in damage to the inner ear.
- Repeated and sustained sound exposure above the level of approximately 85 dBA may cause the hair cells and associated nerve fibres to degenerate and may become permanent [1].

17.3 Balance, Imbalance and Vertigo

Introduction

Vertigo is a feeling of movement in space and this could be objective when the surrounding objects appear to turn in relation to the individual or subjective, the reverse. Vertigo is a specific term, unlike dizziness which is a non-specific term describing an array of symptoms such as lightheadedness, faintness, unsteadiness, falling and passing out among others. Vertigo accounts for 52 % of all cases [16, 17] and up to 56.4 % in the elderly [18].

Physiology

Balance and imbalance

Balance or the sensation of equilibrium is maintained by visual, vestibular and somatosensory functions of the sensory systems and integrated sensory inputs within the central nervous system. Sensory receptors of the vestibular system reside in the inner ear. The semicircular canals respond to angular acceleration and the saccule and utricle to linear acceleration. These structures are connected to the vestibular nuclei in the brain stem by the eighth cranial nerve. Visual acuity, depth perception and peripheral vision and proprioception play important roles. The midline structures of the cerebellar hemispheres also play an important role in balance by modulating motor activity and co-ordination. Decreased sensory input and slowing down of motor responses result in imbalance or disequilibrium.

Dizziness has been classified into four subtypes: vertigo, presyncope, disequilibrium and lightheadedness [19]. Vertigo has been categorised as to the cause: (1) peripheral vestibulopathy and (2) central neurological. There is some uncertainty of the term 'central' for according to some it also includes causes proximal to the vestibular end organ as central, but others consider involvement of the eighth nerve with, for instance, neurofibroma as peripheral [20]. The central causes are much less common than the peripheral causes. In a study of 652 occurrences of vertiginous syndrome, 38.7 % was due to benign positional vertigo, 31.9 % labyrinthitis, 17.4 % Meniere's disease and 12.1 % other vestibular disorders [21].

Pathophysiology

The peripheral causes result from dysfunction of the vestibular end organ – the semicircular canals, utricle, saccule and the eighth nerve. The central causes are caused by involvement of the vestibular pathways which spread out from the vestibular nuclei in the medulla to the vestibular portions of the cerebellum, oculomotor nuclei, to the integration centres in the midbrain, thalamus and the multisensory vestibular cortical areas in the temporoparietal cortex (Fig. 17.1). The vestibular nucleus is made up of four subdivisions. Axons are sent from the medial vestibular nucleus via the ipsilateral and contralateral medial longitudinal fasciculi to the nuclei of the nerves III, IV and VI and also establish contact with three other adjacent nuclei (not shown in the diagram) which control aspects of eye movements. The medial longitudinal fasciculi rostrally reach the III cranial nucleus and caudally extend to the cervical part of the spinal cord as the medial vestibulo-spinal tract; the lateral vestibulo-spinal tract arises from the lateral vestibular nucleus.

Box 17.2. Key Points. Vertigo, Balance and Imbalance

- Vertigo is a feeling of movement in space and this could be objective or subjective.
- Balance or the sensation of equilibrium is maintained by visual, vestibular and somatosensory functions of the sensory systems and integrated sensory inputs within the central nervous system.
- Vertigo has been categorised as to the cause: (1) peripheral vestibulopathy and (2) central neurological.
- The peripheral causes result from dysfunction of the vestibular end organ – the semicircular canals, utricle, saccule and the eighth nerve.
- The central causes are caused by involvement of the vestibular pathways which spread out from the vestibular nuclei in the medulla to the vestibular portions of the cerebellum, oculomotor nuclei, to the integration centres in the midbrain, thalamus and the multisensory vestibular cortical areas in the temporoparietal cortex.

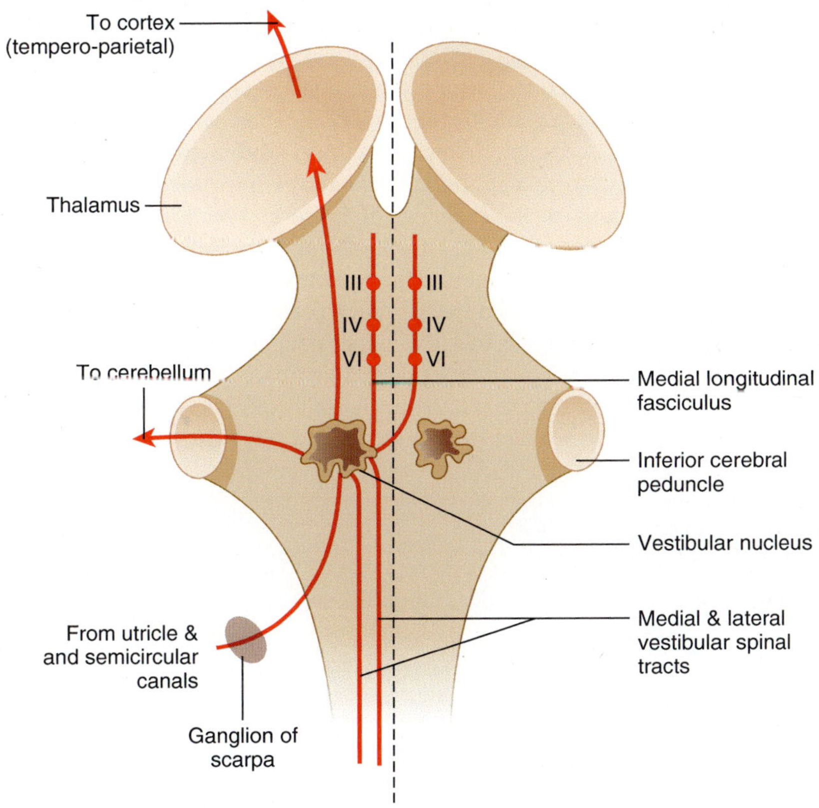

Fig. 17.1 Central vestibular pathways

17.4 Tinnitus

Introduction

Tinnitus is characterised by the perception of sound in the ears or in the head. Tinnitus is common in the elderly and its prevalence increases with age. In the elderly, it is most commonly associated with hearing loss [22].

Pathophysiology

There are two distinctive types of tinnitus: subjective and objective. Subjective tinnitus is caused by abnormal neural activity that is not evoked by sound and is audible only to the affected individual [23, 24]. Objective tinnitus is caused by sounds generated in the body and are clearly audible to the affected person and to the listener [23, 24]. Objective tinnitus is sound created somewhere in the body [23] and has usually a muscular or vascular cause. The fundamental pathophysiology of subjective tinnitus is unclear. There are a number of forms of subjective tinnitus. This results from abnormal neural activity generated in the ear, auditory nerve or the central nervous system [25]. The anatomical location or locations of physiological abnormality of chronic subjective tinnitus is rarely in the ear but more often found in the auditory nervous system [23, 25]. It has been proposed that the changes are within the auditory pathways, the auditory cortex and the emotional limbic system [26]. Involvement of these structures may explain some of the symptoms of some forms of tinnitus such as hyperacusis, phonophobia and depression [27]. There are indications that the pathophysiology of unilateral and bilateral tinnitus is different [25]. Most forms of subjective tinnitus are from changes brought about by expression of neural plasticity, a form of reprogramming of the brain (auditory cortex) caused by deprivation of input from the auditory periphery [25]. Lack of output from the damaged cochwlea alters the tonotopic organisation of the auditory cortex, the region that corresponds to the area of cochlear damage called the lesion projection zone (LPZ). The LPZ following cochlear damage shows an increase in the spontaneous firing rate and increase in the frequency representations of the neurons that border the damaged region [24]. Tinnitus neurophysiology thus is related to the injurious cortical adaptation to the deprival of input from the sensory periphery [24, 25] (Fig. 17.2).

Box 17.3. Key Points. Tinnitus

- Tinnitus is characterised by the perception of sound in the ears or in the head.
- There are two distinctive types of tinnitus: subjective and objective.
- Objective tinnitus is sound created somewhere in the body and has usually a muscular or vascular cause [22, 23].
- Subjective tinnitus results from abnormal neural activity generated in the ear, auditory nerve or the central nervous system. The anatomical location or locations of physiological abnormality of chronic subjective tinnitus is rarely in the ear but more often found in the auditory nervous system [22, 24].
- Lack of output from the damaged cochlea alters the tonotopic organisation of the auditory cortex, the region that corresponds to the area of cochlear damage and is called the lesion projection zone (LPZ) [24].

- Tinnitus neurophysiology thus is related to the injurious cortical adaptation to the deprival of input from the sensory periphery [24, 25].

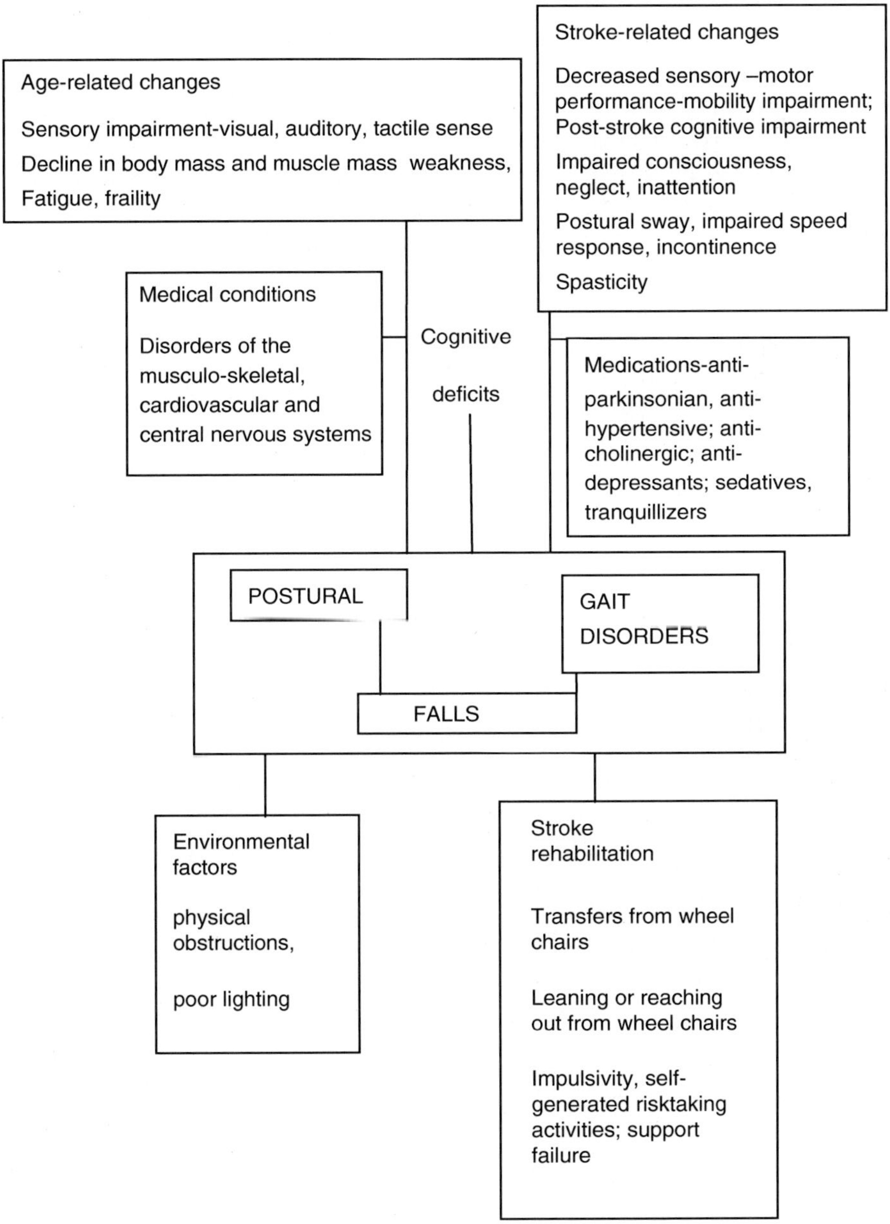

Fig. 17.2 Pathophysiology of falls

17.5 Related Disorders

17.5.1 Falls in the Elderly: Evaluation and Management

Introduction

According to the Kellogg International Working Group on prevention of falls [28, 29], a fall is defined as an event when an individual finds himself on the ground and is not the result of a violent blow or an event such as a stroke or epileptic seizure. The prevalence of falls has been shown to dramatically increase with advancing age, and after the age of 80–85 years, it has been evaluated to be at 50 %[30]. Approximately one of three Australians aged more than 65 years living in the community [31] and up to 65 % of the nursing home residents fall each year, and women are twice more likely to fall than men. One in three persons aged 65 years and over would experience at least one fall [29, 32], and 9 % of individuals aged 65 years and over are seen in the emergency with falls and 5–6 % have sustained a fracture [33].

Pathophysiology

Falls result from a single or a combination of environmental and medical factors that interact with physiological related changes which increase with age. It is mandatory that those treating falls have a clear understanding of postural control. The efficiency of physiological systems for postural control diminishes with age. Postural stability or balance is maintained by continued adjustments to sensory outputs, visual, vestibular and somatosensory [34], which tend to diminish with ageing and play an important role in causing falls in the elderly. Postural instability is due to decreased sensory input, slowing down of the motor responses and weakness of support [35]. In old age, the integrated sensory inputs [36] together with the slower rate of central processing [37, 38] lead to difficulties in co-ordination of reflexes and voluntary movements.

Loss of visual acuity, peripheral vision, depth perception and contrast sensitivity occurs with ageing [39]. Impaired vision could lead to impaired ability to cope with environmental demands, loss of balance and falls [40]. Proprioceptive loss increases the threshold to movement detection and impaired sense of vibration in the legs leading to increase in postural sway [41]. The vestibular system is also affected by ageing. Components of the sensorimotor system, medications and diseases also contribute to balance problems. Neurological factors include disease processes such as stroke [42] and Parkinson's disease [43]. Vestibular and proprioceptive changes have been singled out [44] and up to 50 % of the falls are due to extrinsic factors.

There is a close association between postural stability, gait and falls. Over the past decade, it has been recognised that cognition and gait are connected [45], and considerable importance has been attributed to cognition [46, 47]. However, it is unclear whether cognition is global (i.e. dementia) or whether it is a specific cognitive function [48]. Several studies have shown that in the elderly with dementia, there is an association of gait and balance abnormalities [49, 50]. The higher cognitive processes are referred to as executive function (EF) which integrates, controls and organises other cognitive abilities [51] and involves components such as problem solving, task planning and reasoning [51]. In older adults with no overt cognitive impairment, EF deficits may increase risk of falls [52, 53].

Attention is a specific type of EF [45] and attention-related cognitive deficits decrease postural stability in cognitively impaired elderly with history of falls [54]. Attention mechanisms are necessary to select processing to accomplish a task, and selection by location takes precedence over object-based attention although both may be intact [55]. Fallers tend to fall because of deficits in visual spatial attention which cause problems with planning and guiding movements, and they have a limited focus of attention compared to non-fallers [56].

Falls are closely associated with syncope, and in a study of 188 older patients who attended the emergency department after a fall, 26 % reported syncope [57]. There exists an overlap between syncope and falls although they are often considered as two different diagnoses with two separate aetiologies [58]. In the elderly with syncope due to cardiovascular causes, their successful intervention not only controls syncopal occurrences but includes reductions in falls [59].

There have been several studies since 2004 relating to the association between vitamin D insufficiency and falls and vitamin D supplementation results in reduction of falls. Vitamin D deficiency is very frequent in the elderly [60, 61]. Vitamin D deficiency (<20 ng/ml) was seen in 54 % of patients tested, previously unrecognised in a study of older adults with gait imbalance and falls [62]. Vitamin D deficiency is associated with muscle weakness resulting in poor balance and gait predisposing to falls [63, 64]. Unexplained or recurrent falls are often due to syncope [65]. The explanation for the effectiveness of vitamin D is attributed to the action of vitamin D on muscle and the nervous system function [66] by improving postural balance and navigation abilities [63]. It has been shown that vitamin D has direct effects on muscle strength modulated by specific vitamin D receptors present in the human muscle [67, 68]. Furthermore, it appears to stabilise postural equilibrium and this is largely due to improvement of attention capacities and is unrelated to any muscle action [63]. There are vitamin D receptors in the brain which appear to regulate development and homeostasis of the nervous system and skeletal muscle [69].

In stroke changes in stability, balance, muscle strength and co-morbidities are precipitating factors for falls. Studies have shown that postural sway, cognitive and behavioural deficits and moderate to severe disability on admission were common in patients who fall [70]. Components of the sensorimotor system also contribute to balance problems. Among fallers, vertigo and antihypertensive drug intake were predictors of falls. Vertigo is common in the elderly more so in the stroke patient and is a significant predictor of falls [71]. Stroke and vascular disease of the labyrinth are leading causes of central vestibular disturbances [71].

Box 17.4. Key Points. Falls

- Falls increase with age, 50 % at age 80–85 years [29].
- Falls result from a single or a combination of environmental and medical factors that interact with physiological-related changes which increase with age.
- The efficiency of physiological systems for postural control diminishes with age.
- Loss of visual acuity, peripheral vision, depth perception and contrast sensitivity occurs with ageing [39].
- There is a close association between postural stability, gait and falls.
- Over the past decade, it has been recognised that cognition and gait are connected [45].
- Attention is a specific type of executive function (EF), and attention-related cognitive deficits decrease postural stability in cognitively impaired elderly with history of falls [45, 54].
- Vitamin D deficiency is associated with muscle weakness resulting in poor balance and gait predisposing to falls [63, 64].
- Components of the sensorimotor system also contribute to balance problems.
- Stroke and vascular disease of the labyrinth are leading causes of central vestibular disturbances [71].

Multiple Choice Questions (MCQs)

1. The following are true in relation to hearing loss in the elderly, EXCEPT:
   A. Four different types of presbycusis are sensory presbycusis, neural presbycusis, strial presbycusis and cochlear conductive presbycusis.
   B. Age-related changes occur in the cochlea resulting in sensorineural hearing loss affecting high-frequency behaviours.
   C. Degenerative changes occur in the semicircular canals, utricle and saccule with advancing age.
   D. By the age of 70 years, there is an 80 % loss of vestibular hair and nerve cells which gives rise to a reduction in the function of the vestibular system.
2. The following in relation to falls in the elderly are true, EXCEPT:
   A. Fractures occur in 50 % of falls.
   B. More than 90 % of hip fractures are result of falls and most occur over the age of 70 years.
   C. If a person has fallen more than twice in a 6th-month period, evaluation for a treatable cause should be considered.
   D. Fear of falling has been identified in 10–12 % of fallers.

3. The following are true in relation to falls in the elderly, EXCEPT:
   A. In persons over 75 years, falls are the most frequent cause of accidental injury.
   B. Syncope is a frequent cause for falls.
   C. Falls are relatively uncommon in Parkinson's disease.
   D. Postural hypotension is a high-risk factor for falls.
4. A 72-year-old woman was seen in the clinic with a history of recurrent falls. According to the daughter, her mother lives alone and was coping well. Over the past 3–4 months, she has had 5–6 falls within her house. She has had no loss of consciousness, jerky movements of her limbs nor incontinent of urine. On examination, the blood pressure was normal with no postural drop. The nervous system was generally intact. Her gait was normal. She however had mild cognitive impairment. What will you do?
   A. Request for a bone mineral density (BMD) test
   B. Provide a hip protector
   C. Do a home safety check
   D. Request for a CT scan of the brain

Extended Matching Questions (EMQs)

Theme: Recurrent falls

A. Lewy body dementia (LBD)
B. Normal pressure hydrocephalus (NPH)
C. Progressive supranuclear paralysis (PSP)
D. Parkinson's disease (PD)
E. Multisystem atrophy (MSA)
F. Binswanger's disease (BD)
G. Lacunar state

Can be used once, more than once or not at all

1. A 67-year-old man was seen with an unsteady gait, frequent falls and urinary incontinence. According to the wife who had accompanied him, he was complaining that his feet seem stuck to the ground and walked broad based and shuffling at times over the past 4–5 months. Initially, he had frequency of urine and now had become incontinent. Furthermore, he was forgetful and had change in behaviour, mood fluctuating from amiability to frank hostility. CT scan of the brain is shown below.

CT scan of the brain of patient 1

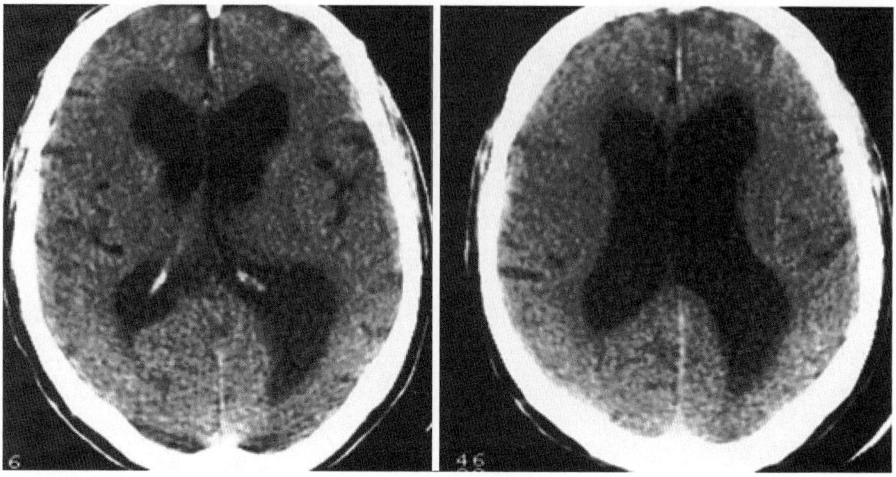

2. A 72-year-old man presented to the clinic accompanied by his wife. According to her, there has been a progressive decline in his mental ability. His mental state fluctuated: lucid at times and confused at other times. He had difficulty in judging distances; as a result, he has had repeated falls. He hallucinates seeing people and things that are not there.
3. A 64-year-old man, a widower, lived with his daughter. According to her, his walking had become awkward and developed stiffness with loss of balance and has had several falls. He had lost interest in his usual activities and was forgetful. Neurological examination revealed axial more than appendicular rigidity and paralysis of downward gaze.
4. According to the wife, a 68-year-old man had considerably slowed down over the past 3–4 months. He was slow in rising from the chair and turning in bed. He walked with a shuffle and has had several falls. Neurological examination revealed a mask-like face and a resting tremor of his left hand. There was rigidity of the limbs but no weakness. The reflexes were normal. He had a stoop and walked with a shuffle.
5. A 64-year-old man when seen was said to have become slow in movement, stiff with loss of balance resulting in repeated falls over the past 5–6 months. Over the months, there had been a worsening of his symptoms. He complained of dizziness, urinary incontinence and impotence. His sleep was disturbed and he often had nightmares. His blood pressure on examination was 130/80 mmHg lying down and 90/60 mmHg standing.

Answers to MCQs

1 = D; 2 = D; 3 = C; 4 = C
EMQ 1 = B; 2 = A; 3 = C; 4 = D;5 = E

References

Anatomical and Physiological Changes with Ageing-EAR

1. Liu XZ, Yan D. Aging and hearing loss. J Pathol. 2007;211(2):188–97 (abstract).
2. Niwa H, Yanagita N. Presbyacusis. Nippon Ronen Igakkai Zasshi. 1990;27(5):545–9 (abstract).
3. Belal A. Prebyacusis: physiological or pathological. J Laryngol Otol. 1975;89:1011–25.
4. Weinstein BE. Geriatric audiology. New York: Thieme Medical Publishers; 2000.
5. Rosenwasser H. Otic problems in the aged. Geriatrics. 1964;1911:17.
6. Schuknecht HF, Gacek MR. Cochlear pathology in presbyacusis. Ann Otol Rhinol Laryngol. 1993;1021:16.
7. Browning GG. Clinical otology and audiology. London: Arnold; 2001.
8. Rosenhall U, Rubin W. Degenerative changes in the human vestibular sensory epithelia. Acta Otolaryngol. 1975;79:67–81.

Common ear Problems in the Elderly

9. Herlost KG, Humphrey C. Hearing impairment and mental state in the elderly living at home. Br Med J. 1980;281:903–5.
10. Britt H, Miller GC, Charles J, Pan Y, Valenti L, Henderson L, et al. General practice activity in Australia 2005–06. Canberra: Institute of Health and Welfare; 2007.
11. Angell SL, YYan D, Telischi F, Malkany TJ, Ouyang XM, Du LL, et al. Etiologic diagnosis of sensorineural hearing loss in adult. Otolaryngol Head Neck Surg. 2005;132:890–5.
12. Balasubramaniam T. Presbyacusis. Website: http://www.drtbalu.com/presbyacusis.html.
13. Bergman M. Aging and the perception of speech. Baltimore: University Park Press; 1980.
14. Sensear. 2009. www.sensear.com/noise-induced-hearingloss.php. Retrieved 20 June 2014.
15. Thorne PR, Ameratunge SN, Stewart J, Reid N, Williams W, et al. Epidemiology of noise-induced hearing loss. N Z Med J. 2008;121(1280):33–44.

Imbalance and Vertigo

16. Hanley K, Dowd T, Crosindine N. A systematic review of vertigo in primary care. Br J Clin Pract. 2001;51:666–71.
17. Colledge NR, Barr-Hamilton M, Lewis SJ, Sellar RJ, Wilson JA. Evaluation of investigation to diagnosis of the cause of dizziness in elderly people in community and controlled study. Br Med J. 1996;313:788–92.
18. Bird JC, Beynon GJ, Prevost AT, Baguley DM. Analysis of referral patterns for dizziness in the primary care setting. Br J Gen Pract. 1998;48:1828–32.
19. Drachman DA, Hart CW. A approach to the dizzy patient. Neurology. 1992;22:341–54.
20. Troost T. Dizziness and vertigo in vertebrobasilar disease. Stroke. 1990;11:301–3, 413–5.
21. Charles J, Fahridin S, Britt H. The BEACH program. Australian GP Statistical Classification Centre. University of Sydney; 2007

Tinnitus

22. Davis A, El Rafaie A. Epidemiology of tinnitus. In: Tyler R, editor. Tinnitus handbook. San Diego: Singular Publishing Group. 2000. p. 1–23.
23. Richmond BS. Tinnitus: prevalence, causes and treatment approaches. Geriatric Times 2003; vol. iv. website: http://www.cmellc.com/geriatrictimes/g030821.html.
24. Benson AG, McGuire JF, Djalilian HR, Hanks KM, McGuire JF. Inner ear, tinnitus Overview. eMedicine Otolaryngology and Facial plastic surgery. 2008. website: http://emedicine.medscape.com/article/856916-overview. Accessed 4/8/2009.

25. Moller AR. Tinnitus: presence and future. Prog Brain Res. 2007;166:3–16 (abstract).
26. Lockwood AH, Salvi RJ, Coad ML, Towsley ML, Wack DS, Murphy BW, et al. The functioning neuroanatomy of tinnitus: evidence for limbic system, tinnitus and neural plasticity. Neurology. 1998;50(1):114–24.
27. Moller AR. Pathophysiology of tinnitus. Otolaryngol Clin North Am. 2003;36(2):249–66 (abstract).

Falls

28. Gibson MJ, Andres K, Isaacs B, Radebaugh T, Worm-Petersen J. Prevention of falls in later life. Dan Med Bull S. 1987;34(Supp 4):1–24.
29. Tinetti ME, Speechley M, Ginter SF. Risk factors for falls among the elderly persons in the community. N Engl J Med. 1988;319(26):1701–7.
30. Tinetti ME, Williams CS. Falls injuries and the risk of admission to a nursing home. N Engl J Med. 1997;337:1279–94.
31. Lord S, Ward J, Williams P, Anstey K. An epidemiological study of falls in older community-dwelling women. The Randwick falls and fractures study. Aust J Public Health. 1993;17:240–5.
32. Graafmans WC, Ooms ME, Hofstee HM, Bezemer PD, Bouter LM, Lips P, et al. Falls in the elderly: a study of risk factors and risk profiles. Am J Epidemiol. 1996;143:1129–36.
33. Bischoff HA, Stahelin HB, Dick W, Akos R, Knecht M, Salis C, et al. Effects of vitamin D and calcium supplementation on falls: a randomized controlled trial. J Bone Miner Res. 2003;18:343–51.
34. Lee D, Lishman R. Vision in movement and balance. New Sci. 1975;9:59–61.
35. Baloh RW, Fife TD, Zwerling L, Socotch T, Jacobson K, Bell T, et al. Comparison of static and dynamic posturography in young and older normal people. J Am Geriatr Soc. 1994;42: 404–16.
36. Manchester D, Woollacott M, Zoderbauer-Hylton N, Marino O. Visual, vestibular and somatosensory contributions to balance control in older adults. J Gerontol. 1989;44:M118–27.
37. Stelmach GE, Worringham CJ. Sensation for deficits related to postural stability implications for falling in the elderly. Clin Geriatr Med. 1984;1:679–94.
38. Woollacott M, Shunway-Cook SA, Nashner L. Aging and postural control. Changes in sensory organization in muscular co-ordination. Int J Aging Hum Dev. 1986;23:97–114.
39. Spirduso WW. Physical dimensions of aging. Champaign: Human Kinetics; 1995.
40. Gerson LW, Jarjoura D, McCord G. Risk of imbalance in elderly people with impaired hearing or vision. Age Ageing. 1989;18:31–4.
41. Brockelhurst JC, Robertson D, James-Groin P. Clinical correlates of sway in old age-sensory modalities. Age Ageing. 1982;11:1–10.
42. Nagaratnam N, Leung H, Bou-Haider P. Lacunar stroke proclivity for falls. Int J Clin Pract. 2004;58:83–6.
43. Ashburn A, Stack E, Pickering PM, Ward CD. A community –dwelling sample of people with Parkinson's disease: characteristic of fallers and non-fallers. Age Ageing. 2001;30:47–52.
44. Overstall PW. Epidemiology and pathophysiology of falls. In: Katara MS, editor. Fits, faints and falls in old age. Lancaster: MTP Press; 1985. p. 15–26.
45. Segev-Jacubovski O, Herman T, Yogev-Seligman G, Mirelman A, Giladi N, Hausdirff JM, et al. The interplay between gait, falls and cognition: can cognitive therapy reduce fall risk? Expert Rev Neurother. 2011;11(7):1057–75.
46. Horak FB. Postural orientation and equilibrium: what do we need to know about neural control of balance to prevent falls? Age Ageing. 2006;35 suppl 2:ii7–11.
47. Atkinson HH, Rosano C, Simmonsick EM, Williamson JD, Davis C, Ambrosius WT, et al. Cognitive function speed decline and comorbidities: the health aging and body composition study. J Gerontol A Biol Med Sci. 2007;62:844–50.
48. Muir SW, Gopaul K, Odasso MMM. The role of cognitive impairment in fall risk among older adults: a systematic review and meta-analysis. Age Ageing. 2012;41(3):299–308.

49. Allan IM, Ballard CG, Burn DJ, Kenny RA. Prevalence and severity of gait disorders in Alzheimer's and non-Alzheimer's dementias. J Am Geriatr Soc. 2005;53:1681–7.
50. Nadkarni NK, Mawji E, Mcllroy WE, Black SE. Spatial and temporal gait parameters in Alzheimer's disease and aging. Gait Posture. 2009;30:542–4.
51. Stuss DT, Alexander MP. Executive functions and the frontal lobes : a conceptual view. Psychol Res. 2000;63:289–98.
52. Herman T, Mirelman A, Giladi N, Schweiger A, Hausdorff JM. Executive control deficits as a prodrome to falls in healthy older adults: a prospective study linking thinking, walking and falling. J Gerontol A Biol Sci Med Sci. 2010;65(10):1086–92 (abstract).
53. Mirelman A, Herman T, Brozgol M, Dorfmn M, Sprecher E, Schweiger A, et al. Executive function and falls in older adults: new findings from a five-year prospective study link fall risk to cognition. PLoS One. 2012;7(6):240297. doi:10.1371/journal.pone.0040297. Epub 2012 Jun 29 (abstract).
54. Hauer K, Pfisterer M, Weber C, Wezler N, Keigel M, Oster P. Cognitive impairment decreases postural control during dual tasks in geriatric patients with history of falls. J Am Geriatr Soc. 2003;51:1638–44.
55. Soto D, Blanco MJ. Spatial attention and object –based attention : a comparison within a single task. Vision Res. 2004;44:69–81.
56. Nagamutsu LS, Liu-Ambrose TYL, Carolan P, Handy TC. Are impairments in visual-spatial attention a critical factor for increased risk in seniors? An event –related potential study. Neuropsychologia. 2009;47:2749–55.
57. Davies AJ, Kenny CA. Falls presenting to the accident and emergency department. Types of presentation and risk factor profile. Age Ageing. 1996;25:362–6.
58. Shaw FE, Kenny RA. The overlap between syncope and falls in the elderly. Postgrad Med J. 1997;73(864):635–9.
59. Kenny RA. Syncope in the elderly. J Cardiovasc Electrophysiol. 2003;14(S9):S74–7 (abstract).
60. Horlick MF, Matsuoka LY, Wartsmann J. Age, vitamin D and solar ultraviolet. Lancet. 1989;2:1104–5.
61. Sakuma M, Endo N. Muscle and bone health as a risk factor of fall among the elderly. Vitamin D for prevention of fall and fracture. Clin Calcium. 2008;18(6):816–20 (abstract).
62. Dharmarajan TS, Akula M, Kuppachi S, Norkus EP. Vitamin D deficiency in community older adults with falls of gait imbalance: an under-recognized problem in the inner city. J Nutr Elder. 2005;25:7–19 (abstract).
63. Anneweiler C, Montero-Odasso M, Schott AM, Berut G, Fantino B, Beauchet O. Fall prevention and vitamin D in the elderly: an overview of the key role of the non-bone effects. J Neuroeng Rehabil. 2010;7:50.
64. Gerdheim P, Ringsberg KA, Obrant KJ, Akesson K. Association between 25-hydroxy vitamin D levels, physical activity, muscle strength and function in the prospective population based OPRA study of elderly women. Osteoporos Int. 2005;16:1425–31.
65. Dey AB, Stout NR, Kenny RA. Cardiovascular syncope is the most common cause of drop attacks in the elderly. Pacing Clin Electrophysiol. 1997;20:818–9.
66. Dhesi JK, Jackson SH, Bearne LM, Moniz C, Hurley MV, Swift CG, et al. Vitamin D supplemental improve neuromuscular function in older people with fall. Age Ageing. 2004;33:589–95.
67. Bischoff-Ferrari HA, Borcbers M, Gudat F, Durmuller V, Stahelin HB, Dick W. Vitamin D receptor expression in human muscle decreases with age. J Bone Miner Res. 2004;19:265–9.
68. Glerup H, Mikkelsen K, Poulsen L, Hass E, Overbocks S, Thomsen J, et al. Hypovitaminosis D myopathy without biochemical signs of osteomalacic bone involvement. Calcif Tissue Int. 2000;66:419–24.
69. Nagagawa K. Effect of vitamin D on the nervous system and the skeletal muscle. Clin Calcium. 2006;16(2):1182–7 (abstract).
70. Nyberg L, Gustafson Y. Patient falls in stroke rehabilitation. Stroke. 1995;26:838–42.
71. Aizen E, Shugaer I, Lenger R. Risk factors and characteristics of falls during inpatient rehabilitation of elderly patients. Arch Gerontol Geriatr. 2007;44:1–12.

Oral Issues and Related Disorders in the Elderly

18

18.1 Oral Changes with Ageing

With ageing, structural changes occur in the oral and perioral tissues [1] which include the lips, oral mucosa, teeth, gingivae and associated structures such as tongue and the bone that support the teeth and the muscles of the jaw and their functional activity [2]. There is dryness of the lips and oral mucosa with loss of elasticity with development of fissures in the corners of the mouth. In the tongue, there is loss of papillae (glossitis) with formation of fissures [3] and sublingual varicosities, atrophy of the taste buds and of the salivary glands [1]. The teeth show changes in colour and tooth wear with occlusal and incisional attrition. With age, there is a decrease in the pulp cell density with increase in the dentinal thickness [4].

18.2 Oral Issues in the Elderly

Introduction

There are 390 million people aged over 60 years with oral issues recorded in 1998 WHO Report and this figure is estimated to double in 2025 [5], and by 2050 there will be 2 billion people over the age of 60 years, 80 % living in the developing countries [1]. The average person over the age of 65 years visits his physician at least six times in the year, whereas he is seen by the dentist probably once a year [6]. Basic health services are an indispensable part of primary health care. Oral health is an essential component to an elderly's general health and quality of life [7]. Oral health is often neglected in the elderly and affects the quality of life [2]. High levels of tooth loss, dental caries and the prevalence rates of periodontal disease, xerostomia and oral precancer and cancer have been evident in older people with poor oral health globally [8]. Chewing, eating habits and nutritional intake can compromise oral health. Furthermore, systemic diseases or their treatment can lead to risk of oral disease. Periodontitis may heighten the susceptibility to systemic disease [9]. Oral organisms have been the source of infection of the

N. Nagaratnam et al., *Diseases in the Elderly: Age-Related Changes and Pathophysiology*, DOI 10.1007/978-3-319-25787-7_18

meninges, endocardium, mediastinum, vertebrae, prosthetic joints and hepatobiliary system [10]. In the United States, 12 % of the population over the age of 60 years consume 30 % of all prescription medicine; many of them can have a negative impact on oral health [11].

18.2.1 Caries

Caries is disintegration or decay of the substance of teeth (enamel or dentine). With the older adult living longer and able to retain more of the teeth, they are at risk of developing caries. Caries, attrition and abrasion increase with ageing [12]. For these patients, the prevention and treatment of caries will become an essential part of their oral health needs.

Pathophysiology
Over the years, it was accepted that dental caries forms through an interaction of acid-forming bacteria, carbohydrate [13] and a host of other factors relating to the teeth and saliva. The bacteria in the mouth converts all foods especially starch and sugar into acids. Acid, bacteria, debris and saliva form a sticky substance, the plaque [14]. The plaque if not removed calcifies to form calculus commonly called tartar. The acids in the plaque dissolve the enamel surface to form cavitations. Today, it is acknowledged that dental caries is much more complex and is caused interaction between the tooth structure, biofluid [15], dietary, saliva and genetic factors [16]. Biofilm/fluid bacteria live in microcolonies encapsulated in a matrix of extracellular polymeric substances [17]. The microbial aetiology has been of interest, and it has been shown that the bacteria are normal and cause the disease when their numbers and pathogenicity alter in response to environmental conditions [16–18]. The interplay between dietary habits, saliva and many biological determinants influences biofilm metabolism and composition [17]. Occlusive surfaces in the interproximal areas below contact points and marginal gingivae [17], the molar teeth and the pits and fissures of permanent posterior teeth are the most vulnerable for carious lesions in more than 90 % of cases [19].

18.2.2 Periodontitis

Periodontitis is a chronic bacterial infection resulting in progressive destruction of the tissues that support the teeth, the gingiva, the cementum, the alveolar bone and the periodontal ligaments [20]. Periodontitis has worldwide prevalence and affects individuals of all ages but is most common in the elderly. In the United States, up to 70 % of adults have at least mild periodontitis, and gingivitis is highly prevalent [21].

Pathophysiology
The formation of the dental plaque at the gumline causes gingivitis which is limited to the covering gingival tissues [22]. With the destruction of the gingival fibres, the

gum tissues separate from the tooth forming a periodontal pocket with root exposure and gingival recession resulting in increased tooth mobility which may lead to tooth loss [16]. A number of factors increase the rate and severity of periodontal destruction [22], poor nutrition and diseases such as diabetes and genetic susceptibility. In older adults, several risk factors apart from those have been identified, such as tobacco smoking, presence of certain anaerobes in the microbiota, gingival bleeding and social issues [20].

18.2.3 Tooth Wear

Tooth wear caused by factors other than tooth decay can be part of normal ageing process, and hence it is not surprising to find older adults having more tooth wear. In one study, it was found that the proportion of pathological tooth wear in the 65 years and older people to be three times that seen in people aged 26–30 years [23].

Pathophysiology
Tooth wear is the result of processes such as abrasion, attrition, erosion, demastication and possibly a further process, abfraction (abrasion and fracture), and tooth wear can result from any combination of these [24, 25]. It is estimated that on average, tooth wear is about 30 u per year or about 0.3 postodontic treatment. The types most commonly seen in dental practice are abrasion and erosion [26].

Abrasion is produced by interaction between teeth and materials, for instance, aggressively brushing the teeth, foreign objects or bruxism [26]. Wedge-shaped lesions on the teeth are frequently cited as symptoms of abrasion from toothbrushing [27]. Attrition is loss of tooth tissue as a result of tooth-to-tooth contact, for instance, grinding the teeth (bruxism). In addition to tooth wear, consequences of attrition include fractured teeth and dental treatment.

Regurgitation, coke-swishing and fruit mulling are the major causes of erosion [26]. Erosion is loss of hard dental tissue due to the presence of acids not involving bacteria. Acidic foods and beverages cause thinning of the enamel, loss of surface characteristics and exposure of dentine [27]. There is considerable evidence that the major cause is regurgitation erosion due to a variety of factors including gastro-oesophageal reflux disorder (GORD) [28]. Regurgitation of gastric contents (GORD) reduces the pH of the oral cavity. Erosions appear as hollowed or cupped lesions and gradually link to form larger lesions and occur on smooth occlusal or incisal tooth surfaces [29]. Erosion of the enamel exposes the underlying softer dentine. The extent of the erosion will depend on the frequency of the exposure as well as the duration of the disease. Stained teeth suggest acid erosion and wear are inactive, whereas stain-free tooth suggests erosion process is active [30]. The modifiable risk factors are food with high acid content, yoghurt, citrus fruits, pickles, vinegar and intrinsic acids – from gastro-oesophageal reflux.

18.2.4 Oral Cancer

Oral cancer is any cancerous tissue growth in the mouth, and primary cancers may originate from any of the anatomical structures: the lips, the oral mucosa, the gums, the tongue and the bone that support the teeth. Men are affected twice as often as women. Smoking and other forms of tobacco use account for 75 % of oral cancers. Another risk factor is alcohol. In the United States, overall 10.5 adults per 100,000 will develop oral cancer and increases with age peaking between 60 and 70 years [31]. Oral cancers account for nearly 8000 deaths per year, and more than half of these occur at an age of 65 years and over [2].

Pathophysiology
Oral cancers may be of varied histological types, and the most common oral cancer is the squamous cell cancer which originates in the mucosa that lines the mouth and lips.

18.2.5 Edentulism

Edentulism is tooth loss which can be partial or complete. The United States National Institute of Dentition and Craniofacial Research [32] found that people over the age of 65 years had an average of 18.9 remaining teeth, and 27.2 % were totally toothless. The same report found older seniors, females, blacks seniors, those with low income and those with less education were more severely affected. Edentulism increased with age and ranges from 8.4 % in the 55–64 years age group to 19.7 % in the 75 years and older with 31.5 % being females and 9.6 % males [33]. However, the prospect of losing teeth with ageing is diminishing in developed countries because of better access to dental care, effective treatment and better nutrition. A research group found nine risk indications for tooth loss and these include age, male gender, smoking, lack of professional management, poor oral hygiene, diabetes, hypertension, cancer and anterior tooth type [34]. The most important cause of tooth loss in developed countries is periodontitis.

Box 18.1. Key Points. Oral Issues and Related Disorders

- With ageing, structural changes occur in the oral and perioral tissues [1].
- Dental caries is complex and is caused by interaction between the tooth structure, biofluid, dietary, saliva and genetic factors [16].
- Biofilm/fluid bacteria live in microcolonies encapsulated in a matrix of extracellular polymeric substances [17].
- Periodontitis is a chronic bacterial infection resulting in progressive destruction of the tissues that support the teeth the gingiva, the cementum, the alveolar bone and the periodontal ligaments [20].
- Tooth wear caused by factors other than tooth decay can be part of normal ageing process, and hence it is not surprising to find older adults having more tooth wear [23].
- The prospect of losing teeth with ageing is diminishing in developed countries.

Multiple Choice Questions

1. The following are true in relation to dental caries, EXCEPT:
   A. Dental caries is caused by interaction between the tooth structure, biofluid, dietary, saliva and genetic factors.
   B. Biofilm/fluid bacteria live in microcolonies encapsulated in a matrix of extracellular polymeric substances.
   C. The molar teeth and the pits and fissures of permanent posterior teeth are the most vulnerable for carious lesions in more than 90 % of cases.
   D. It is accepted that dental caries forms through an interaction of acid-forming bacteria, carbohydrate and a host of other factors relating to the teeth and saliva.
2. The following are true in relation to the teeth, EXCEPT:
   A. Tooth wear is the result of processes such as abrasion, attrition, erosion and demastication.
   B. Regurgitation, coke swishing and fruit mulling are the major causes of erosion.
   C. Poor nutrition and diseases such as diabetes increase the rate and severity of periodontal destruction.
   D. In erosion, stained tooth suggests acid erosion and wear are active, whereas stain-free tooth suggests erosion is inactive.

Answers to MCQs

1 = D; 2 = D

References

1. Al-Drees AM. Oral and perioral physiological changes with ageing. Pakistan Oral Dental J. 2010;30(1):26–30.
2. Guiglia R, Musciotto A, Compilato D, Procaccini M, Russo LL, Ciavarella D, et al. Aging and oral health: effects in hard and soft tissues. Curr Pharm Des. 2010;16(6):619–30 (abstract).
3. Klein DR. Oral soft tissue changes in geriatric patients, symposium on considerations for oral health care in the aging patient. Dental Society of the State of New York; 1980. p. 56.
4. Murray PE, Stanley HR, Matthews JB, Sloan AJ, Smith AJ. Age related odontometric changes of human teeth. Oral Surg Oral Med Oral Pathol Oral Radiol Endod. 2002;93(4):474–82.
5. WHO. http://www.int/oral_health/action/groups/in/index.html.
6. Chauncey HH, Feldman RS, Weyker AH. Oral aspects of aging. Am J Fam Physician. 1983; 28(1):147–52.
7. Dolan TA, Atchison KA. Implications of access, utilization and need for oral health care by the non-institutionalised and institutionalized elderly on the dental delivery system. J Dent Educ. 1993;57(12):876–87.
8. Petersen PE, Yamamoto T. Improving the oral health of older people: the approach of the WHO Global Oral Health Programme. Community Dent Oral Epidemiol. 2005;33(2):81–92.
9. Page RC. The pathobiology of periodontal diseases may affect systemic diseases: inversion of a paradigm. Ann Periodontol. 1998;3(1):108–20 (abstract).
10. Shay K. Infectious complications of dental and periodontal diseases in the elderly population. Clin Infect Dis. 2002;34:1215–23.

11. Niessen LC, Fedele DJ. Aging successfully: oral health for the prime of life. Compend Contin Educ Dent. 2002;23(10 Suppl):4–11.
12. Tofino PME, Cepeda GLA. Ageing and oral cavity. Pract Odontol. 1989;10(3):33–6.
13. Miller W. The presence of bacterial plaques on the surface of teeth and their significance. Dent Cosmos. 1902;44:425–46.
14. William LJ. A contribution to the study of pathology of enamel. Dent Cosmos. 1897; 39:169–96.
15. Fejerskov O, Nyvad B. Is dental caries an infectious disease? Diagnostic and treatment consequences for the practitioner. In: Schon I, editor. Norde Dentistry 2003 Year book. Copenhagen: Quintessence Publishing; 2003. p. 41–151.
16. Zero T, Fontana M, Martinez-Mier EA, Ferriera-Zandona A, Ando M, Gomzalez-Cabezas C, et al. The biology, prevention, diagnosis and treatment of dental caries. J Am Dent Assoc. 2009;140 suppl 1:25S–34.
17. Fejerskov O. Changing paradigms in concepts on dental caries: consequences for oral health care. Caries Res. 2004;35:183–91.
18. Marsh PD. Are dental diseases examples of ecological catastrophes? Microbiology. 2003;149(Pt 2):279–94.
19. Beltran-Aquilar ED, Barker LR, Canto MT, Dye B, Gooch BF, Griffin SO, et al. Surveillance for dental caries, dental sealants, tooth retention, edentulism and enamel fluorosis. United States 1988–1994 and 1999-2—2. MMWR Surveill Summ. 2005;54(3):1–43.
20. Ellen RP. Considerations for physicians caring for the older adults with periodontal disease. Clin Geriatr Med. 1992;8(3):599–616 (abstract).
21. Jeffcoat MK. Prevention of periodontal diseases in adults: strategies for the future. Prev Med. 1994;23(5):704–8 (abstract).
22. Kinane DF, Marshall GJ. Periodontal manifestations of systemic disease. Aust Dent J. 2001;46(1):2–12 (abstract).
23. Smith BG, Robb ND. The prevalence of tooth wear in 1007 dental patients. Oral Rehab. 1993;23(4):232–9.
24. De Baat C, van Nieuw Amerongen A. Tooth wear. Classification and terminology. Ned Tijdschr Tandheelkd. 1997;104(4):138–41 (abstract).
25. Imfeld T. Dental erosion. Definition and classification and links. Eur J Oral Sci. 1996; 104(2 (Pt 2)):151–5.
26. Abrahamsen TC. The worn dentition-pathognomonic patterns of abrasion and erosion. Int Dent J. 2005;55(4 Suppl 1):268–76 (abstract).
27. Moffitt AR. Tooth wear and erosion Update on patient care. Inside Densistry. http://www.dental-professional.com/Nrews_Articles.aspx?NewsID=News044.
28. Smith BG, Bartlett DW, Robb ND. The prevalence etiology and management of tooth wear in the United Kingdom. J Prosthet Dent. 1997;78(1):367–72 (abstract).
29. Bartlett D. A new look at erosive tooth wear in elderly people. J Am Den Ass. 2007; 135(Supp (7)):21S–5.
30. Bartlett DW, Shah PA. A critical review of non-caries cervical (wear) lesions and the role of abfract erosion and abrasion. J Dent Res. 2006;8594:306–12.
31. National Institute of Dentition and Craniofacial Research (NICDR) Update; 2013.
32. National Institute of Dentition and Craniofacial Research (NICDR) Update 20 Dec 2008.
33. NSW Health. http://www.health.nsw.gov.au/public-health/chorep/ora/ora_den_stat.htm.
34. Al-Shamnari KF, Al-Kabbaz AK, Al-Ansari JM, Neiva R, Wang HL. Risk indications for tooth loss due to periodontal disease. J Periodontol. 2005;76:1910–8.

Connective Tissue Disorders and Vasculitis in the Elderly

19

19.1 Age-Related Changes

It is well known that immune function wanes with age. The ageing of the immune system is known as immunosenescence and is characterised by a reduced humoral response as well as a decrease in cell-mediated immune function [1]. Immunosenescence affects both innate and adaptive immunity [2]. In the elderly, alterations occur in the innate/natural and clonal type immunity and the former is largely preserved [3, 4], whereas the clonic component undergoes appreciable alterations [3, 4]. The mechanism mediated by the antibody called humoral immune response is brought about by antibodies that bind to the antigens and promote their destruction. In another mechanism, the lymphocytes together with the macrophages cause the destruction of the pathogenic organisms and is called cellular immune response. The susceptibility of the elderly to infectious diseases, autoimmunity and cancer and in their decreased responsiveness to vaccination is directly or indirectly related to age-related changes of the immune system [3]. Most of the parameters are largely under genetic control [5]. The genetic component appears to control the functioning of the innate/inflammatory and clonotypic responses and necessarily the inflammatory state in late life [6, 7]. The major driving force of immunosenescence seems to be the lifelong chronic antigen load [3, 8] and leads to chronic inflammatory status and which characterises ageing [9], resulting in damage to the organs late in life and is deleterious for longevity [3]. Chronic antigenic overload (virus, bacteria, fungi, toxins, mutated cells) results in a pro-inflammatory condition that continuously stimulates innate immunity and seems to incline towards the onset of age-related disease where immune and autoimmune factors play an important role [9]. The immune activity of the innate immune system in later life is evident by the presence of elevated markers of inflammation such as TNF-alpha and interleukin-6 (IL-6) [10].

N. Nagaratnam et al., *Diseases in the Elderly: Age-Related Changes and Pathophysiology*, DOI 10.1007/978-3-319-25787-7_19

19.2 Connective Tissue Disorders

Introduction

Connective tissue disorders form a wide spectrum of disorders including systemic lupus erythematosus (SLE), systemic sclerosis (SSc), Sjogren's syndrome (SS), mixed connective diseases, giant cell arteritis, polymyalgia rheumatica and polyarteritis nodosa. All are immune-complex-mediated auto-immune conditions. The connective tissue disorders occur at all ages but higher in prevalence in the young adults [11]. SLE is an auto-immune condition characterised by multisystem involvement [12, 13]. In the elderly with SLE, the female/male ratio is 2:1 and 10–20 % of the cases occur [12, 14, 15]. The diagnosis is often delayed in the late onset [16, 17]. There is evidence to suggest that incidence of progressive SSc in the elderly is more common than in younger age group [18]. The incidence in patients over 75 years with systemic sclerosis is around 20 per million per year, and the peak incidence in white females is between 65 and 75 years and in white males over 75 years [19]. The prevalence of SS is about 3 % in people above the age of 50 years and primary SS in elderly people is subclinical, benign and relatively common [20]. Approximately 40 % of xerostomia in the elderly is due to Sjogren's syndrome and the elderly account up to 20 % of Sjogren's syndrome [21].

19.2.1 Systemic Lupus Erythematosus (SLE)

Pathophysiology

In both innate and adaptive immunity, immunopathologically notable cells include the dendritic cells, macrophages, neutrophils, lymphocytes as well as non-immune cells such as epithelial, endothelial and tubular cells, and they have significant role in the pathogenesis of SLE [22]. The pathogenesis of SLE is characterised by interplay of several factors, such as multiple genes, gender, sex hormones and environmental triggers resulting in immunodysregulation [23]. It involves multitude of cells and includes the involvement of apoptotic cells and innate and adaptive immune responses [24]. In SLE, immune responses against endogenous nuclear antigens are distinctive, and the autoantigens released by the apoptotic cells are presented by the dendritic cells to T cells activating them [24]. Activated T cells in turn interact with B cells to produce antibodies to these self-constituents by secreting cytokines [24]. In normal healthy individuals, the excessive production of antibodies is prevented by an idiotype network which is defective in SLE [23]. Immune complexes and complement activation pathways lead to tissue injury and damage [23, 24], and the pathological changes that occur include vasculopathy, vasculitis, immune complex deposition and inflammation [23]. The endothelial cells are directly or indirectly affected by the anti-endothelial cell antibodies, antiphospholipid antibodies and the anti-double-strand antibodies causing inflammatory damage to the vessel wall [25].

19.2.2 Systemic Sclerosis (SSc)

Pathophysiology
The pathogenesis of systemic sclerosis (SSc) is characterised by immune and endothelial activation, vascular dysfunction and overproduction of extracellular matrix [26, 27]. The role of cellular and humoral immunity has been highlighted following genetic and serological approaches to the understanding of the pathogenesis of SSc. Endothelial activation is followed by extravasation of inflammatory cells, initially monocytes and latterly lymphocytes [28]. Activation of fibroblasts follows from complex interactions among the endothelial cells, lymphocytes, macrophages and a number of mediators such as cytokines, chemokines and growth factors [27]. The resulting fibroblastic proliferation leads to obliteration of the lumen of the vessels with damage in the microvasculature of the various internal organs and the skin due to ischaemia [28]. It has been suggested that reactive oxygen species (ROS) and apoptosis are involved in SSc, and furthermore there is a genetic susceptibility to the disease [26, 27].

19.2.3 Sjogren's Syndrome

Pathophysiology
Sjogren's syndrome (SS) is an autoimmune disorder characterised by lymphocytic infiltration and destruction of the salivary and lacrimal glands [29]. The infiltrating cells cause not only glandular destruction by cell-mediated mechanisms but also activate pathways by secreting cytokines [29]. The inability to secrete adequately is likely due to glandular decrease in the release of neurotransmitters and decrease response of the residual glandular cells by cytokines, autoantibodies and metalloproteinases [30]. Cytokines are also involved in the dysregulation of apoptosis, and during the lymphocyte-independent stage, apoptotic autoantigens are generated [31]. This is followed by the lymphocyte-dependent stage when an immune attack may cause further cell destruction and salivary dysfunction [31].

Box 19.1. Key Points. Connective Tissue Disorders

- All connective disorders are immune-complex-mediated auto-immune conditions.
- They occur at all ages though the prevalence is higher in the young [11].
- The susceptibility of the elderly to auto-immune and infectious diseases and cancer is directly or indirectly related to age-related changes to the immune system [3].
- The immune activity of the innate immune system in later life is evident by the presence of elevated markers of inflammation [10].
- Most of the parameters are under genetic control [15].

- The pathogenesis of SLE is characterised by interplay of several factors, hormones and such as multiple genes, gender, sex hormones and environmental triggers resulting in immunodysregulation. Both innate and adaptive immunity have a significant role in the pathogenesis of SLE [23].
- The pathogenesis of systemic sclerosis (SSc) is characterised by immune and endothelial activation, vascular dysfunction and overproduction of extracellular matrix [26, 27].
- Sjogren's syndrome (SS) is an autoimmune disorder characterised by lymphocytic infiltration and destruction of the salivary and lacrimal glands [29].

19.3 Vasculitis

Introduction

Vasculitis constitutes a heterogenous group of diseases characterised by inflammation and necrosis [32] of the blood vessels and may affect the large, medium, small arteries, arterioles, veins and venules. The incidence of vasculitis is increasing. In a study of selected vasculitides in the United States, the combined prevalence was over 30/100,000 population. Of the specific vasculitis studied, giant cell arteritis of the elderly was the commonest (20/1,000,000) [33]. The overall frequency of primary systemic small vessel vasculitis (PSV) was 19.9/million [34, 35] and was shown to increase with age, the incidence greatest in the elderly and peaking in the 65–74 years group [34]. The overall incidence of PSV was 48.9/million in the older and 17.2/million in the younger age group [35]. Microscopic polyangiitis was common in the older and Wegener's granulomatosis in the younger [35]. ANCA vasculitis in patients over the age of 75 years or older is associated with a higher mortality and related to the presence of renal involvement, and the elderly have a greater risk of dying within the first 6 months of diagnosis [36].

Pathophysiology

Various classifications have been proposed, and because there is a marked overlap in the clinical and pathological features, most classifications are found to be inadequate [37] and there is no universally accepted classification. The involvement of different end organs, the kidney, lung, central nervous system and gastrointestinal tract, and the spectrum of clinical presentation and the varying types of inflammatory cells involved make classification baffling [38]. However, an important progress is the appreciation of vessel size, the distinction between primary and secondary vasculitis (Box 19.2) and pathogenic markers [39]. A useful classification is one based on the size of the vessel, namely, small vessel, small to medium size and medium to large vessel size [40], affected although overlap is common. Another is based on the vascular histology on the type of cellular infiltration in and around the affected vessels. Primary systemic vasculitis in practice can be classified according to the affected vessel size, histological features and clinical presentation [41] (Table 19.1).

Table 19.1 Classification of primary vasculitic disorders in the elderly

Size of vessels involved[a]	Disorders	Histopathology
Large sized	Temporal arteritis Takayasu arteritis	Granulomatous Granulomatous
Medium sized	Polyarteritis nodosa	Necrotizing vasculitis Granulomatous necrotizing glomerulonephritis
Small-sized ANCA positive	Kawasaki Microscopic polyangiitis Churg-Strauss syndrome Wegener's granulomatosis	Necrotizing vasculitis Eosinophilic and granulomatous Granulomatous
Small-sized ANCA negative	Cryoglobulinemia Henoch-Scholein purpura Secondary vasculitides	Cryoglobulin immune deposits

[a]Large-sized vessels – aorta and largest branches to the head and neck; medium-sized vessels – e.g. coronary, renal, hepatic and mesenteric; small-sized vessels – capillaries, arterioles, venules

Box 19.2. Secondary Vasculitis

Infection-related vasculitis
Drug hypersensitivity-related vasculitis
Vasculitis secondary to connective tissue disorders
Malignancy-related vasculitis
Hypocomplementemic urticaria vasculitis
Post-organ transplant vasculitis

Information source: Hom [48]

Three immunopathological categories of vasculitis have been proposed [37]: (1) circulating anti-GBM antibodies cross-reacting with alveolar basement membrane producing pulmonary renal syndromes, (2) granular deposits of immunoglobulin and complement on vessel walls and glomeruli in small vessel vasculitis and (3) few if any deposits are seen in the target tissues as in Churg-Strauss syndrome, Wegener's granulomatosis, microscopic polyangiitis and in renal-limited pauci-immune crescentic glomerular nephritis [37]. The detection of anti-neutrophil cytoplasm autoantibodies (ANCA) has made it possible for small-vessel vasculitis to be further classified as ANCA-associated and non-ANCA-associated vasculitis. The ANCA-associated vasculitides are a group of disorders which include Wegener's granulomatosis, microscopic polyangiitis and Churg-Strauss syndrome.

The American College of Rheumatology (ACR) in 1990 [42] published a criteria for the diagnosis of polyarteritis nodosa, Churg-Strauss syndrome, Wegener's granulomatosis, hypersensitivity vasculitis, Henoch-Schonlein purpura, giant cell arteritis and Takayasu arteritis [43]. ACR criteria are useful for classification for some forms of vasculitis and useful in clinical practice although in many instances in practice there is overlapping in diagnoses and in particular in patients with small vessel vasculitis and classical polyarteritis [44]. The Chapel Hill Consensus Conference (CHCC) [45] has clarified some of the controversies in the nomenclature of systemic vasculitides [46]. CHCC defines ten vasculitides based on vessel size (large, medium and small). The ACR classification criteria and CHCC are the most widely used to distinguish different forms of vasculitis [44].

There are several mechanisms involved in the vascular inflammation, namely, immune-complex disease, antibody-mediated disease, antibody-dependent cellular cytotoxicity and endothelial activation among others.

(i) Immune Complex Disease
Circulating immune (antigen-antibody) complexes are removed from the circulation by mononuclear phagocytic system. The factors that determine whether the immune complexes formed will lead to tissue deposition and disease are not clear [47]. Possible factors are (1) the size of the immune complexes (small size binds less avidly to phagocytic cells) (2) and the mononuclear phagocytic system (overloaded or dysfunction) [47]. The immune complexes reach the vessel wall through increased vascular permeability and are deposited in the wall of the vessel. The Fc portions of the immunoglobulins IgG and IgM activate complement and initiate T- and B-cell responses with cytokine activation and recruitment of neutrophils [48]. The consequences of immune-complex injury are dominated by acute necrotizing vasculitis, microthrombi and superimposed ischemic necrosis accompanied by inflammation of the affected organ [47]. Figure 19.1 shows a vasculitic skin rash following *Campylobacter jejuni* infection in an elderly patient. Skin biopsy showed extravascular red blood cells, oedema and endothelial swelling of the capillaries peri-vascular infiltration. Immunofluorescence revealed granular deposits of IgM (traces) and C3 (1+) in occasional vessels of the superficial venous plexus, granular deposits of C3 in the dermo-epidermal junction and extensive deposits of fibrinogen (3+) in and around the vessels. These findings are consistent with immune-complex vasculitis.

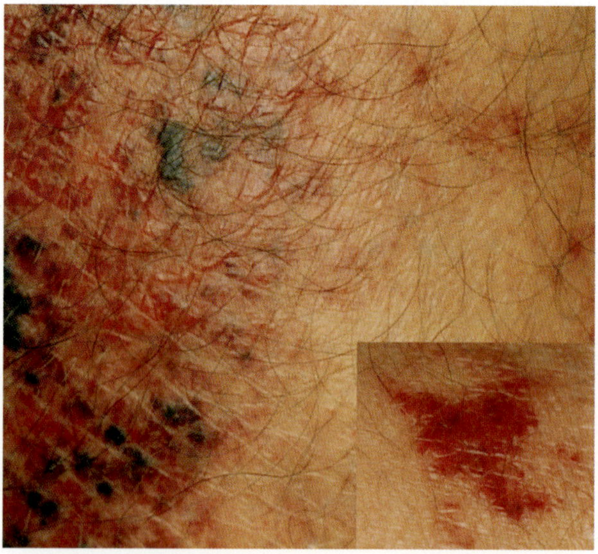

Fig. 19.1 Vasculitic rash with fading violaceous areas and dark infarct spots

(ii) Antibody-mediated disease
Specific antibodies that bind to the granulocytic cells lead to endothelial cell cytolysis and subsequent activation of natural killer cells [48]. The activated neutrophils adhere to the endothelium and stimulate lysis of the endothelial cells in the presence of TNF-alpha and trigger degranulation of the neutrophils and necrotizing vasculitis with granuloma formation [48]. Anti-neutrophil cytoplasmic antibodies (ANCAs) have been found in Wegener granulomatosis (WG), Churg-Strauss syndrome (CSS) and microscopic polyarteritis nodosa (MPA). The ANCAs can be divided by immunofluorescence into those that produce cytoplasmic (C-ANCA) or perinuclear (P-ANCA) patterns [48]. The Churg-Strauss syndrome, Wegener's granulomatosis and microscopic polyangiitis constitute the anti-neutrophil cytoplasmic antibody (ANCA)-associated systemic vasculitides (AASV) [49].

(iii) Antibody-dependent cellular cytotoxicity
Endothelial dysfunction can be triggered by infectious agents, immune complexes and anti-endothelial antibodies [50]. The endothelium controls vascular permeability and cell adhesion molecules and secretes a large range of proinflammatory cytokines [48]. Anti-endothelial cell antibodies demonstrate complement-dependent cytotoxicity against endothelial cells and play a role in vascular damage in a number of vasculitic syndromes. The dysregulated adhesion molecules cause uncontrolled inflammation, and thrombosis and vessel occlusion lead to the clinical manifestations of vasculitis [50].

Box 19.3. Key Points. Vasculitis in the Elderly

- A useful classification is based on the size of the vessel [40].
- Several mechanisms are involved in the vascular inflammation, immune-complex disease, antibody-mediated disease, antibody-dependent cellular cytotoxicity and endothelial activation among others.
- Endothelial dysfunction can be triggered of by infectious agents, immune complexes and anti-endothelial antibodies [50].
- The consequences of immune complex injury are dominated by acute necrotizing vasculitis, microthrombi and superimposed ischaemic necrosis accompanied by inflammation of the affected organ [47].

Multiple Choice Questions (MCQs)

1. The following pathophysiological mechanisms in vasculitis are true, EXCEPT:
   A. Immune-complex injuries are dominated by acute necrotizing vasculitis and microthrombi-superimposed ischaemic necrosis.
   B. Anti-neutrophil cytoplasmic antibodies (ANCAs) have been found in Henoch-Scholein purpura and Takayasu's arteritis.
   C. Endothelial dysfunction can be triggered by infectious agents, immune complexes and anti- endothelial antibodies.
   D. Anti-endothelial cell antibodies demonstrate complement-dependent cytotoxicity against endothelial cells and play a role in vascular damage in a number of vasculitic syndromes.

2. The following are true in the pathogenesis of systemic lupus erythematosus (SLE), EXCEPT:
   A. Non-immune cells such as epithelial, endothelial and tubular cells do not have a significant role.
   B. Immune complexes and complement activation pathways lead to tissue injury and damage.
   C. Inflammatory damage to the endothelial cells of the vessel wall is caused by antibodies such as anti-endothelial and anti-phospholipid among others.
   D. In SLE, immune response against endogenous nuclear antigen is distinctive.
3. The following statements are true in relation to systemic sclerosis (SSc) and Sjogren's syndrome (SS), EXCEPT:
   A. The pathogenesis of systemic sclerosis is characterised by immune and endothelial activation.
   B. It is the fibroblastic proliferation that leads to obstruction of the vessels in SSc.
   C. Sjogren's syndrome is characterised by neutrophilic infiltration and destruction of the salivary and lacrimal glands.
   D. The infiltrating cells cause not only glandular destruction by cell-mediated mechanisms but also by activating pathways by secreting cytokines.

Answers to MCQs

1 = B, 2 = A, 3 = C

References

Age-Related Changes

1. Weiskopf D, Weinberger B, Grubeck-Loebenstein B. The aging immune system. Transpl Int. 2009;22(11):1041–50 (abstract).
2. Ongradi J, Stercz B, Kovesdi V, Vertes L. Immunosenescence and vaccination of the elderly. I Age-related immune impairment. Acta Microbiol Immunol Hung. 2009;56(3):199–210 (abstract).
3. Burkle A, Casell G, Franceschi C, Mariani E, Sansoni P, Sansoni A, et al. Pathophysiology of ageing, longevity and age related disease. Immun Ageing. 2007;4:4. doi:10.1186/1742-4933-4-4.
4. Franceschi CS, Bonafe M. Centenarians as a model for healthy aging. Biochem Soc Trans. 2003;3192:457–61 (abstract).
5. Franceschi CS, Valensin F, Fagnoni C, Barbi C, Bonafe M. Biomarkers of immunosenescence within an voluntary perspective: the challenge of heterogeneity and the role antigenic load. Exp Gerontol. 1999;34:911–21.
6. Capri M, Salvioli S, Sevini F, Valesin S, Celani L, Monti D, et al. The genetics of human longevity. Ann N Y Acad Sci. 2006;1007:252–7.
7. Candore G, Colonna-Romano G, Balistreri CR, Malaguarnera M, Capri M, Vasto S, et al. Breaking of longevity: role of innate immune system. Rejuvenation Res. 2006;9:143–8.
8. Campisi J. The biology of replicative senescence. Eur J Cancer. 1997;33(5):703–9 (abstract).
9. Vasto S, Colonna-Romano G, Larbi A, Wikby A, Caruso C, Powelec G. Role of persistent CMV infection in conferring T cell immunity in the elderly. Immun Ageing. 2007;4:2. doi:10.1186/1742-4933-42.
10. Bruunsgaard H, Pedersen M, Pedersen BK. Aging and proinflammatory cytokines. Curr Opin Hematol. 2001;8:131–6.

Connective Tissue Disorders

11. Gaubitz M. Epidemiology of connective tissue disorders. Rheumatology (Oxford). 2006;45(Suppl):iii3–4. doi:10.1093/rheumatology/kel282.
12. Rovensky J, Tuchynova A. Systemic lupus erythematosus in the elderly. Autoimmun Rev. 2008;7(3):235–9 (abstract).
13. Ho CT, Mok CC, Lau CS, Wong RW. Late-onset systemic lupus erythematosus in southern Chinese. Ann Rheum Dis. 1998;57(7):437–40 (abstract).
14. Lazaro D. Elderly-onset systemic lupus erythematosus: prevalence clinical course and treatment. Drugs Aging. 2007;24(9):701–15 (abstract).
15. Arnaud L, Mathian A, Boddaert J, Amoura Z. Late-onset systemic lupus erythematosus: epidemiology diagnosis and treatment. Drugs Aging. 2012;29(3):181–9 (abstract).
16. Tomic-Lucic A, Petrovic R, Radak-Perovic M, Milovanovic D, Milovanovic S, et al. Late onset systemic lupus erythematosus: clinical features and prognosis. Clin Rheumatol. 2013;32(7):1093–8 (abstract).
17. Font J, Pallares L, Cervera R, Lopez-Soto A, Navarro M, Bosch Z, et al. Systemic lupus erythematosus in the elderly. Clinical and immunological characteristics. Ann Rheum Dis. 1991;50(10):702–5.
18. Dalziel JA, Wilcock GH. Evidence to suggest the incidence of progressive systemic sclerosis in the elderly is more common than with the younger age group. Postgrad Med J. 1979; 55(84):192–5.
19. Mayes MD, Lacey JU, Beebee-Dimmer J, Gillepsie BW, Cooper B, Liang TJ, et al. Prevalence incidence survival and disease characteristics of systemic sclerosis in a large US population. Arthritis Rheum. 2003;48:246–55.
20. Drosus AA, Andonopoulos AP, Costopouls JS, Papadimitriou CS, Montsopoulos HM. Prevalence of primary systemic sclerosis in elderly population. Br J Rheumatol. 1988;27(2):123–7.
21. Hashimi AC. Xerostomia secondary to Sjogren's syndrome in the elderly: recognition and management. Drugs Aging. 2005;22(11):887–9 (abstract).
22. Kow NY, Mak A. Costimulatory pathways: physiology and potential therapeutic manipulation in systemic lupus erythromatosus. Clin Develop Immun. http://dx.doi.org/10.1155/2013/245928.
23. Mok CC, Lau CS. Pathogenesis of systemic lupus erythematosus. J Clin Pathol. 2003;56:481–90.
24. Bertsias G, Cervera R, Boumpas DJ. Systemic lupus erythrematosus: pathogenesis and clinical features. http://www.euler.org/my/hpcondData/files/sample%20_nod%2017 pdf. Accessed 28 Apr 2015.
25. Cieslik P, Hrycek A, Klucinski P. Vasculopathy and vasculitis in systemic lupus erythematosus. Pol Arch Med Wewn. 2008;118(1–2):57–63 (abstract).
26. Denton CP. Pathogenesis of systemic sclerosis (scleroderma). UpToDate http://www.update.com/contents/pathogensis-of-systemic-sclerosis-scleroderma. Accessed 27 Apr 2015.
27. Yamamoto T. Scleroderma-pathophysiology. Eur J Dermatol. 2009;19(1):14–24 (abstract).
28. Chatterjea S. Systemic scleroderma. http://www.clevelandclinicmeded.com/medicalpubs/diseasemanagement/rheumatology/systemicsclerosis/Default.htm. Accessed 27 Apr 2015.
29. Garcia-Carrasco M, Fuentes-Alexandro S, Escarcega RO, Salgado G, Riebeling C, Cervera R. Pathophysiology of Sjogren's syndrome. Arch Med Res. 2006;37(8):921–32.
30. Fox RI, Stern M. Sjogren's syndrome: mechanisms of pathogenesis involve interaction of immune and neurosensory systems. Scand J Rheumatol Suppl. 2002;116:3–13 (abstract).
31. Borchers AT, Naguwa SM, Keen CL, Gershwin ME. Immunopathogenesis of Sjogren's syndrome. Clin Rev Allergy Immunol. 2003;25(1):89–104.

Vasculitis in the Elderly

32. Watts RA, Scott DG. Vasculitis. Baillieres Clin Rheumatol. 1995;9(3):529–54.
33. About vasculitis. http://www.2.ccf.org/inssys/vasculitis.htmwebsite. Accessed 6 Sept 2009.
34. Watts RA, Lane SE, Bentham G, Scott DG. Epidemiology of systemic vasculitis : a ten year study in the United Kingdom. Arthritis Rheum. 2000;43(2):414–9.

35. Panagiotakis SH, Perysinakio GS, Kritikos H, Vassilopoulos D, Vrentzos G, Linardakis M, et al. The epidemiology of primary systemic vasculitides involving small vessels in Crete (southern Greece): a comparison of older versus younger adult patients. Clin Exp Rheumatol. 2007;27(3):409–15.
36. Hoganson DD, From AM, Michet CT. Antineutrophil cytoplasmic antibodies vasculitis in the elderly. J Clin Rheumatol. 2008;14(2):78–81.
37. D'Agate V. Anti-neutrophil cytoplasmic antibodies and vasculitis: much more than a disease marker. J Clin Invest. 2002;119(7):919–21.
38. Watts R, Lane S, Hanstek T, Hauser T, Hellmich B, Koldingsnes W, et al. Development and validation of a consensus methodology for the classification of the ANCA-associated vasculitis and polyarteritis nodosa for epidemiological study. Ann Rheum Dis. 2011;66:222–7.
39. Watts RA, Scott DG. Classification and epidemiology of vasculitides. Baillieres Clin Rheumatol. 1997;11(2):191–217 (abstract).
40. Carlson JA, Cavaliere LF, Grant-kels JM. Cutaneous vasculitis: diagnosis management. Clin Dermatol. 2006;24:414–29.
41. Guillevin L, Pagnoux C, Guilpain P. Classification of systemic vasculitides. Presse Med. 2007;36(5 (Pt 2)):845–53 (abstract).
42. Leavitt RY, Fauci AS, Bloch DA, Michel BA, Hunder GG, Arend NP, et al. The American College of Rheumatology 1990 Criteria for the classification of Wegener's granulomatosis. Arthritis Rheum. 1990;33(8):1101–7.
43. Hunder GG, Arend WP, Bloch DA, Caabresse LH, Fauci AS, Fries F, et al. The American College of Rheumatology 1990 criteria for classification of vasculitis. Introduction. Arthritis Rheum. 1990;33:1065–7.
44. Kallenberg CG. The last classification of vasculitis. Clin Rev Allergy Immunol. 2008; 35(1-2):5–10.
45. Jennette JC, Falk RJ, Andrassy K, Bacon PA, Chung J, Gross WI, et al. Nomenclature of systemic vasculitides proposal of an international consensus conference. Arthritis Rheum. 1994; 37:187–92.
46. Saleh A, Stone JH. Classification and diagnostic criteria in systemic vasculitis. Best Pract Res Clin Rheumatol. 2005;19(2):209–21.
47. Kumar V, Cotran RS, Robbins SL. Basic pathology. 5th ed. Philadelphia: WB Saunders Company; 1992.
48. Hom C. Vasculitis and thrombophlebitis. e medicine. 30 Mar 2006. http://www.emedicine.com/ped/topic2390.htm.
49. Kallenberg CGM. Antineutrophil cytoplasmic autoantibody-associated small vessel vasculitis. Curr Opin Rheumatol. 2007;19:17–24.
50. Sindy JS, Haynes BF. Cytokines and adhesion molecules in the pathogenesis of vasculitis. Curr Rheumatol Rep. 2000;2(5):402–10 (abstract).

Index

N. Nagaratnam et al., *Diseases in the Elderly: Age-Related Changes and Pathophysiology*, DOI 10.1007/978-3-319-25787-7

Printed by Printforce, the Netherlands